QUALITATIVE ANALYSIS AND SYNTHESIS OF RECURRENT NEURAL NETWORKS

PURE AND APPLIED MATHEMATICS

A Program of Monographs, Textbooks, and Lecture Notes

EXECUTIVE EDITORS

Earl J. Taft
Rutgers University
New Brunswick, New Jersey

Zuhair Nashed
University of Delaware
Newark, Delaware

EDITORIAL BOARD

M. S. Baouendi
University of California,
San Diego

Jane Cronin
Rutgers University

Jack K. Hale
Georgia Institute of Technology

S. Kobayashi
University of California,
Berkeley

Marvin Marcus
University of California,
Santa Barbara

W. S. Massey
Yale University

Anil Nerode
Cornell University

Donald Passman
University of Wisconsin,
Madison

Fred S. Roberts
Rutgers University

David L. Russell
Virginia Polytechnic Institute
and State University

Walter Schempp
Universität Siegen

Mark Teply
University of Wisconsin,
Milwaukee

MONOGRAPHS AND TEXTBOOKS IN PURE AND APPLIED MATHEMATICS

1. K. Yano, Integral Formulas in Riemannian Geometry (1970)
2. S. Kobayashi, Hyperbolic Manifolds and Holomorphic Mappings (1970)
3. V. S. Vladimirov, Equations of Mathematical Physics (A. Jeffrey, ed.; A. Littlewood, trans.) (1970)
4. B. N. Pshenichnyi, Necessary Conditions for an Extremum (L. Neustadt, translation ed.; K. Makowski, trans.) (1971)
5. L. Narici et al., Functional Analysis and Valuation Theory (1971)
6. S. S. Passman, Infinite Group Rings (1971)
7. L. Dornhoff, Group Representation Theory. Part A: Ordinary Representation Theory. Part B: Modular Representation Theory (1971, 1972)
8. W. Boothby and G. L. Weiss, eds., Symmetric Spaces (1972)
9. Y. Matsushima, Differentiable Manifolds (E. T. Kobayashi, trans.) (1972)
10. L. E. Ward, Jr., Topology (1972)
11. A. Babakhanian, Cohomological Methods in Group Theory (1972)
12. R. Gilmer, Multiplicative Ideal Theory (1972)
13. J. Yeh, Stochastic Processes and the Wiener Integral (1973)
14. J. Barros-Neto, Introduction to the Theory of Distributions (1973)
15. R. Larsen, Functional Analysis (1973)
16. K. Yano and S. Ishihara, Tangent and Cotangent Bundles (1973)
17. C. Procesi, Rings with Polynomial Identities (1973)
18. R. Hermann, Geometry, Physics, and Systems (1973)
19. N. R. Wallach, Harmonic Analysis on Homogeneous Spaces (1973)
20. J. Dieudonné, Introduction to the Theory of Formal Groups (1973)
21. I. Vaisman, Cohomology and Differential Forms (1973)
22. B.-Y. Chen, Geometry of Submanifolds (1973)
23. M. Marcus, Finite Dimensional Multilinear Algebra (in two parts) (1973, 1975)
24. R. Larsen, Banach Algebras (1973)
25. R. O. Kujala and A. L. Vitter, eds., Value Distribution Theory: Part A; Part B: Deficit and Bezout Estimates by Wilhelm Stoll (1973)
26. K. B. Stolarsky, Algebraic Numbers and Diophantine Approximation (1974)
27. A. R. Magid, The Separable Galois Theory of Commutative Rings (1974)
28. B. R. McDonald, Finite Rings with Identity (1974)
29. J. Satake, Linear Algebra (S. Koh et al., trans.) (1975)
30. J. S. Golan, Localization of Noncommutative Rings (1975)
31. G. Klambauer, Mathematical Analysis (1975)
32. M. K. Agoston, Algebraic Topology (1976)
33. K. R. Goodearl, Ring Theory (1976)
34. L. E. Mansfield, Linear Algebra with Geometric Applications (1976)
35. N. J. Pullman, Matrix Theory and Its Applications (1976)
36. B. R. McDonald, Geometric Algebra Over Local Rings (1976)
37. C. W. Groetsch, Generalized Inverses of Linear Operators (1977)
38. J. E. Kuczkowski and J. L. Gersting, Abstract Algebra (1977)
39. C. O. Christenson and W. L. Voxman, Aspects of Topology (1977)
40. M. Nagata, Field Theory (1977)
41. R. L. Long, Algebraic Number Theory (1977)
42. W. F. Pfeffer, Integrals and Measures (1977)
43. R. L. Wheeden and A. Zygmund, Measure and Integral (1977)
44. J. H. Curtiss, Introduction to Functions of a Complex Variable (1978)
45. K. Hrbacek and T. Jech, Introduction to Set Theory (1978)
46. W. S. Massey, Homology and Cohomology Theory (1978)
47. M. Marcus, Introduction to Modern Algebra (1978)
48. E. C. Young, Vector and Tensor Analysis (1978)
49. S. B. Nadler, Jr., Hyperspaces of Sets (1978)
50. S. K. Segal, Topics in Group Kings (1978)
51. A. C. M. van Rooij, Non-Archimedean Functional Analysis (1978)
52. L. Corwin and R. Szczarba, Calculus in Vector Spaces (1979)
53. C. Sadosky, Interpolation of Operators and Singular Integrals (1979)
54. J. Cronin, Differential Equations (1980)
55. C. W. Groetsch, Elements of Applicable Functional Analysis (1980)

56. *I. Vaisman*, Foundations of Three-Dimensional Euclidean Geometry (1980)
57. *H. I. Freedan*, Deterministic Mathematical Models in Population Ecology (1980)
58. *S. B. Chae*, Lebesgue Integration (1980)
59. *C. S. Rees et al.*, Theory and Applications of Fourier Analysis (1981)
60. *L. Nachbin*, Introduction to Functional Analysis (R. M. Aron, trans.) (1981)
61. *G. Orzech and M. Orzech*, Plane Algebraic Curves (1981)
62. *R. Johnsonbaugh and W. E. Pfaffenberger*, Foundations of Mathematical Analysis (1981)
63. *W. L. Voxman and R. H. Goetschel*, Advanced Calculus (1981)
64. *L. J. Corwin and R. H. Szczarba*, Multivariable Calculus (1982)
65. *V. I. Istrățescu*, Introduction to Linear Operator Theory (1981)
66. *R. D. Järvinen*, Finite and Infinite Dimensional Linear Spaces (1981)
67. *J. K. Beem and P. E. Ehrlich*, Global Lorentzian Geometry (1981)
68. *D. L. Armacost*, The Structure of Locally Compact Abelian Groups (1981)
69. *J. W. Brewer and M. K. Smith, eds.*, Emmy Noether: A Tribute (1981)
70. *K. H. Kim*, Boolean Matrix Theory and Applications (1982)
71. *T. W. Wieting*, The Mathematical Theory of Chromatic Plane Ornaments (1982)
72. *D. B. Gauld*, Differential Topology (1982)
73. *R. L. Faber*, Foundations of Euclidean and Non-Euclidean Geometry (1983)
74. *M. Carmeli*, Statistical Theory and Random Matrices (1983)
75. *J. H. Carruth et al.*, The Theory of Topological Semigroups (1983)
76. *R. L. Faber*, Differential Geometry and Relativity Theory (1983)
77. *S. Barnett*, Polynomials and Linear Control Systems (1983)
78. *G. Karpilovsky*, Commutative Group Algebras (1983)
79. *F. Van Oystaeyen and A. Verschoren*, Relative Invariants of Rings (1983)
80. *I. Vaisman*, A First Course in Differential Geometry (1984)
81. *G. W. Swan*, Applications of Optimal Control Theory in Biomedicine (1984)
82. *T. Petrie and J. D. Randall*, Transformation Groups on Manifolds (1984)
83. *K. Goebel and S. Reich*, Uniform Convexity, Hyperbolic Geometry, and Nonexpansive Mappings (1984)
84. *T. Albu and C. Năstăsescu*, Relative Finiteness in Module Theory (1984)
85. *K. Hrbacek and T. Jech*, Introduction to Set Theory: Second Edition (1984)
86. *F. Van Oystaeyen and A. Verschoren*, Relative Invariants of Rings (1984)
87. *B. R. McDonald*, Linear Algebra Over Commutative Rings (1984)
88. *M. Namba*, Geometry of Projective Algebraic Curves (1984)
89. *G. F. Webb*, Theory of Nonlinear Age-Dependent Population Dynamics (1985)
90. *M. R. Bremner et al.*, Tables of Dominant Weight Multiplicities for Representations of Simple Lie Algebras (1985)
91. *A. E. Fekete*, Real Linear Algebra (1985)
92. *S. B. Chae*, Holomorphy and Calculus in Normed Spaces (1985)
93. *A. J. Jerri*, Introduction to Integral Equations with Applications (1985)
94. *G. Karpilovsky*, Projective Representations of Finite Groups (1985)
95. *L. Narici and E. Beckenstein*, Topological Vector Spaces (1985)
96. *J. Weeks*, The Shape of Space (1985)
97. *P. R. Gribik and K. O. Kortanok*, Extremal Methods of Operations Research (1985)
98. *J.-A. Chao and W. A. Woyczynski, eds.*, Probability Theory and Harmonic Analysis (1986)
99. *G. D. Crown et al.*, Abstract Algebra (1986)
100. *J. H. Carruth et al.*, The Theory of Topological Semigroups, Volume 2 (1986)
101. *R. S. Doran and V. A. Belfi*, Characterizations of C*-Algebras (1986)
102. *M. W. Jeter*, Mathematical Programming (1986)
103. *M. Altman*, A Unified Theory of Nonlinear Operator and Evolution Equations with Applications (1986)
104. *A. Verschoren*, Relative Invariants of Sheaves (1987)
105. *R. A. Usmani*, Applied Linear Algebra (1987)
106. *P. Blass and J. Lang*, Zariski Surfaces and Differential Equations in Characteristic $p > 0$ (1987)
107. *J. A. Reneke et al.*, Structured Hereditary Systems (1987)
108. *H. Busemann and B. B. Phadke*, Spaces with Distinguished Geodesics (1987)
109. *R. Harte*, Invertibility and Singularity for Bounded Linear Operators (1988)
110. *G. S. Ladde et al.*, Oscillation Theory of Differential Equations with Deviating Arguments (1987)
111. *L. Dudkin et al.*, Iterative Aggregation Theory (1987)
112. *T. Okubo*, Differential Geometry (1987)

113. *D. L. Stancl and M. L. Stancl*, Real Analysis with Point-Set Topology (1987)
114. *T. C. Gard*, Introduction to Stochastic Differential Equations (1988)
115. *S. S. Abhyankar*, Enumerative Combinatorics of Young Tableaux (1988)
116. *H. Strade and R. Farnsteiner*, Modular Lie Algebras and Their Representations (1988)
117. *J. A. Huckaba*, Commutative Rings with Zero Divisors (1988)
118. *W. D. Wallis*, Combinatorial Designs (1988)
119. *W. Więsław*, Topological Fields (1988)
120. *G. Karpilovsky*, Field Theory (1988)
121. *S. Caenepeel and F. Van Oystaeyen*, Brauer Groups and the Cohomology of Graded Rings (1989)
122. *W. Kozlowski*, Modular Function Spaces (1988)
123. *E. Lowen-Colebunders*, Function Classes of Cauchy Continuous Maps (1989)
124. *M. Pavel*, Fundamentals of Pattern Recognition (1989)
125. *V. Lakshmikantham et al.*, Stability Analysis of Nonlinear Systems (1989)
126. *R. Sivaramakrishnan*, The Classical Theory of Arithmetic Functions (1989)
127. *N. A. Watson*, Parabolic Equations on an Infinite Strip (1989)
128. *K. J. Hastings*, Introduction to the Mathematics of Operations Research (1989)
129. *B. Fine*, Algebraic Theory of the Bianchi Groups (1989)
130. *D. N. Dikranjan et al.*, Topological Groups (1989)
131. *J. C. Morgan II*, Point Set Theory (1990)
132. *P. Biler and A. Witkowski*, Problems in Mathematical Analysis (1990)
133. *H. J. Sussmann*, Nonlinear Controllability and Optimal Control (1990)
134. *J.-P. Florens et al.*, Elements of Bayesian Statistics (1990)
135. *N. Shell*, Topological Fields and Near Valuations (1990)
136. *B. F. Doolin and C. F. Martin*, Introduction to Differential Geometry for Engineers (1990)
137. *S. S. Holland, Jr.*, Applied Analysis by the Hilbert Space Method (1990)
138. *J. Oknínski*, Semigroup Algebras (1990)
139. *K. Zhu*, Operator Theory in Function Spaces (1990)
140. *G. B. Price*, An Introduction to Multicomplex Spaces and Functions (1991)
141. *R. B. Darst*, Introduction to Linear Programming (1991)
142. *P. L. Sachdev*, Nonlinear Ordinary Differential Equations and Their Applications (1991)
143. *T. Husain*, Orthogonal Schauder Bases (1991)
144. *J. Foran*, Fundamentals of Real Analysis (1991)
145. *W. C. Brown*, Matrices and Vector Spaces (1991)
146. *M. M. Rao and Z. D. Ren*, Theory of Orlicz Spaces (1991)
147. *J. S. Golan and T. Head*, Modules and the Structures of Rings (1991)
148. *C. Small*, Arithmetic of Finite Fields (1991)
149. *K. Yang*, Complex Algebraic Geometry (1991)
150. *D. G. Hoffman et al.*, Coding Theory (1991)
151. *M. O. González*, Classical Complex Analysis (1992)
152. *M. O. González*, Complex Analysis (1992)
153. *L. W. Baggett*, Functional Analysis (1992)
154. *M. Sniedovich*, Dynamic Programming (1992)
155. *R. P. Agarwal*, Difference Equations and Inequalities (1992)
156. *C. Brezinski*, Biorthogonality and Its Applications to Numerical Analysis (1992)
157. *C. Swartz*, An Introduction to Functional Analysis (1992)
158. *S. B. Nadler, Jr.*, Continuum Theory (1992)
159. *M. A. Al-Gwaiz*, Theory of Distributions (1992)
160. *E. Perry*, Geometry: Axiomatic Developments with Problem Solving (1992)
161. *E. Castillo and M. R. Ruiz-Cobo*, Functional Equations and Modelling in Science and Engineering (1992)
162. *A. J. Jerri*, Integral and Discrete Transforms with Applications and Error Analysis (1992)
163. *A. Charlier et al.*, Tensors and the Clifford Algebra (1992)
164. *P. Biler and T. Nadzieja*, Problems and Examples in Differential Equations (1992)
165. *E. Hansen*, Global Optimization Using Interval Analysis (1992)
166. *S. Guerre-Delabrière*, Classical Sequences in Banach Spaces (1992)
167. *Y. C. Wong*, Introductory Theory of Topological Vector Spaces (1992)
168. *S. H. Kulkarni and B. V. Limaye*, Real Function Algebras (1992)
169. *W. C. Brown*, Matrices Over Commutative Rings (1993)
170. *J. Loustau and M. Dillon*, Linear Geometry with Computer Graphics (1993)
171. *W. V. Petryshyn*, Approximation-Solvability of Nonlinear Functional and Differential Equations (1993)

172. *E. C. Young*, Vector and Tensor Analysis: Second Edition (1993)
173. *T. A. Bick*, Elementary Boundary Value Problems (1993)
174. *M. Pavel*, Fundamentals of Pattern Recognition: Second Edition (1993)
175. *S. A. Albeverio et al.*, Noncommutative Distributions (1993)
176. *W. Fulks*, Complex Variables (1993)
177. *M. M. Rao*, Conditional Measures and Applications (1993)
178. *A. Janicki and A. Weron*, Simulation and Chaotic Behavior of α-Stable Stochastic Processes (1994)
179. *P. Neittaanmäki and D. Tiba*, Optimal Control of Nonlinear Parabolic Systems (1994)
180. *J. Cronin*, Differential Equations: Introduction and Qualitative Theory, Second Edition (1994)
181. *S. Heikkilä and V. Lakshmikantham*, Monotone Iterative Techniques for Discontinuous Nonlinear Differential Equations (1994)
182. *X. Mao*, Exponential Stability of Stochastic Differential Equations (1994)
183. *B. S. Thomson*, Symmetric Properties of Real Functions (1994)
184. *J. E. Rubio*, Optimization and Nonstandard Analysis (1994)
185. *J. L. Bueso et al.*, Compatibility, Stability, and Sheaves (1995)
186. *A. N. Michel and K. Wang*, Qualitative Theory of Dynamical Systems (1995)
187. *M. R. Darnel*, Theory of Lattice-Ordered Groups (1995)
188. *Z. Naniewicz and P. D. Panagiotopoulos*, Mathematical Theory of Hemivariational Inequalities and Applications (1995)
189. *L. J. Corwin and R. H. Szczarba*, Calculus in Vector Spaces: Second Edition (1995)
190. *L. H. Erbe et al.*, Oscillation Theory for Functional Differential Equations (1995)
191. *S. Agaian et al.*, Binary Polynomial Transforms and Nonlinear Digital Filters (1995)
192. *M. I. Gil'*, Norm Estimations for Operation-Valued Functions and Applications (1995)
193. *P. A. Grillet*, Semigroups: An Introduction to the Structure Theory (1995)
194. *S. Kichenassamy*, Nonlinear Wave Equations (1996)
195. *V. F. Krotov*, Global Methods in Optimal Control Theory (1996)
196. *K. I. Beidar et al.*, Rings with Generalized Identities (1996)
197. *V. I. Arnautov et al.*, Introduction to the Theory of Topological Rings and Modules (1996)
198. *G. Sierksma*, Linear and Integer Programming (1996)
199. *R. Lasser*, Introduction to Fourier Series (1996)
200. *V. Sima*, Algorithms for Linear-Quadratic Optimization (1996)
201. *D. Redmond*, Number Theory (1996)
202. *J. K. Beem et al.*, Global Lorentzian Geometry: Second Edition (1996)
203. *M. Fontana et al.*, Prüfer Domains (1997)
204. *H. Tanabe*, Functional Analytic Methods for Partial Differential Equations (1997)
205. *C. Q. Zhang*, Integer Flows and Cycle Covers of Graphs (1997)
206. *E. Spiegel and C. J. O'Donnell*, Incidence Algebras (1997)
207. *B. Jakubczyk and W. Respondek*, Geometry of Feedback and Optimal Control (1998)
208. *T. W. Haynes et al.*, Fundamentals of Domination in Graphs (1998)
209. *T. W. Haynes et al.*, Domination in Graphs: Advanced Topics (1998)
210. *L. A. D'Alotto et al.*, A Unified Signal Algebra Approach to Two-Dimensional Parallel Digital Signal Processing (1998)
211. *F. Halter-Koch*, Ideal Systems (1998)
212. *N. K. Govil et al.*, Approximation Theory (1998)
213. *R. Cross*, Multivalued Linear Operators (1998)
214. *A. A. Martynyuk*, Stability by Liapunov's Matrix Function Method with Applications (1998)
215. *A. Favini and A. Yagi*, Degenerate Differential Equations in Banach Spaces (1999)
216. *A. Illanes and S. Nadler, Jr.*, Hyperspaces: Fundamentals and Recent Advances (1999)
217. *G. Kato and D. Struppa*, Fundamentals of Algebraic Microlocal Analysis (1999)
218. *G. X.-Z. Yuan*, KKM Theory and Applications in Nonlinear Analysis (1999)
219. *D. Motreanu and N. H. Pavel*, Tangency, Flow Invariance for Differential Equations, and Optimization Problems (1999)
220. *K. Hrbacek and T. Jech*, Introduction to Set Theory, Third Edition (1999)
221. *G. E. Kolosov*, Optimal Design of Control Systems (1999)
222. *N. L. Johnson*, Subplane Covered Nets (2000)
223. *B. Fine and G. Rosenberger*, Algebraic Generalizations of Discrete Groups (1999)
224. *M. Väth*, Volterra and Integral Equations of Vector Functions (2000)
225. *S. S. Miller and P. T. Mocanu*, Differential Subordinations (2000)

226. R. Li et al., Generalized Difference Methods for Differential Equations: Numerical Analysis of Finite Volume Methods (2000)
227. H. Li and F. Van Oystaeyen, A Primer of Algebraic Geometry (2000)
228. R. P. Agarwal, Difference Equations and Inequalities: Theory, Methods, and Applications, Second Edition (2000)
229. A. B. Kharazishvili, Strange Functions in Real Analysis (2000)
230. J. M. Appell et al., Partial Integral Operators and Integro-Differential Equations (2000)
231. A. I. Prilepko et al., Methods for Solving Inverse Problems in Mathematical Physics (2000)
232. F. Van Oystaeyen, Algebraic Geometry for Associative Algebras (2000)
233. D. L. Jagerman, Difference Equations with Applications to Queues (2000)
234. D. R. Hankerson et al., Coding Theory and Cryptography: The Essentials, Second Edition, Revised and Expanded (2000)
235. S. Dăscălescu et al., Hopf Algebras: An Introduction (2001)
236. R. Hagen et al., C*-Algebras and Numerical Analysis (2001)
237. Y. Talpaert, Differential Geometry: With Applications to Mechanics and Physics (2001)
238. R. H. Villarreal, Monomial Algebras (2001)
239. A. N. Michel et al., Qualitative Theory of Dynamical Systems, Second Edition (2001)
240. A. A. Samarskii, The Theory of Difference Schemes (2001)
241. J. Knopfmacher and W.-B. Zhang, Number Theory Arising from Finite Fields (2001)
242. S. Leader, The Kurzweil-Henstock Integral and Its Differentials (2001)
243. M. Biliotti et al., Foundations of Translation Planes (2001)
244. A. N. Kochubei, Pseudo-Differential Equations and Stochastics over Non-Archimedean Fields (2001)
245. G. Sierksma, Linear and Integer Programming, Second Edition (2002)
246. A. A. Martynyuk, Qualitative Methods in Nonlinear Dynamics: Novel Approaches to Liapunov's Matrix Functions (2002)
247. B. G. Pachpatte, Inequalities for Finite Difference Equations (2002)
248. A. N. Michel and D. Liu, Qualitative Analysis and Synthesis of Recurrent Neural Networks (2002)

Additional Volumes in Preparation

QUALITATIVE ANALYSIS AND SYNTHESIS OF RECURRENT NEURAL NETWORKS

Anthony N. Michel
University of Notre Dame
Notre Dame, Indiana

Derong Liu
University of Illinois
Chicago, Illinois

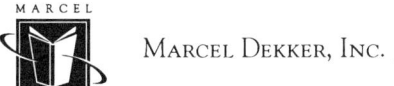

MARCEL DEKKER, INC.　　　　　　NEW YORK · BASEL

ISBN: 0-8247-0767-2

This book is printed on acid-free paper.

Headquarters
Marcel Dekker, Inc.
270 Madison Avenue, New York, NY 10016
tel: 212-696-9000; fax: 212-685-4540

Eastern Hemisphere Distribution
Marcel Dekker AG
Hutgasse 4, Postfach 812, CH-4001 Basel, Switzerland
tel: 41-61-261-8482; fax: 41-61-261-8896

World Wide Web
http://www.dekker.com

The publisher offers discounts on this book when ordered in bulk quantities. For more information, write to Special Sales/Professional Marketing at the headquarters address above.

Copyright © 2002 by Marcel Dekker, Inc. All Rights Reserved.

Neither this book nor any part may be reproduced or transmitted in any form or by any means, electronic or mechanical, including photocopying, microfilming, and recording, or by any information storage and retrieval system, without permission in writing from the publisher.

Current printing (last digit):
10 9 8 7 6 5 4 3 2 1

PRINTED IN THE UNITED STATES OF AMERICA

Preface

In the present book we concern ourselves exclusively with the qualitative analysis and synthesis of recurrent artificial neural networks. There is an abundance of papers, monographs, and books that address qualitative properties of such networks. However, whereas in these works, the analysis of the networks is frequently incidental to the achievement of some other principal goal, in the present book the network itself is the primary object of inquiry. Works in which the primary object of study is the recurrent neural network itself are rare. Consequently, many of the qualitative attributes and limitations of such networks have been ignored and are therefore obscure.

In the present book we present a systematic analysis of artificial recurrent neural networks which addresses limitations to the qualitative behavior (and thus, to the performance) of the networks. These limitations are either due to the *inherent properties of the networks*, or they are *incurred during the implementation process of a network* (e.g., by VLSI, specialized digital hardware, opto-electronic means, simulations, or some other methods). While our objective is to present results that are as universal as possible, we do not intend to undertake an encyclopedic effort involving the many variants of recurrent neural networks encountered in the literature. Such an attempt would be futile, and more importantly, undesirable, since it would lead us astray from our main objective. Instead, to fix ideas and provide motivation, we concentrate on a small number of important and representative classes of neural networks, using specific applications as needed. These include analog (i.e., continuous-time) Hopfield neural networks (with sigmoidal activation functions); analog Hopfield neural networks with infinite gain amplifiers (i.e., variable structure systems); analog Hopfield-type neural networks having saturation nonlinearities for activation functions; some generalizations to the analog Hopfield neural network, including Cohen-Grossberg networks; discrete Hopfield neural networks (i.e., asynchronous discrete-time networks with sign functions serving as activation functions); Hopfield-type synchronous discrete-time neural networks with sigmoidal functions, saturation functions, and sign functions serving as activation functions; and linear systems operating on a closed hypercube (both continuous-time and discrete-time cases). When required to ascertain network performance, we usually employ applications to associative memories, using the Outer Product Method, the Projection Learning Rule, the Eigenstructure Method, or a perceptron based training method to synthesize the networks.

Some of the more important issues that we address in the qualitative analysis of the networks considered are discussed in the following.

Since the variable structure systems and the linear systems operating on a closed hypercube exhibit discontinuous dynamics, we give careful consideration to questions concerning existence, uniqueness, and continuation of solutions of the differential equations describing these networks. Also, for the networks under study, we establish conditions which guarantee the existence of isolated (i.e., discrete) equilibria; which give upper bounds for the total number of equilibria; and which give upper bounds for the number of asymptotically stable equilibria. Further, we establish results which enable us to locate systematically all the equilibria and ascertain the *local* stability properties of the equilibria of a network. Also, we present results which

PREFACE

provide estimates of the domains of attraction of the asymptotically stable equilibria in a given network. We also establish estimates of trajectory bounds, and rates of convergence to asymptotically stable equilibria for some of the networks considered. Moreover, we give conditions under which a given neural network has only one equilibrium.

For the networks under study, we establish conditions (using appropriate energy functions) which guarantee that a given network is *globally* stable (i.e., that all the motions of the network tend to an asymptotically stable equilibrium). The state space in which a globally stable network operates is partitioned by the domains of attraction of the asymptotically stable equilibria of the network. Such a partition establishes an equivalence relation which serves as the theoretical foundation for a variety of applications, including applications to associative memories.

Prespecified asymptotically stable equilibria of a recurrent neural network, which are used to store information or data, are called *stable memories* while the remaining (undesirable) asymptotically stable equilibria of the network are referred to as *spurious states*. For some of the networks that we consider, we establish conditions on the network parameters which tend to reduce the number of spurious states. This has the effect of increasing the storage capacity of a network.

We address the following important problem which arises during the *implementation process* of an artificial neural network: Given a neural network with a desired set of operating points (e.g., in associative memories, a desired set of stable memories), and given an associated neural network with *perturbations in the parameters* of the original (unperturbed) network, determine conditions which ensure that the perturbed neural network will possess a set of operating points (with identical stability properties) which are near the operating points of the original unperturbed neural network. Determine estimates of the distances between the operating points of the unperturbed neural network and the corresponding operating points of the perturbed neural network. Results of this type give an indication of the size of inaccuracies of the network operating points due to network parameter perturbations.

We address the following important problem which may also arise during the *implementation process* of a recurrent artificial neural network: Given a neural network with a desired set of operating points (and with no time delays in the interconnections), and given an associated neural network with *time delays*, determine conditions which ensure that for all time delays that are less than some upper bound, the operating points of the neural network with time delays coincide with the operating points of the corresponding network without delays and exhibit similar qualitative behavior (e.g., in associative memories, the network with delays should possess asymptotically stable equilibria which coincide with the asymptotically stable equilibria of the corresponding network without delays). Determine estimates for the upper bound for the permissible time delays.

We address the following important problem which may also arise during the *implementation process* of an artificial recurrent neural network: Devise synthesis techniques (for associative memories) which incorporate *constraints on the interconnecting structure* of a network (e.g., prespecified *sparsity constraints*, arising for instance, in the case of cellular neural networks).

In concluding, we note that in the present book we do not address questions concerning the existence and the qualitative properties of periodic motions (limit cycles) in artificial neural networks. (Rather, throughout, we are interested in questions concerning the non-existence of periodic motions in such networks.)

The present book is intended for researchers and graduate students in applied mathematics, the physical sciences, and any of the engineering disciplines who are interested in artificial neural networks. It is assumed that the reader has a background in linear algebra, real analysis, and differential equations. The book is suitable as a graduate text and as a reference source.

PREFACE

A great deal of the material presented in this book is based on research which we conducted with several colleagues and former students, including J. A. Farrell, Z. Feng, D. L. Gray, Lj. T. Grujić, L. Hou, J.-H. Li, D. Liu, Z. Lu, W. Porod, J. Si, H.-F. Sun, K. Wang, H. Ye, and G. Yen.

We appreciate the efforts and patience of Ms. Connie C. Zhang in the typing and extensive correcting of the manuscript.

Anthony N. Michel

Derong Liu

Contents

Preface		i
1 Introduction		**1**
1.1	Issues to be Addressed in the Present Book	3
1.2	Some Neural Network Models	6
1.3	Qualitative Analysis of Analog Hopfield-Type Neural Networks: Global Results	9
1.4	Stability Analysis of Linear Systems Operating on a Closed Hypercube	12
1.5	Qualitative Analysis of Hopfield-Type Neural Networks: Local Results	13
1.6	Qualitative Effects of Parameter Perturbations	17
1.7	Qualitative Effects of Time Delays	19
1.8	Some Synthesis Methods for Associative Memories	22
1.9	Effects of Interconnection Constraints	26
	Bibliography	27
2 Some Neural Network Models		**33**
2.1	Introduction	33
2.2	Analog Hopfield Neural Network Model	40
2.3	Discrete Hopfield Neural Network Model	44
2.4	Generalizations of the Hopfield Model	48

CONTENTS

- 2.5 Analog Hopfield Neural Networks with Infinite Gain Amplifiers 50
- 2.6 Linear Systems Operating on a Closed Hypercube . . 52
- 2.7 Summary 58
- 2.8 Notes and References 62
- Bibliography 62

3 Qualitative Analysis of Analog Hopfield-Type Neural Networks: Global Results 69

- 3.1 Generalized Analog Hopfield Neural Network Model: System (L) 70
- 3.2 Notation and Some Preliminaries 71
- 3.3 Assumptions for the Generalized Hopfield Model . . . 75
- 3.4 Main Results (Generalized Hopfield Model) 80
- 3.5 Analog Hopfield Neural Network Model with Infinite Gain Amplifiers: System (N) 85
- 3.6 Definition and Properties of the Solutions of System (N) 87
- 3.7 Qualitative Properties of the Equilibrium Points and of the Output Vectors of System (N) 97
- 3.8 Qualitative Analysis of System (N) in Terms of an Energy Function 100
- 3.9 Summary 109
- 3.10 Notes and References 111
- Bibliography 112

4 Stability Analysis of Linear Systems Operating on a Closed Hypercube: System (M) 115

- 4.1 Linear Continuous-Time Systems Operating on a Closed Hypercube: System (M) 116

4.2	Notation	117
4.3	Definition and Properties of the Solutions of System (M)	118
4.4	Qualitative Properties of the Equilibrium Points of System (M)	122
4.5	Qualitative Analysis of System (M) in Terms of an Energy Function	128
4.6	Linear Discrete-Time Systems Operating on a Closed Hypercube	131
4.7	Global Asymptotic Stability of Linear Continuous-Time Systems Operating on a Closed Hypercube	144
4.8	Global Asymptotic Stability of Linear Discrete-Time Systems Operating on a Closed Hypercube	152
4.9	Summary	159
4.10	Notes and References	161
	Bibliography	161

5 Qualitative Analysis of Hopfield-Type Neural Networks: Local Results — 165

5.1	Notation	166
5.2	Some Background Material	167
5.3	Analog Hopfield Model Viewed as an Interconnected System	170
5.4	Stability Analysis of the Single Neuron Subsystems	175
5.5	Qualitative Analysis of the Analog Hopfield Neural Network Model: Local Results	180
5.6	Analysis of Synchronous Discrete-Time Hopfield-Type Neural Networks	206
5.7	Analysis of Analog Hopfield Neural Networks with Saturation Nonlinearities as Activation Functions	216

	5.8	Summary	224
	5.9	Notes and References	228
		Bibliography	229

6 Qualitative Effects of Parameter Perturbations — 233

- 6.1 Introduction 233
- 6.2 Notation 235
- 6.3 Robust Stability: Perturbed Systems with Fixed Equilibria 236
- 6.4 Robust Stability: Perturbed Systems with Perturbed Equilibria 241
- 6.5 Analysis of Neural Networks with Sigmoidal Activation Functions 250
- 6.6 Analysis of Neural Networks with Hard Limiter Activation Functions 259
- 6.7 Summary 265
- 6.8 Notes and References 269
- Bibliography 270

7 Qualitative Effects of Time Delays — 271

- 7.1 Introduction 271
- 7.2 Preliminaries (Hopfield Neural Networks) 275
- 7.3 Global Stability of Hopfield Neural Networks with Delays 278
- 7.4 Local Stability Results for Hopfield Neural Networks with Delays 285
- 7.5 An Example for the Hopfield Neural Networks 289
- 7.6 Preliminaries (Cohen-Grossberg Neural Networks) . . 291

CONTENTS   xi

- 7.7 Global Stability of Cohen-Grossberg Neural Networks with Multiple Delays 294
- 7.8 Local Stability Results for Cohen-Grossberg Neural Networks with Multiple Delays 302
- 7.9 Nonlinear Systems with Arbitrary Bounded Delays .. 307
- 7.10 Nonlinear Systems with Fixed Bounded Delays 313
- 7.11 Stability Analysis of Time-Delay Neural Networks with Nonsymmetric Interconnecting Structure 322
- 7.12 Robust Stability Analysis of Time-Delay Neural Networks 331
- 7.13 Examples 333
- 7.14 Summary 335
- 7.15 Notes and References 342
- Bibliography 343

8 Some Synthesis Methods for Associative Memories 347

- 8.1 Introduction: The Outer Product Method and the Projection Learning Rule 347
- 8.2 Some Extensions to the Projection Learning Rule ... 355
- 8.3 The Eigenstructure Method 360
- 8.4 Some Extensions to the Eigenstructure Method 369
- 8.5 Synthesis of Recurrent Neural Networks Based on the Perceptron Training Algorithm 373
- 8.6 Some Extensions to the Perceptron Based Training Algorithm 388
- 8.7 Illustrative Examples 395
- 8.8 Summary 414
- 8.9 Notes and References 419
- Bibliography 420

9 Effects of Interconnection Constraints — 425

- 9.1 Introduction . . . 425
- 9.2 The Eigenstructure Method in the Synthesis of Sparsely Interconnected Neural Networks . . . 427
- 9.3 The Perceptron Based Training Algorithm in the Synthesis of Sparsely Interconnected Neural Networks . . . 435
- 9.4 Synthesis of Cellular Neural Networks for Associative Memories . . . 438
- 9.5 Illustrative Examples . . . 450
- 9.6 Summary . . . 469
- 9.7 Notes and References . . . 471
- Bibliography . . . 471

Index — 475

Chapter 1

Introduction

Artificial neural networks were inspired by the functioning of the brain and attempts to mimic certain biological systems. As such, artificial neural networks constitute massive interconnections of elements, the neurons, whose inputs consist of appropriately weighted sums of the neuron outputs, along with suitable bias terms, when necessary. The neurons are represented by appropriate functions, called activation functions.

The many different types of artificial neural networks that have been considered in the literature fall generally into one of two categories: feedforward neural networks (i.e., neural networks with no feedback) and recurrent neural networks (i.e., neural networks endowed with feedback loops). Perhaps the most widely known and applied example of the former is the multi-layer perceptron for which the Back Propagation Algorithm is used to "train" the network, while the most popular example of the latter is the Hopfield neural network for which the Outer Product Method is used to "train" the network.

Although strict adherence to formal definitions in the classification of artificial neural networks does not appear to be in place at this time, the term *"feedback neural network"* seems to apply generally to single layer, fully interconnected feedback networks. Most of the neural networks that we consider in the present book fall into this category. However, in the last chapter, we will concern ourselves with networks that are endowed with intentional sparsity constraints (resulting in networks that are not fully interconnected), and it is for this reason that we will apply in the present book the term *"recurrent neural network"* to the networks addressed herein. No matter what term is used, however, such networks constitute important classes of large-scale dynamical systems with interesting qualitative properties.

There are certainly numerous papers, monographs, and books that address qualitative properties of recurrent neural networks (see, e.g., [1], [5], [8], [9], [13]–[16], [30], [46], [51]). However, in these works, the qualitative analysis is usually incidental to achieving some other principal goal. Works in which the primary object of inquiry is the recurrent neural network itself are rare, with the consequence that the *qualitative limitations* that are either *inherent in such networks*, or are *incurred during the implementation process* of such networks (be it by VLSI, specialized digital hardware, opto-electronic means, or even simulations) have been ignored and are therefore obscure.

In the present book, we will present a systematic analysis of artificial recurrent neural networks which addresses limitations to the qualitative behavior (and thus, to the performance) of such networks that are due, either to the inherent properties of the networks, or are incurred during the implementation process of such networks. While our objective is to present results that are as universal as possible, we do not intend to undertake an encyclopedic effort involving the many variants of recurrent neural networks encountered in the literature. Such an attempt would be futile, and more importantly, undesirable, since it would lead us astray from our main objective. Instead, to fix ideas and provide motivation, we will concentrate on a small number of important and representative classes of neural networks, using specific applications, as needed. These include analog (i.e., continuous-time) Hopfield neural networks and Hopfield-type synchronous discrete-time neural networks with sigmoidal functions and saturation nonlinearities as activation functions; discrete Hopfield neural networks (i.e., asynchronous discrete-time networks) with the sign function serving as activation functions; analog Hopfield neural networks with sigmoidal functions having infinite gain (i.e., systems with variable structure); the Grossberg model (as a generalization of the analog Hopfield model); and linear systems operating on a closed hypercube (both the continuous-time and the discrete-time case). When required to ascertain network performance, we will usually employ applications to associative memories (using the Outer Product Method, the Projection Learning Rule, the Eigenstructure Method, or a perceptron based training method to synthesize the networks).

In the present book we will not address questions concerning the existence and the qualitative properties of periodic motions (limit cycles) in artificial neural networks. Rather, throughout, we will be interested in questions concerning the non-existence of such motions in the networks considered.

1.1 Issues to be Addressed in the Present Book

In the following, we comment in some detail on the specific issues that will be addressed in the present book.

a) For the case of analog Hopfield neural networks with sigmoidal functions having infinite gains and for linear systems operating on a closed hypercube, the differential equations describing these networks exhibit discontinuous dynamics, and therefore, careful considerations will be given to questions concerning the existence, uniqueness, and continuation of solutions of such equations.

b) For the networks under study, precise conditions will be established which guarantee the existence of isolated equilibria; which give upper bounds for the number of equilibria; and which give upper bounds for the number of asymptotically stable equilibria. Also, algorithms will be established which systematically locate all the equilibria and ascertain their stability properties. Furthermore, methods will be presented which provide estimates for the domains of attraction of the asymptotically stable equilibria. Also, conditions will be established under which a given neural network has only one equilibrium.

c) For the networks under study, precise conditions will be established which guarantee that a given network is globally stable, i.e., that all the motions of a network tend to an equilibrium. Under these conditions, the state space in which a network operates is partitioned by the domains of attraction of the asymptotically stable equilibria of the network. This partition in turn establishes an equivalence relation which is suitable in a variety of applications, including classification of data, pattern recognition, and others.

d) Prespecified asymptotically stable equilibria of a recurrent neural network which are used to store information, or data, are called *stable memories* while the remaining (undesirable) asymptotically stable equilibria of the network are referred to as *spurious states*. For some of the networks that we consider, we will establish conditions on the network parameters which tend to reduce the number of spurious states. This has the effect of increasing the storage capacity of a network.

e) We will address the following important problem which may arise during the implementation process of a recurrent artificial neural network: Given a neural network with a desired set of operating points (e.g., in associative memories, a desired set of stable memories), and given an associated neural network with perturbations in the parameters of the original (unperturbed) network, determine conditions which will ensure that the perturbed neural network will possess a set of operating points (with identical stability properties) which are near the operating points of the original unperturbed neural network. Determine estimates of the distances between the operating points of the unperturbed neural network and the corresponding operating points of the perturbed neural network.

f) We will address the following important problem which may also arise during the implementation process of a recurrent artifi-

1.1. ISSUES TO BE ADDRESSED

cial neural network: Given a neural network with a desired set of operating points (and with no time delays in the interconnections), and given an associated neural network with time delays, determine conditions which ensure that for all time delays that are less than some upper bound, the operating points of the neural network with time delays will coincide with the operating points of the corresponding network without delays, exhibiting similar qualitative behavior (e.g., in associative memories, the network with delays should possess asymptotically stable equilibria which coincide with the asymptotically stable equilibria of the corresponding network without delays). Determine estimates for the upper bound for the permissible time delays.

g) We will address the following important problem which may also arise during the implementation process of a recurrent artificial neural network: Devise synthesis techniques (for associative memories) which incorporate constraints on the interconnecting structure of a network (e.g., prespecified sparsity constraints, arising for instance, in the case of cellular neural networks).

The issues addressed above have significant practical implications. For example, consideration of item (a) above is important in the modeling (and well-posedness) of recurrent neural networks, while items (b) and (d) provide information concerning the capacity of a network to store information and item (c) ensures the proper functioning of the network in the first place. Finally, the issues addressed in items (e), (f), and (g) above, have significant implications in the implementation process of networks (especially VLSI implementations). Thus, parameter perturbations will in general result in inaccuracies of the network operating points (stable memories), transmission delays will in general impose limitations on the size of a network, and interconnection constraints will in general result in a reduction in the storage capacity of a network.

In the remainder of this chapter, we provide a summary of some of the contents of this book.

1.2 Some Neural Network Models

There are numerous models of recurrent neural networks that have been considered in the literature. In Chapter 2 we will single out and discuss several of these.

For historic reasons, we will first introduce the *McCulloch-Pitts model* [29], given by

$$\begin{cases} v_i(k+1) = \text{sgn}(u_i(k)), & 1 \leq i \leq n \\ u_i(k) = \sum_{j=1}^{n} T_{ij} v_j(k) + I_i, & 1 \leq i \leq n \end{cases} \quad (1.2.1)$$

where each neuron is represented by the sign function,

$$\text{sgn}(\theta) = \begin{cases} 1, & \theta > 0 \\ -1, & \theta < 0, \end{cases} \quad (1.2.2)$$

u_i denotes the input to the ith neuron, v_i represents the output of the ith neuron, T_{ij} specifies the interconnection strength between the jth and ith neurons, and I_i represents the external input to neuron i. The states in (1.2.1) switch *asynchronously*.

Next, we address in some detail the *analog Hopfield neural network model* [10], [11], including its implementation [30], described by equations of the form

$$\begin{cases} C_i(du_i/dt) = -1/R_i + \sum_{j=1}^{n} t_{ij} v_j + w_i \\ v_i = g_i(\lambda u_i), \; i = 1, \cdots, n \end{cases} \quad (1.2.3)$$

where, as before, u_i and v_i denote neuron inputs and outputs, respectively, w_i denotes the external input to the ith neuron, $C_i > 0$ and $R_i > 0$ are capacitances and resistances, respectively, and $t_{ij} \in \Re$ represent neuron interconnection weights determined by conductances. Each neuron is represented by a sigmoidal function. The specific example of sigmoidal function that we frequently use is given by

$$v_i = g_i(\lambda u_i) = (2/\pi)\tan^{-1}\left((\pi/2)\lambda u_i\right). \quad (1.2.4)$$

We rewrite (1.2.3) in vector form as

$$\begin{cases} \dot{x} = -Ax + Ty + I \\ y = S(x) \end{cases} \quad (1.2.5)$$

1.2. SOME NEURAL NETWORK MODELS

where $S(x) = (s_1(x_1), \cdots, s_n(x_n))^T$, $s_i(x_i) = g_i(\lambda u_i)/C_i$, and $x = (x_1, \cdots, x_n)^T$, $A = \text{diag}[a_1, \cdots, a_n]$, $T = [T_{ij}]$, and $I = (I_1, \cdots, I_n)^T$ are defined in the obvious way.

A *variant* of (1.2.5) that we will also address are networks described by equations of the form (see [2], [24]),

$$\begin{cases} \dot{x} = -Ax + Ty + I \\ y = \text{sat}(x) \end{cases} \quad (1.2.6)$$

where $\text{sat}(x) = (\text{sat}(x_1), \cdots, \text{sat}(x_n))^T$ and where

$$\text{sat}(x_i) = \begin{cases} 1, & x_i > 1 \\ x_i, & -1 \leq x_i \leq 1 \\ -1, & x_i < -1. \end{cases} \quad (1.2.7)$$

To approximate the analog Hopfield neural network by digital computer simulations or by means of specialized digital hardware, we will also address in Chapter 2 the *synchronous discrete-time Hopfield neural network model* [31], [33] described by equations of the form

$$u_i(k+1) = \sum_{j=1}^n T_{ij} v_j(k) - a_i u_i(k) + I_i, \quad i = 1, \cdots, n \quad (1.2.8)$$

where all symbols are defined similarly as in (1.2.5).

We will also consider in Chapter 2 two *generalizations to the analog Hopfield neural network model*. The first of these is described by equations of the form [18]

$$\dot{x} = -H(x)(-Tx + S(x) - I) \quad (1.2.9)$$

where x, T, $S(x)$ and I are defined similarly as in (1.2.5) and $H(x)$ is an $n \times n$ matrix-valued function. The second of these, known as the *Cohen-Grossberg model* (see [4]) is described by equations of the form

$$\dot{x}_i = -a_i(x_i)\left[b_i(x_i) - \sum_{j=1}^n t_{ij} s_j(x_j)\right], \quad i = 1, \cdots, n \quad (1.2.10)$$

where x_i, t_{ij} and $s_j(x_j)$ are defined similarly as in (1.2.3) and (1.2.5), $a_i(\cdot)$ is a bounded, positive and continuous function, and the function $b_i(\cdot)$ is continuous.

Some of the synthesis procedures for the analog Hopfield neural network work best for very large amplifier gains, i.e., when in (1.2.3) [resp., (1.2.4)] λ is arbitrarily large. This case is also addressed in Chapter 2. Under the present assumptions, the analog Hopfield neural network assumes the form of the variable structure system given by (see [19])

$$\frac{dx}{dt} = F(x) \qquad (1.2.11)$$

with

$$F(x) = -Ax + TS(x) + I \qquad (1.2.12)$$

where $S(x) = (s_1(x_1), \cdots, s_n(x_n))^T$ and each $s_i(\cdot)$ denotes the sign function [see (1.2.2)], and where the remaining symbols are defined as in (1.2.5). Under appropriate assumptions, the output values of the neurons in the above model agree with the *discrete asynchronous Hopfield model* given by

$$v_i^+ = \begin{cases} 1, & \text{if } \sum_{j=1}^n T_{ij}v_j + I_i > 0 \\ -1, & \text{if } \sum_{j=1}^n T_{ij}v_j + I_i < 0 \end{cases} \qquad (1.2.13)$$

where all symbols are defined similarly as in (1.2.1).

The preceding neural network models are concerned with the analog Hopfield neural network model, generalizations and variants to this model, and synchronous and asynchronous digital networks which are counterparts to the analog Hopfield neural networks. The last class of neural networks that we will consider in Chapter 2 differs significantly from the networks described thus far. The continuous-time networks of this class are described by equations of the form [20]

$$\frac{dx}{dt} = Tx + I \qquad (1.2.14)$$

with the constraints

$$-1 \leq x_i \leq 1, \ i = 1, \cdots, n \qquad (1.2.15)$$

1.3. HOPFIELD GLOBAL RESULTS

while the discrete counterpart of these networks is described by equations of the form [36]

$$x((k+1)h) = F(\Phi x(kh) + \Gamma) \qquad (1.2.16)$$

where $F(x) = (F_1(x_1), \cdots, F_n(x_n))^T$, where each $F_i(\cdot)$ denotes the saturation function [see (1.2.7)], where

$$\Phi = [\Phi_{ij}] = \exp(hT) \qquad (1.2.17)$$

and where

$$\Gamma = I \cdot \left(\int_0^h \exp(\eta T) d\eta \right). \qquad (1.2.18)$$

Independent of the continuous-time system (1.2.14), we will also concern ourselves with discrete-time systems described by difference equations of the form

$$x(k+1) = \text{sat}(Tx(k) + I). \qquad (1.2.19)$$

This system is related to (1.2.16), letting $T = \Phi$, $I = \Gamma$, and $h = 1$.

1.3 Qualitative Analysis of Analog Hopfield-Type Neural Networks: Global Results

In Chapter 3 we will first investigate global qualitative properties of the *generalized analog Hopfield neural networks* described by equations of the form (1.2.9) (see [18]). Using an energy function of the form

$$E(x) = -\frac{1}{2}x^T T x + \sum_{i=1}^{n} \int_0^{x_i} s_i(\rho) d\rho - x^T I, \qquad (1.3.1)$$

where all symbols in (1.3.1) are defined in (1.2.9). We will show that under reasonable assumptions, the following results are true for system (1.2.9):

i) for any $x \in (-1,1) \times \cdots \times (-1,1) = (-1,1)^n$, there is a unique solution $\varphi(\cdot, 0, x)$ for (1.2.9);

ii) along a non-equilibrium solution of (1.2.9), the energy function E decreases monotonically, and therefore, no non-constant periodic solutions exist for (1.2.9);

iii) each solution exists on $\Re^+ = [0, \infty)$;

iv) each non-equilibrium solution of (1.2.9) converges to an equilibrium of (1.2.9) as $t \to \infty$ [i.e., the network (1.2.9) is *globally stable*]; and

v) there are only finitely many equilibrium points for (1.2.9).

We will further show that under mild assumptions, the following statements are equivalent:

i') $\tilde{x}$ is a stable equilibrium of (1.2.9);

ii') $\tilde{x}$ is a local minimum of the energy function E;

iii') $J(\tilde{x}) > 0$, i.e., the Jacobian matrix for system (1.2.9) evaluated at $x = \tilde{x}$ is positive definite; and

iv') $\tilde{x}$ is asymptotically stable.

Results of the type given above can be used in a variety of applications. For example, the global stability property of system (1.2.9) [refer to item iv) above] enables us to partition the state space of (1.2.9), using the domains of attraction of the asymptotically stable equilibria of (1.2.9). Such a partition in turn determines an equivalence relation for system (1.2.9), which in turn can be used in classification problems, including applications to associative memories. We will demonstrate this in Chapter 8.

In Chapter 3 we will also investigate the global (and some local) qualitative properties of the class of neural networks described by the variable structure systems given by (1.2.11), (1.2.12) (see [19]). For such systems we will establish results along the following lines:

i) We will introduce an appropriate notion of solution for system (1.2.11), (1.2.12) [which includes the concept of *sliding mode* (see [45])] and we will show that for any initial condition, there exists such a solution and that all solutions can be extended to the infinite time interval.

1.3. HOPFIELD GLOBAL RESULTS

ii) We will make precise the notion of equilibrium point for system (1.2.11), (1.2.12), and we will show that in each of 2^n regions [which are separated by the surfaces of discontinuities, M, of the right hand side of equation (1.2.11)], there exists at most one asymptotically stable equilibrium point.

iii) We will show that if in one of the above regions, call it G, there is an equilibrium point, say x_0, then G is contained in the domain of attraction of x_0.

iv) We will show that there is a one-to-one correspondence between the asymptotically stable equilibrium points in $\Re^n - M$ and the stable output vectors of (1.2.11), (1.2.12) [the ranges of the components of S (which are functions) make up the output vectors of (1.2.11), (1.2.12)].

Furthermore, under the assumptions that $T = [T_{ij}]$ is symmetric and the diagonal elements of T are non-negative, we will use an energy function of the form

$$E(\xi) = -\frac{1}{2}\xi^T T\xi - \xi^T I + c$$

to establish the following properties of (1.2.11), (1.2.12):

i') The set of local minima of E is contained in the set of stable output vectors of (1.2.11), (1.2.12). These two sets turn out to be equal if $T_{ii} = 0$, $1 \leq i \leq n$.

ii') Solutions of system (1.2.11), (1.2.12) are not in a sliding mode.

iii') If T is positive semidefinite, then along each output sequence [i.e., along each sequence of output vectors of (1.2.11), (1.2.12)], the energy function decreases monotonically, and system (1.2.11), (1.2.12) does not exhibit periodic solutions.

iv') If T is not positive semidefinite, then statement iii') is true with respect to asynchronous solutions of (1.2.11), (1.2.12).

As in the case for the results described earlier for system (1.2.9), the above results can be used (as will be shown in Chapter 8) to establish synthesis procedures for system (1.2.11), (1.2.12) (e.g., with

1.4 Stability Analysis of Linear Systems Operating on a Closed Hypercube

In Chapter 4 we will investigate local and global qualitative properties of continuous-time neural networks described by linear differential equations defined on a hypercube, described by (1.2.14), (1.2.15) (see [20]). For such systems, we will first formulate a definition of solution which incorporates the notion of solution in a *saturated mode* and we will study some of the properties of such solutions. We will show in particular that system (1.2.14), (1.2.15) possesses for every initial conditions a unique solution which exists over the infinite time interval $[t_0, \infty)$.

Next, we will introduce the concept of equilibrium for (1.2.14), (1.2.15) and we will establish an algorithm which enables us to determine in a systematic manner the locations of all equilibria of (1.2.14), (1.2.15) and their stability properties.

Next, we will show that system (1.2.14), (1.2.15) has at most 3^n equilibrium points and that at most 2^n of these are asymptotically stable.

Next, we will introduce an energy function for system (1.2.14), (1.2.15) of the form

$$E(x) = -\frac{1}{2} x^T T x - x^T I.$$

Assuming that T is symmetric, we will show that there is a one-to-one correspondence between the set of local minima of E and the set of asymptotically stable equilibria of system (1.2.14), (1.2.15).

Next, we will show that along each solution of (1.2.14), (1.2.15), the energy function E decreases monotonically, and therefore, system (1.2.14), (1.2.15) does not exhibit periodic solutions.

In Chapter 4 we also will investigate local and global qualitative properties of discrete-time neural networks described by linear

1.5. HOPFIELD LOCAL RESULTS 13

difference equations defined on a hypercube, described by (1.2.19) (see [36]). For such systems we will establish results which are very similar to the ones described above for system (1.2.14), (1.2.15). In doing so, we will make use of an energy function for system (1.2.19) of the form
$$E(x) = -x^T(T + E_n)x - 2x^T I,$$
under the assumption that T is symmetric (E_n denotes the $n \times n$ identity matrix).

In applications to optimization problems, neural networks with globally asymptotically stable equilibria have been employed. In Chapter 4 we will also establish sufficient conditions for the global asymptotic stability of the continuous-time neural network (1.2.14), (1.2.15) (assuming without loss of generality that $I = 0$) and of the discrete-time neural network (1.2.19) (assuming $I = 0$) [12], [23].

1.5 Qualitative Analysis of Hopfield-Type Neural Networks: Local Results

In Chapter 5 we will first show that a Hopfield neural network (1.2.3) can always be expressed by an equivalent system of equations,
$$\dot{x}_i = -a_i x_i + \sum_{j=1}^{n} T_{ij} G_j(x_j) + I_i(t), \quad i = 1, \cdots, n \quad (\Sigma_i)$$
having the property that a given equilibrium $u = u^* = (u_1^*, \cdots, u_n^*)^T$ of (1.2.3) (with $w_i \equiv 0$) is transformed to the equilibrium $x = 0$ of (Σ_i) (with $I_i(t) \equiv 0$). In (Σ_i), G_j is a real, continuous, monotonically increasing function satisfying the conditions $G_i(0) = 0$, $x_i G_i(x_i) > 0$ for $x_i \neq 0$, and
$$\sigma_{i1} x_i^2 < x_i G_i(x_i) < \sigma_{i2} x_i^2, \quad -r_i < x_i < r_i. \quad (1.5.1)$$
In our analysis we view (Σ_i) to be an *interconnected system* (see [7], [35], [43]) consisting of an interconnection of n *free subsystems* described by equations of the form
$$\dot{p}_i = -a_i p_i + T_{ii} G_i(p_i) + I_i(t), \quad i = 1, \cdots, n, \quad (\mathcal{S}_i)$$

with the *system interconnecting structure* given by

$$h_i(x_1, \cdots, x_n) = \sum_{j=1, j \neq i}^{n} T_{ij} G_j(x_j), \quad i = 1, \cdots, n. \tag{1.5.2}$$

Rewriting (Σ_i) in vector form as

$$\dot{x} = -Ax + TG(x) + I(t) \tag{$\mathcal{S}$}$$

we speak under the present viewpoint of an *interconnected system* ($\mathcal{S}$) *with decomposition* (Σ_i).

Our aim in Chapter 5 will be to analyze system ($\mathcal{S}$) in terms of the qualitative properties of the subsystems ($\mathcal{S}_i$) (representing the individual neurons with their associated dynamics) and the system interconnecting structure (representing the interactions of the neurons). To accomplish this, we will first conduct a stability analysis of the free subsystems ($\mathcal{S}_i$) under the assumption that $I_i(t) \equiv 0$ (see [32]). For such systems, we will establish sufficient conditions for the asymptotic stability, exponential stability, instability, and complete instability of the equilibrium $p_i = 0$.

Next, we will use *scalar Lyapunov functions* that consist of a weighted sum of quadratic Lyapunov functions for the free subsystems, given by

$$v(x) = \sum_{i=1}^{n} \frac{1}{2} \alpha_i x_i^2, \tag{1.5.3}$$

to establish sufficient conditions for asymptotic stability (resp., exponential stability) of the equilibrium $x = 0$ of system ($\mathcal{S}$), under the assumption that $I(t) \equiv 0$ (see [32]). These results involve three basic ingredients. The first of these characterizes the qualitative properties of the free subsystems; the second specifies constraints on the interconnecting structure of ($\mathcal{S}$); and the third combines information from the first two to form a *test matrix* with certain desired definiteness properties. A *sample result* that we will prove in Chapter 5 follows.

Assume that the following hypotheses hold for system ($\mathcal{S}$):

1) $I_i(t) \equiv 0$, $i = 1, \cdots, n$;

1.5. HOPFIELD LOCAL RESULTS

2) there are $a_{ij} \in \Re$, $i,j = 1,\cdots,n$, such that

$$x_i T_{ij} G_j(x_j) \leq |x_i||a_{ij}||x_j|$$

for all $|x_i| < r_i$, $|x_j| < r_j$, $i,j = 1,\cdots,n$; and

3) there exists an n-vector $\alpha^T = (\alpha_1,\cdots,\alpha_n)$, $\alpha_i > 0$, $i = 1,\cdots,n$, such that the $n \times n$ test matrix $S = [s_{ij}]$ given by

$$s_{ij} = \begin{cases} \alpha_i(-a_i + a_{ii}), & i = j \\ (\alpha_i a_{ij} + \alpha_j a_{ji})/2, & i \neq j \end{cases}$$

is negative definite.

Then the equilibrium $x = 0$ of the interconnected system $(\mathcal{S})$ with decomposition (Σ_i) is *asymptotically stable*.

When the off-diagonal elements of a test matrix are non-negative, we are able to simplify results of the type described above by invoking the properties of M-matrices (see [6], [35]). A *sample result* of this type which we will prove in Chapter 5 requires that hypothesis 3) above be replaced by the following assumption (see [32]):

3′) the successive principal minors of the $n \times n$ *test matrix* $D = [d_{ij}]$ are all positive, where

$$d_{ij} = \begin{cases} a_i - \delta_i T_{ii}, & i = j \\ -|T_{ij}|\sigma_{j2}, & i \neq j \end{cases}$$

where $\delta_i = \sigma_{i2}$ when $T_{ii} > 0$, $\delta_i = \sigma_{i1}$ when $T_{ii} < 0$, and σ_{i1}, σ_{i2} are defined in (1.5.1).

Next, by invoking the *comparison principle* [for the stability theory of ordinary differential equations (see, e.g., [17], [37], [39])], and by invoking the use of *vector Lyapunov* functions, $V(x) = (v_1(x),\cdots,v_n(x))^T$ (whose components are scalar Lyapunov functions for the subsystems), we will establish in Chapter 5 several additional results for asymptotic and exponential stability of the equilibrium $x = 0$ of system $(\mathcal{S})$. These results, as well as the results discussed above, are in many instances equivalent (see [32]).

Using the stability results described above, we will also establish in Chapter 5 *estimates for trajectory bounds* (see [32]). Results of this type provide a measure of the rate of convergence of trajectories sufficiently close to the asymptotically stable equilibrium $x = 0$ of $(\mathcal{S})$ under the following additional hypothesis:

4) assume there exist $\lambda_i > 0$, $i = 1, \cdots, n$ and $\varepsilon > 0$ such that

$$\left(\frac{a_i}{\sigma_{i2}} - T_{ii}\right) - \sum_{j=1, j \neq i}^{n} \left(\frac{\lambda_j}{\lambda_i}\right) |T_{ij}| \geq \varepsilon > 0, \ i = 1, \cdots, n.$$

The estimates for trajectory bounds that we will establish are of the form

$$\begin{aligned}\|\varphi(t, t_0, x_0)\| &\triangleq \sum_{i=1}^{n} \lambda_i |\varphi_i(t, t_0, x_0)| \\ &\leq (\alpha - k/c)e^{-c(t-t_0)} + k/c, \ t \geq t_0 \geq 0,\end{aligned} \quad (1.5.4)$$

provided that $\alpha > k/c$ and $\|x_0\| = \sum_{i=1}^{n} \lambda_i |x_{i0}| \leq \alpha$. In (1.5.4), k is determined by $\sum_{i=1}^{n} \lambda_i |I_i(t)| \leq k$ for all $t \geq t_0 \geq 0$; the λ_i, $i = 1, \cdots, n$ are given in hypothesis 4); c is determined by $c = \varepsilon \delta$, where $\varepsilon > 0$ is given in hypothesis 4) and δ is defined by $\delta = \min_{i} \sigma_{i1}$.

In Chapter 5 we will also demonstrate how to determine an *estimate of the domain of attraction* of the equilibrium $x = 0$ of system $(\mathcal{S})$ when this equilibrium is asymptotically stable (see [32]). For example, we will show that if the assumptions 1), 2), and 3) given earlier are true, then the set C_λ is a subset of the domain of attraction of the equilibrium $x = 0$ of the neural network $(\mathcal{S})$, where

$$C_\lambda = \left\{x \in \Re^n : v(x) = \sum_{i=1}^{n} \alpha_i v_i(x_i) < \lambda\right\}$$

where

$$\lambda = \sum_{i=1}^{n} \left(\alpha_i r_i^2\right),$$

where α_i is given in 3), and r_i is given in 2).

We will also establish *instability* and *complete instability* results for system $(\mathcal{S})$ (see [32]). These results are similar in form and spirit

1.6. EFFECTS OF PARAMETER PERTURBATIONS

as the stability results addressed thus far. Also, we will address stability under structural perturbations of the analog Hopfield neural network, and we will revisit such networks when the neuron gains become arbitrarily large (see [32]).

In Chapter 5 we will also perform an analysis for *synchronous discrete-time Hopfield-type neural networks* described by equations of the form (1.2.8). For such systems, we will establish results that are analogous to many of the results that were discussed above, using the same methodology used in analyzing the analog Hopfield neural network model (see [33]).

Finally, we will conclude Chapter 5 with an analysis of the analog Hopfield-type neural network model having saturation nonlinearities as activation functions, described by equations of the form (1.2.6). For such networks, we will establish results that enable one to locate in a systematic manner the locations and to ascertain the stability properties of all the equilibria. The method of analysis that we will employ to accomplish this is similar to that used in establishing the results for linear systems operating on a closed hypercube, (1.2.14), (1.2.15), described earlier in Section 1.4 (see [25]).

For all networks that we will consider in Chapter 5, we will generally impose no restrictions (such as symmetry) on the interconnection matrix T, and in cases when restrictions are required, this will be explicitly stated.

1.6 Qualitative Effects of Parameter Perturbations

In Chapter 6 we will investigate the effects of parameter perturbations on neural networks that can be described by equations of the form

$$\dot{x} = -Bx + TS(x) + I. \tag{S}$$

Such parameter errors may include perturbations ΔT, ΔB, ΔS, and ΔI, resulting in a *perturbation model* which we will assume to be of the form (see [26], [38], [47])

$$\dot{x} = -(B + \Delta B)x + (T + \Delta T)[S(x) + \Delta S(x)] + (I + \Delta I). \quad (\tilde{S})$$

We will assume that in (S) and ($\tilde{S}$), the activation functions are either *sigmoidal functions* (see [47]) or *hard limiters* represented by saturation functions (see [26]). In the former case, system (S) is the *analog Hopfield neural network model* represented by Eq. (1.2.5) while in the latter case, system (S) is represented by (1.2.6).

We will consider first systems with *sigmoidal activation functions*. We will define such systems as being *robust* if for every asymptotically stable equilibrium x_e of system (S), there is an asymptotically stable equilibrium $\tilde{x}_e$ of ($\tilde{S}$) which is near x_e and the distance between x_e and $\tilde{x}_e$, given by $|x_e - \tilde{x}_e|$, can be made as small as desired by requiring that

$$\max\{\|\Delta B\|, \|\Delta T\|, |\Delta I|, |\Delta S(x_e)|, |\Delta S'(x_e)|\}$$

be sufficiently small. [Here $\Delta S'(x) = (\Delta s'_1(x_1), \cdots, \Delta s'_n(x_n))^T$ and $\Delta s'_i(x_i) = d\Delta s_i(x_i)/dx_i$.]

We will show that system (S) (with sigmoidal activation functions) is is robust if for every asymptotically stable equilibrium x_e of (S), x_e is asymptotically stable with respect to the linearization of system (S). This condition can be verified by testing the Hurwitz stability of the coefficient matrix

$$-B + TS'(x_e)$$

for each asymptotically stable equilibrium x_e (see [47]).

We will show that when the above condition is satisfied [i.e., when system (S) is robust], Brouwer's fixed-point theorem (see [44]) can be used to obtain the following estimate of the distance between the equilibrium x_e of (S) and the corresponding perturbed equilibrium $\tilde{x}_e$ of system ($\tilde{S}$),

$$|x_e - \tilde{x}_e|_\infty \leq c \cdot \max\{\|\Delta B\|_\infty, \|\Delta T\|_\infty, |\Delta S(x_e)|_\infty, |\Delta I|_\infty\} \quad (1.6.1)$$

when in the right-hand side of inequality (1.6.1), the maximal number is sufficiently small. In (1.6.1), $c = 2(2 + R_0 + \|T\|_\infty)\|A^{-1}\|_\infty$ with

$R_0 \geq |x_e|_\infty$ and $A = -B + TS'(x_e)$ (see [47]). (For $x \in \Re^n$, $|x|_\infty = \max_i \{|x_i|\}$ and for $P \in \Re^{n \times n}$, $\|P\|_\infty$ denotes the norm of P induced by the vector norm $|\cdot|_\infty$.)

Next, we will consider in Chapter 6 systems (S) with *hard limiter activation functions* (saturation functions) under the assumption that $\Delta S(x) = 0$ and that only bipolar vectors (i.e., vectors belonging to $B^n = \{x \in \Re^n : x_i = 1 \ x_i = -1\}$) are considered as candidates for stable memories (see [26]). For $x \in \Re^n$, let

$$\delta(x) = \min_{1 \leq i \leq n} \{|x_i|\}$$

and for $\alpha = (\alpha_1, \cdots, \alpha_n)^T \in B^n$, let $F(\alpha) = \{x \in \Re^n : x_i \alpha_i > 1\}$. Suppose that $\alpha^1, \cdots, \alpha^m$ are desired stable memories of system (S) corresponding to the asymptotically stable equilibria $\beta^1, \cdots, \beta^m$, respectively [i.e., $\alpha^j = \text{sat}(\beta^j)$, $j = 1, \cdots, m$]. Let

$$\nu = \min_{1 \leq j \leq m} |\delta(\beta^j)| > 1. \tag{1.6.2}$$

We will show in Chapter 6 that $\alpha^1, \cdots, \alpha^m$ are also stable memory vectors of system (S̃) provided that

$$\|B^{-1}\Delta B\|_\infty + \|B^{-1}\Delta T\|_\infty + |B^{-1}\Delta I|_\infty < \nu - 1. \tag{1.6.3}$$

Now suppose that α is a stable memory and β is a corresponding asymptotically stable equilibrium for system (S). After perturbation, the new asymptotically stable equilibrium point $\overline{\beta}$ is given by

$$\overline{\beta} = (B + \Delta B)^{-1}[(T + \Delta T)\alpha + (I + \Delta I)]. \tag{1.6.4}$$

We will show in Chapter 6 that when condition (1.6.3) is satisfied, $\overline{\beta} \in F(\alpha)$ implies that α is still a stable memory of system (S̃) (see [26]).

1.7 Qualitative Effects of Time Delays

During the implementation process of artificial recurrent neural networks (especially by VLSI), transmission delays may unavoidably be introduced. Since in globally stable recurrent neural networks without time delays, oscillations can occur after the introduction of delays, it is important to take into account the effects of time delays in the qualitative analysis of such networks (see, e.g., [3], [28], [38], [42], [48]–[50]).

In Chapter 7 we will first present *global* and *local stability results* for *Hopfield neural networks with identical delays*, described by equations of the form (see [28], [48])

$$\dot{x}(t) = -Cx(t) + T_0 S(x(t)) + T_1 S(x(t-\tau)) + I \qquad (1.7.1)$$

and for *Cohen-Grossberg neural networks with multiple delays* described by equations of the form (see [49])

$$\dot{x}(t) = -A(x(t))\left[B(x(t)) - T_0 S(x(t)) - \sum_{k=1}^{K} T_k S(x(t-\tau_k))\right]. \qquad (1.7.2)$$

We will assume that both of these networks are endowed with symmetric interconnecting structure.

We first show that if for a given set of parameters, the Hopfield neural network described by

$$\dot{x}(t) = -Cx(t) + TS(x(t)) + I \qquad (1.7.3)$$

with $T = T_0 + T_1$, is globally stable, then the corresponding network (1.7.1), with delay $\tau > 0$, will also be globally stable, provided that (see [48])

$$\tau \beta \|T_1\| < 1 \qquad (1.7.4)$$

where

$$\beta \stackrel{\triangle}{=} \max_{x \in \Re^n} |S'(x)|, \ S'(x) = \text{diag}\left[\frac{ds_1}{dx_1}(x_1), \cdots, \frac{ds_n}{dx_n}(x_n)\right],$$

and $\|\cdot\|$ in (1.7.4) denotes the matrix norm induced by the Euclidean vector norm.

We will also show that if for a given set of parameters, the Cohen-Grossberg neural network described by

$$\dot{x}(t) = -A(x(t))[B(x(t)) - TS(x(t))] \qquad (1.7.5)$$

1.7. EFFECTS OF TIME DELAYS

with $T = T_0 + \sum_{k=1}^{K} T_k$, is globally stable, then the corresponding network (1.7.2), with delays $\tau_k > 0$, $k = 1, \cdots, K$, will also be globally stable, provided that (see [49])

$$\sum_{k=1}^{K} \tau_k \beta \|T_k\| < 1 \tag{1.7.6}$$

where

$$\beta \triangleq \max_{x \in \Re^n} |A(x) S'(x)|$$

and where $S'(x)$ and $\|\cdot\|$ are defined as before.

The above results state that in the case of Hopfield neural networks and Cohen-Grossberg neural networks, the global behavior of networks with and without time delays is similar, provided that the delays are sufficiently small.

Next we will also establish *local stability results* for Hopfield neural networks with delays, still assuming that the networks have symmetric interconnecting structure. Specifically, we will show that when system (1.7.1) satisfies condition (1.7.4) [in which case (1.7.1) is globally stable], then the following statements are equivalent (see [48]):

1) $x_e \in \Re^n$ is a stable equilibrium of (1.7.1);

2) x_e is an asymptotically stable equilibrium of (1.7.1);

3) x_e is a local minimum of the energy functional $E(x_t)$ [used to prove conditions (1.7.4)] given by

$$E(x_t) = -y^T(t) T y(t) + 2 \sum_{i=1}^{n} \int_0^{y_i(t)} c_i s_i^{-1}(\sigma) d\sigma - 2 y^T(t) I$$
$$+ \int_{t-\tau}^{t} [y(w) - y(t)]^T T_1^T f(w-t) T_1 [y(w) - y(t)] dw \tag{1.7.7}$$

where $y(t) = S(x(t))$, c_i denotes the ith diagonal element of the diagonal matrix C, $T = T_0 + T_1$, and $f(\cdot)$ is a continuously differentiable non-negative scalar valued function defined on

$[-\tau, 0]$ [having the property that the time derivative of E along the solutions of (1.7.1) is a non-positive valued function].

4) x_e is a stable equilibrium of (1.7.3);

5) x_e is an asymptotically stable equilibrium of (1.7.3); and

6) x_e is a local minimum of the energy function E given by

$$E(y) = -\frac{1}{2} y^T T y - I^T y + \sum_{i=1}^{n} c_i \int_0^{y_i} s_i^{-1}(\eta) d\eta \qquad (1.7.8)$$

where $y = (y_1, \cdots, y_n)^T$ and $y_i = s_i(x_i)$, $i = 1, \cdots, n$.

The above results show that when the time delay τ is sufficiently small (i.e., when $\tau \beta \|T_1\| < 1$), then a study of the stability properties of the equilibria of a Hopfield neural network with delays [system (1.7.1)] can be reduced to a study of the stability properties of the equilibria of a corresponding Hopfield neural network without delays [system (1.7.3)].

The above statements apply also to Cohen-Grossberg neural networks with multiple delays, system (1.7.2), with condition (1.7.4) replaced by condition (1.7.6).

Next, we will study the stability properties of the equilibria of (1.7.1), assuming that $I = 0$, and assuming that the interconnecting structure of (1.7.1) is not necessarily symmetric. The results that we will establish include small gain, sector, and linearization criteria for stability, estimates for the domain of attraction of an equilibrium, and robust stability results (see [50]).

1.8 Some Synthesis Methods for Associative Memories

In Chapter 8 we will address several synthesis procedures using various types of artificial recurrent neural networks. In doing so, we

1.8. SYNTHESIS METHODS

will first apply the *Outer Product Method* in the synthesis of *asynchronous networks* (networks that switch asynchronously), described by (1.2.1), and given here by

$$\begin{cases} v_i(k+1) = \text{sgn}(u_i(k)), & 1 \le i \le n \\ u_i(k) = \sum_{j=1}^{n} T_{ij} v_j(k) + I_i, & 1 \le i \le n. \end{cases} \quad (1.8.1)$$

This method yields the parameters (see [10], [11], [31])

$$\begin{cases} T = [T_{ij}] = \sum_{i=1}^{m} \alpha^i (\alpha^i)^T \\ I = (I_1, \cdots, I_n)^T = 0 \end{cases} \quad (1.8.2)$$

where $\alpha^i \in B^n$, $i = 1, \cdots, m$, are the prototype patterns to be stored as memory vectors (i.e., asymptotically stable equilibria) in the network (1.8.1). We will argue that the parameters (1.8.2) [obtained for system (1.8.1)] are also applicable to the analog Hopfield neural networks described by

$$\begin{cases} \dot{u}_i = \sum_{j=1}^{n} T_{ij} v_j - b_i u_i + I_i \\ v_i = g(\lambda u_i), & i = 1, \cdots, n \end{cases} \quad (1.8.3)$$

provided that the amplifier gain $\lambda > 0$, is sufficiently high. We will show that when the prototype patterns are not mutually orthogonal, the Outer Product Method will in general not guarantee to store all the desired patterns as equilibria of the synthesized network (see [10], [11], [31]).

Next, we will utilize in Chapter 8 the *Projection Learning Rule* in the synthesis of *synchronous networks* (networks that switch synchronously), described by equations that have the same form as (1.8.1). This rule yields the parameters (see [31], [40], [41])

$$\begin{cases} T = \Sigma \Sigma^\dagger \\ -1 \le I_i \le 1, & i = 1, \cdots, n \end{cases} \quad (1.8.4)$$

where $\Sigma = [\alpha^1 \vdots \cdots \vdots \alpha^m]$ and $\Sigma^\dagger$ denotes the Moore-Penrose pseudoinverse. We will show that the Projection Learning Rule guarantees to store all the desired patterns as equilibrium points in a network; however, not all of these equilibria may be asymptotically stable. We will also show that when all the prototype patterns are mutually orthogonal, the Projection Learning Rule reduces to the Outer Product Method (see [31], [40], [41]).

We will develop in Chapter 8 a third synthesis procedure, called the *Eigenstructure Method*, in the synthesis of linear systems operating on a closed hypercube described by equations of the form (1.2.14), (1.2.15), given by (see [20])

$$\dot{x} = Tx + I, \quad x \in D^n \tag{1.8.5}$$

where $D^n = \{x \in \Re^n : -1 \leq x_i \leq 1, \ i = 1, \cdots, n\}$. In the derivation of this method, we first construct a matrix

$$Y = \left[\alpha^1 - \alpha^m \vdots \cdots \vdots \alpha^{m-1} - \alpha^m \right],$$

followed by a singular value decomposition of Y, to obtain

$$Y = \begin{bmatrix} U_1 \vdots U_2 \end{bmatrix} \begin{bmatrix} D & \vdots & 0 \\ \cdots & \cdots & \cdots \\ 0 & \vdots & 0 \end{bmatrix} \begin{bmatrix} V_1^T \\ \cdots \\ V_2^T \end{bmatrix}.$$

The Eigenstructure Method yields the network parameters (see [20])

$$\begin{cases} T = T^+ - \tau T^- \\ I = \alpha^m - T\alpha^m \end{cases}$$

where $T^+ = U_1 U_1^T$, $T^- = U_2 U_2^T$, and τ is a parameter chosen as $\tau > -1$. We will show that this method guarantees that the synthesized network will store all of the desired patterns as asymptotically stable equilibria of system (1.8.5). We will also show that when choosing $\tau > -1$, the number of spurious states contained in B^n (undesired asymptotically stable equilibria in B^n) will decrease as τ increases (see [20]). We will also apply the Eigenstructure Method described above to various other classes of neural networks discussed in Chapter 2, resp., Section 1.2 (see [18], [19], [25], [36]).

1.8. SYNTHESIS METHODS

In Chapter 8 we will also develop a synthesis procedure for neural networks described by (1.2.6), given by

$$\begin{cases} \dot{x} = -Ax + Ty + I \\ y = \text{sat}(x) \end{cases} \quad (1.8.6)$$

which is based on the perceptron training algorithm (see [22]). We will formulate this design problem as a set of linear inequalities which are amenable to application of the perceptron training algorithm. This approach results in n perceptrons characterized by $W^i = (w_1^i, w_2^i, \cdots, w_{n+1}^i)$, $i = 1, \cdots, n$, such that

$$\begin{cases} W^i \overline{\alpha}^k \geq 0 & \text{if } \alpha_i^k = 1 \\ W^i \overline{\alpha}^k < 0 & \text{if } \alpha_i^k = -1 \end{cases}$$

for $k = 1, \cdots, m$, where $\overline{\alpha}^k = \begin{pmatrix} \alpha^k \\ \cdots \\ 1 \end{pmatrix}$. Choose $A = \text{diag}[a_1, \cdots, a_n]$ with $a_i > 0$. Also, for $i, j = 1, \cdots, n$, choose $T_{ij} = w_j^i$ if $i \neq j$, $T_{ii} = w_i^i + a_i \mu_i$ with $\mu_i > 1$, and $I_i = w_{n+1}^i$. We will show that the perceptron training algorithm described in the above synthesis procedure will always converge to a solution (see [22]).

When the Eigenstructure Method (discussed earlier) and the synthesis method based on the the perceptron training algorithm (discussed above) are both applied to the network described by (1.8.6), we obtain in both cases the parameters $\{A, T, I\}$ from the relationship (see [22])

$$A^{-1}(T\alpha^k + I) \in F(\alpha^k), \quad k = 1, \cdots, m \quad (1.8.7)$$

where $F(\alpha) = \{x \in \Re^n : x_i \alpha^i > 1, i = 1, \cdots, n\}$. However, in the Eigenstructure Method, a special case of (1.8.7) is employed, given by

$$T\alpha^k + I = \mu \alpha^k, \quad k = 1, \cdots, m,$$

with $\mu > 1$. The Eigenstructure Method will always yield a symmetric matrix T, while the perceptron based training algorithm described above will normally lead to a nonsymmetric matrix T (see [22]).

Finally, we will also apply the perceptron based training algorithm proposed above to other networks described in Chapter 2 (see Section 1.2).

1.9 Effects of Interconnection Constraints

In Chapter 9 we will study the effects of interconnecting structure constraints of neural networks on synthesis procedures for associative memories (see [24], [25], [34]). These constraints come in the form of sparsity specifications, and sometimes as symmetry requirements on the interconnection matrix T. To accomplish this, we will utilize an index matrix $S \in \Re^{n \times n}$, defined by $S = [S_{ij}]$, where $S_{ij} = 1$ or 0. This matrix specifies a particular interconnecting structure, with $S_{ij} = 1$ indicating a connection from the jth neuron to the ith neuron, while $S_{ij} = 0$ signifies no such connection. This enables us to define "the restriction of a matrix $W \in \Re^{n \times n}$ to an index matrix S" as $W|S = [h_{ij}] \in \Re^{n \times n}$, where

$$h_{ij} = \begin{cases} W_{ij}, & \text{if } S_{ij} = 1 \\ 0, & \text{otherwise.} \end{cases}$$

With these conventions, the synthesis problem of a neural network will now require that the matrix T satisfies the condition

$$T = T|S$$

for a given index matrix S (see [24], [25], [34]).

We will apply the procedure outlined above to neural networks (1.2.6), rewritten here as

$$\begin{cases} \dot{x} = -Ax + Ty + I, & T = T|S \\ y = \text{sat}(x). \end{cases} \qquad (1.9.1)$$

In particular, we will modify the Eigenstructure Method (developed in Chapter 8) in solving the synthesis problem posed in the preceding. We will show that solutions to this problem will exist as long as $S_{ii} = 1$, $i = 1, \cdots, n$. Thus, if we allow each neuron to have self feedback, we will always be able to determine a solution for the sparse synthesis problem using the Eigenstructure Method for any sparsity constraints and for any number of desired bipolar patterns in the prototype set (see [24], [25], [34]).

The synthesized network with sparsity constraints on the connection matrix T obtained in this manner will in general not possess a symmetric interconnecting structure. In the synthesis of a neural network (1.9.1) with *symmetric* and *sparse interconnection matrix*, we will make use of the robustness analysis results of Chapter 6 (refer to Section 1.6 and see [24], [26], [34]). We will solve this problem also by making use of the perceptron based training algorithm developed in Chapter 8 (see [22]).

Finally, we will apply in Chapter 9 the results discussed above in the synthesis of a specific class of cellular neural networks (see [21], [27]).

Bibliography

[1] NK Bose, P Liang. Neural Networks Fundamentals with Graphs, Algorithms, and Applications. New York, NY: McGraw-Hill, 1996.

[2] LO Chua, L Yang. Cellular neural networks: Theory. IEEE Transactions on Circuits and Systems 35:1257–1272, 1988.

[3] PP Civalleri, M Gilli, L Pandolfi. On stability of cellular neural networks with delay. IEEE Transactions on Circuits and Systems-I: Fundamental Theory and Applications 40:157–165, 1993.

[4] M Cohen, S Grossberg. Absolute stability of global pattern formation and parallel memory storage by competitive neural networks. IEEE Transactions on Systems, Man, and Cybernetics 13:815–826, 1983.

[5] JS Denker. Ed. Neural Networks for Computing. AIP Conference Proceedings, no 151, Snowbird, UT, 1986.

[6] M Fiedler, V Ptak. On matrices with non-positive off-diagonal elements and positive principal minors. Czechoslovak Mathematical Journal 12:382–400, 1962.

[7] LT Grujić, AA Martynyuk, M Ribbens-Pavella. Stability of Large-Scale Systems Under Structural and Singular Perturbations. Kiev, USSR: Nauka Dumka, 1984.

[8] S Haykin. Neural Networks: A Comprehensive Foundation. Upper Saddle River, NJ: Prentice-Hall, 1999.

[9] J Hertz, A Krogh, RG Palmer. Introduction to the Theory of Neural Computation. New York, NY: Addison-Wesley, 1991.

[10] JJ Hopfield. Neural networks and physical systems with emergent collective computational abilities. Proceedings of the National Academy of Sciences USA 79:2554–2558, 1982.

[11] JJ Hopfield. Neurons with graded response have collective computational properties like those of two-state neurons. Proceedings of the National Academy of Sciences USA 81:3088–3092, 1984.

[12] L Hou, AN Michel. Asymptotic stability of systems with saturation constraints. IEEE Transactions on Automatic Control 43:1148–1154, 1998.

[13] C Jeffries. Code Recognition and Set Selection with Neural Networks. Boston, MA: Birkhäuser, 1991.

[14] T Khanna. Foundations of Neural Networks. New York, NY: Addison-Wesley, 1990.

[15] YH Kim, FL Lewis. High-Level Feedback Control with Neural Networks. Singapore: World Scientific, 1998.

[16] B Kosko. Neural Networks and Fuzzy Systems. Englewood Cliffs, NJ: Prentice-Hall, 1992.

[17] V Lakshmikantham, S Leela. Differential and Integral Inequalities, vol 1 and vol 2. New York, NY: Academic Press, 1969.

[18] JH Li, AN Michel, W Porod. Qualitative analysis and synthesis of a class of neural networks. IEEE Transactions on Circuits and Systems 35:976–987, 1988.

[19] JH Li, AN Michel, W Porod. Analysis and synthesis of a class of neural networks: Variable structure systems with infinite gains. IEEE Transactions on Circuits and Systems 36:713–731, 1989.

[20] JH Li, AN Michel, W Porod. Analysis and synthesis of a class of neural networks: Linear systems operating on a closed hypercube. IEEE Transactions on Circuits and Systems 36:1405–1422, 1989.

[21] D Liu. Cloning template design of cellular neural networks for associative memories. IEEE Transactions on Circuits and Systems-I: Fundamental Theory and Applications 44:646–650, 1997.

[22] D Liu, Z Lu. A new synthesis approach for feedback neural networks based on the perceptron training algorithm. IEEE Transactions on Neural Networks 8:1468–1482, 1997.

[23] D Liu, AN Michel. Asymptotic stability of discrete-time systems with saturation nonlinearities with applications to digital filters. IEEE Transactions on Circuits and Systems-I: Fundamental Theory and Applications 39:798–807, 1992.

[24] D Liu, AN Michel. Dynamical Systems with Saturation Nonlinearities: Analysis and Design. Lecture Notes in Control and Information Sciences, vol 195. Berlin, Germany: Springer-Verlag, 1994.

[25] D Liu, AN Michel. Sparsely interconnected neural networks for associative memories with applications to cellular neural networks. IEEE Transactions on Circuits and Systems-II: Analog and Digital Signal Processing 41:295–307, 1994.

[26] D Liu, AN Michel. Robustness analysis and design of a class of neural networks with sparse interconnecting structure. Neurocomputing 12:59–76, 1996.

[27] Z Lu, D Liu. A new synthesis procedure for a class of cellular neural networks with space-invariant cloning template. IEEE Transactions on Circuits and Systems-II: Analog and Digital Signal Processing 45:1601–1605, 1998.

[28] CM Marcus, RM Westervelt. Stability of analog neural networks with delay. Physical Review A 39:347–359, 1989.

[29] WS McCulloch, W Pitts. A logical calculus of the ideas immanent in nervous activity. Bulletin of Mathematical Biophysics 5:115–133, 1943.

[30] C Mead. Analog VLSI and Neural Systems. Reading, MA: Addison Wesley, 1989.

[31] AN Michel, JA Farrell. Associative memories via neural networks. IEEE Control Systems Magazine 10:6–17, 1990.

[32] AN Michel, JA Farrell, W Porod. Qualitative analysis of neural networks. IEEE Transactions on Circuits and Systems 36:229–243, 1989.

[33] AN Michel, JA Farrell, HF Sun. Analysis and synthesis techniques for Hopfield type synchronous discrete time neural networks with applications to content addressable memory. IEEE Transactions on Circuits and Systems 37:1356–1366, 1990.

[34] AN Michel, D Liu. Theory and applications of sparsely interconnected neural networks. Neural, Parallel and Scientific Computations 4:305–324, 1996.

[35] AN Michel, RK Miller. Qualitative Analysis of Large Scale Dynamical Systems, New York, NY: Academic Press, 1977.

[36] AN Michel, J Si, G Yen. Analysis and synthesis of a class of discrete-time neural networks described on hypercubes. IEEE Transactions on Neural Networks 2:32–46, 1991.

[37] AN Michel, K Wang, B Hu. Qualitative Theory of Dynamical Systems–The Role of Stability Preserving Mappings. Second Edition. New York, NY: Marcel Dekker, 2001.

[38] AN Michel, K Wang, D Liu, H Ye. Qualitative limitations incurred in implementations of recurrent neural networks. IEEE Control Systems Magazine 15:52–65, 1995.

[39] RK Miller, AN Michel, Ordinary Differential Equations, New York, NY: Academic Press, 1982.

[40] L Personnaz, I Guyon, G Dreyfus. Information storage and retrieval in spin-glass like neural networks. Journal de Physique Lettres 46:L359–L365, 1985.

BIBLIOGRAPHY

[41] L Personnaz, I Guyon, G Dreyfus. Collective properties of neural networks: New learning mechanism. Physical Review A 34:4217–4228, 1986.

[42] T Roska, C Wu, LO Chua. Stability of cellular neural networks with dominant nonlinear and delay-type templates. IEEE Transactions on Circuits and Systems-I: Fundamental Theory and Applications 40:270–272, 1993.

[43] DD Siljak. Large-Scale Dynamical Systems: Stability and Structure. New York, NY: North Holland, 1978.

[44] MJ Todd. The Computation of Fixed Points and Applications. New York, NY: Springer-Verlag, 1976.

[45] VI Utkin. Variable structure systems with sliding modes. IEEE Transactions on Automatic Control 22:212–222, 1977.

[46] RV Vemuri. Artificial Neural Networks. Los Alamitos, CA: IEEE Computer Society Press, 1992.

[47] K Wang, AN Michel. Robustness and perturbation analysis of a class of artificial neural networks. Neural Networks 7:251–259, 1994.

[48] H Ye, AN Michel, K Wang. Global stability and local stability of Hopfield neural networks with delays. Physical Review E 50:4206–4213, 1994.

[49] H Ye, AN Michel, K Wang. Qualitative analysis of Cohen-Grossberg neural networks with multiple delays. Physical Review E 51:2611–2618, 1995.

[50] H Ye, AN Michel, K Wang. Robust stability of nonlinear time-delay systems with applications to neural networks. IEEE Transactions on Circuits and Systems-I: Fundamental Theory and Applications 43:532–543, 1996.

[51] JM Zurada. Introduction to Artificial Neural Systems. St. Paul, MN: West Publishing Company, 1992.

Chapter 2

Some Neural Network Models

2.1 Introduction

In an article in the *American Scientist* [8], N. R. Franks points out that if 100 army ants (each of which has fewer than 100,000 neurons) are placed on a flat surface, they will walk in circles until they die of exhaustion. On the other hand, a colony of 500,000 such ants (having one-half as many neurons as a typical human brain) is capable of flexible problem solving, far exceeding the capacity of the individual ants. For example, such a colony can build nests in accordance with some sophisticated architecture; it can regulate the temperature within $\pm 1°C$ inside a nest made up of the bodies of ants; it can raid in one day 200 meters through a forest while maintaining a steady compass heading; it appears to follow rules of economic investment theory in matters of colony propagation; and the like. The solutions of relatively complex problems of this type are accomplished through communication among individual ants (and thus, among neurons). Franks notes that the communication among neurons occurs much faster in the case of the human brain than in the case of an ant colony.

The potential of achieving a great deal of processing power by wiring together a large number of very simple and primitive devices (neurons) has captured the imagination of scientists and engineers for some time now. In recent decades, the possibility of implementing such systems (*artificial neural networks*) by electro-optical devices or by very large scale integrated circuits (VLSI) has resulted in substantial research activities that have led to numerous applications.

Artificial neural networks (which only rarely attempt to simulate biological systems) are made up of an interconnection of devices, called *neurons*, and local external inputs. The input/output characteristics of a neuron can be modeled, for example, by a sigmoidal function. The inputs to the neurons consist of weighted sums of the neuron outputs. In applications involving "learning," the interconnection strengths (weights) in a neural network will vary. Usually some dynamic characteristics are associated with each neuron. In principle then, most of the popular neural network models can be implemented by operational amplifiers, capacitors, resistors, and voltage or current sources. Simulations of neural networks (on serial processors) have also received a great deal of attention.

The numerous neural network applications that have been proposed have resulted in a variety of designs ranging from feed-through systems with no feedback (e.g., perceptrons), to systems endowed with local feedback interconnections (e.g., cellular neural networks), to fully interconnected feedback systems. We will confine our attention in the present book to a few important classes of (fully or partially interconnected) recurrent artificial neural networks. From the numerous applications of such networks, we will single out associative memories as a vehicle to fix ideas and explain the subject on hand. It is not our intent to provide a survey of all the different types of recurrent neural networks and their applications that have been considered in the literature. Such an attempt would be futile and would take us too far astray from our principal objectives.

To introduce the subject on hand, we offer in the remainder of the present section some general comments on associative memory, and we briefly consider a few recurrent neural network models. In

2.1. INTRODUCTION

the subsequent sections of the present chapter we consider in greater detail the various recurrent neural network models that will be of interest to us.

A. Associative Memory

Neural networks are candidates for information processing systems because their dynamical behavior exhibits stable states (i.e., asymptotically stable equilibria) that act as basins of attraction toward which neighboring states develop in time. This time evolution of an array of neuron-like elements toward these equilibrium points can be interpreted as the evolution of an imperfect pattern toward the correct (stored) pattern. This is analogous to the storage of information in an associative memory [14], [20]. In other words, the process of association and information retrieval is simulated by the dynamical behavior of a highly interconnected system of nonlinear circuit elements.

In several books (see, for example, [13], [14], [20], [50]) and many papers (see, for example, [2], [7], [9], [15]–[17], [21]–[25], [28], [34], [38]–[40]) the ability of neural networks to implement associative memories (AM) has been discussed. For purposes of comparison, in a digital computer a desired set of information, called a *memory*, is recalled when the correct address of the memory is given. This is called *address addressable memory* (AAM). In contrast, an associative memory is able to recall a full set of the information of the memory when the system (neural network) is excited with a sufficiently large portion of that memory's information, called a *key*. Thus, a full set of the information of the memory is recalled by a portion of the memory's information. For example, if each entry in the bibliography of the present chapter were stored in an associative memory, and the key "neurons with graded response" were given, then the associative memory would respond with the complete set of information corresponding to Ref. [16].

An efficient AM can store a large set of memory patterns and recall each memory pattern when the system (neural network) is excited with a key containing a portion of that memory's information.

In comparison, a complete correct address is required to recall information from an AAM. Moreover, if a sufficient amount of correct memory information is provided, then an AM may be able to correct the erroneous data. On the other hand, an AAM will always provide the correct information if the entire correct address is given, whereas in an AM there are no guarantees that the output will always constitute correct information.

As a specific example, the various Hopfield neural network models have been shown to implement AMs effectively. The approach proposed in [15] and [16] is to design a network (to be discussed later in Chapter 8) in such a way that the memory patterns to be stored are represented by vectors at which an energy function for the network assumes a local minimum. By this design methodology, patterns similar to a given stored pattern will approach this stored pattern, since the circuit is designed such that all of its trajectories seek the local minima of the energy function (corresponding to the asymptotically stable equilibria of the circuit). Thus, if a vector $\hat{x}$ represents a given pattern stored in an AM then the key, $x = \hat{x} + dx$, will elicit the response $\hat{x}$, provided that an appropriate norm of dx (say, $|dx|$) is sufficiently small.

The difficulties involved in the implementation of AMs by neural networks include:

(1) Storing each desired pattern as a vector at which an energy function for the network assumes a local minimum [i.e., storing each desired pattern as an asymptotically stable equilibrium of the network (or, corresponding to an asymptotically stable equilibrium of the network)];

(2) Controlling the extent of the basins of attraction of each stored pattern (i.e., controlling the extent of the domains of attraction of the asymptotically stable equilibrium points of the network); and

(3) Minimizing the number of extraneous stored patterns, called *spurious states* (i.e., minimizing the number of asymptotically stable equilibria in the network that are not used for storing patterns).

2.1. INTRODUCTION

Clearly, the design of such neural networks entails a detailed understanding of the qualitative behavior (e.g., stability properties of equilibria) of such networks. The qualitative analysis of the various classes of recurrent neural networks that we will consider is addressed in Chapters 3–5.

B. Neural Network Models

As we mentioned earlier, a complete discussion of the various neural network models that have been considered is far beyond the scope of the present book. In the present chapter we will focus our attention primarily on fully interconnected recurrent neural networks (also called feedback neural networks).

The term "fully interconnected neural network" refers to network models for which the output of each neuron *may* be connected to the inputs of all the neurons. Perhaps the most important class of neural networks that is not fully interconnected are *feedforward networks* (see, for example, [13], [41], [42], [49], [50]), where the neural elements can be separated into distinct layers. In such cases, the input to the network directly affects the first layer, the output of the first layer affects the second layer, and so forth. Thus, the information flow in feedforward networks is uni-directional (and consequently, such networks are not feedback, resp., recurrent neural networks). Examples of recurrent neural networks that are not fully interconnected include *cellular neural networks* in which the output of a given neuron is allowed to connect only to certain of its neighbors (see, e.g., [3], [26], [35]). We will address such neural networks in Chapter 9.

In 1943, McCulloch and Pitts [29] presented a network of *threshold logic units*, called by this name because such a network is able to assume the binary 1 and -1 values. The time evolution of the output of each unit in such a network is described by the following equation, where T_{ij} and I_i are real numbers,

$$\begin{cases} v_i(k+1) = \text{sgn}(u_i(k)), & 1 \leq i \leq n \\ u_i(k) = \sum_{j=1}^{n} T_{ij} v_j(k) + I_i, & 1 \leq i \leq n. \end{cases} \quad (2.1.1)$$

The sign function sgn(u) is defined to be equal to 1 when u is positive and equal to -1 when u is negative, i.e.,

$$\text{sgn}(u_i(k)) = \begin{cases} 1, & u_i(k) > 0 \\ -1, & u_i(k) < 0. \end{cases} \quad (2.1.2)$$

When $u_i(k) = 0$, then $v_i(k+1) = v_i(k)$. The switching order for this network determines a random process. At any instant of time, each neuron (modeled by the sign function, sgn) has an equally likely chance to evaluate its state according to (2.1.1). Thus the state of the system switches *asynchronously* and the mean rate of change is the same for each neuron. This lack of synchronism is introduced deliberately to improve the modeling of biological systems. We note that the neural network represented by (2.1.1) has n neurons, that the interconnection of the jth neuron to the ith neuron has strength T_{ij}, and that the term I_i represents a firing threshold for the ith neuron.

In demonstrating that their network is capable of solving logic problems, McCulloch and Pitts were able to show that difficult problems can be solved by appropriately interconnecting a network of simple processors. Of course, the inherent difficulty in this work is to determine the appropriate interconnecting structure.

In implementations of AMs for engineering applications, we are usually more interested in solution accuracy and analytic tractability rather than mimicking biological systems accurately. This has led several workers (e.g., [24], [25], [34], [38], [39]) to make use of the synchronous equivalent of (2.1.1) described by equations of the form,

$$\begin{cases} v_i(k+1) = g(u_i(k)), & 1 \leq i \leq n \\ u_i(k) = \sum_{j=1}^{n} T_{ij} v_j(k) + I_i, & 1 \leq i \leq n. \end{cases} \quad (2.1.3)$$

In [24], [25], and [34], g is a continuous, monotonically increasing function called a *sigmoidal function* [see Fig. 2.1.1(a) for an example of the graph of such a function], whereas in [38] and [39], g denotes the sgn function defined in (2.1.2) [see Fig. 2.1.1(c)]. The main difference between systems described by (2.1.1) and (2.1.3), however, is found in their modes of operation: in (2.1.1) the neurons are allowed to switch

2.1. INTRODUCTION

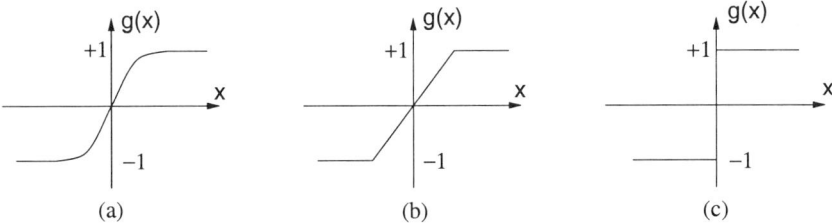

Figure 2.1.1: (a) Sigmoidal input/output characteristics. (b) Saturating linear input/output characteristics. (c) Discontinuous hard limiting input/output characteristics.

asynchronously (to mimic biological systems), whereas in (2.1.3) the neurons evaluate and switch their states *synchronously*.

Next, as pointed out by Hopfield [16], real neurons (and amplifiers) determine continuous input/output relations [see, for example, Fig. 2.1.1(a)] and not the sign function utilized in (2.1.1). Furthermore, due to the presence of capacitances in biological neural networks or in electrical implementations of such networks, the dynamics of neural networks are integrative and must be described by differential equations. Hopfield [16] shows that the continuous-time system described by the following set of equations has computational capabilities similar to those of system (2.1.1),

$$\begin{cases} du_i/dt = \sum_{j=1}^{n} T_{ij}v_j - b_i u_i + I_i \\ v_i = g(u_i), \quad i = 1, \cdots, n. \end{cases} \quad (2.1.4)$$

In (2.1.4), $b_i > 0$, I_i and T_{ij} are real constants and $g(\cdot)$ is a sigmoidal function. Such functions will be defined and explained in greater detail in the next section.

In the remainder of this chapter, we will elaborate further on the neural networks discussed above and we will introduce additional classes of artificial recurrent neural networks.

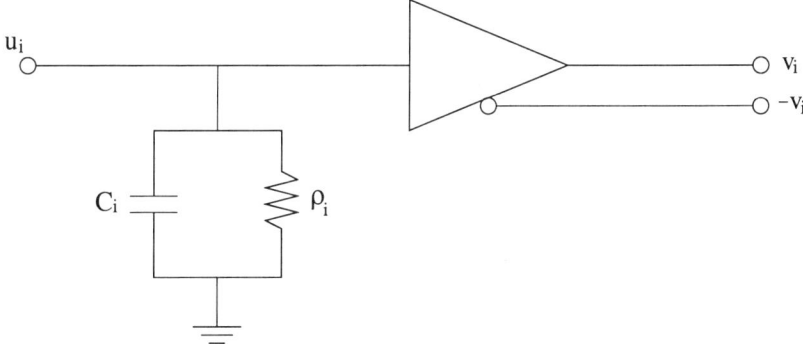

Figure 2.2.1: The ith neural cell in the analog Hopfield model.

2.2 Analog Hopfield Neural Network Model

In [16], Hopfield considers electronic circuits of the type given in Figs. 2.2.1 and 2.2.2 as models for neural systems. In such circuits, there are n identical nonlinear amplifiers. If we do not consider the input capacitance and input resistance, the input-output relation of the ith amplifier is assumed to be given, e.g., by the expression

$$v_i = g_i(\lambda u_i) = \frac{2}{\pi}\tan^{-1}\left(\frac{\pi}{2}\lambda u_i\right) \tag{2.2.1}$$

where u_i denotes the input, v_i represents the output, and the parameter λ is the *gain* of the nonlinear amplifiers. It is assumed that the response time of each amplifier is negligible compared to the time constant determined by the input capacitance and the input resistance. The ith nonlinear amplifier can be illustrated as in Fig. 2.2.1. Note that in the case of each nonlinear amplifier, provisions are made that the amplifier may also serve as an inverter, to make possible sign changes in the amplifier output signals (see Fig. 2.2.1).

Expression (2.2.1) is an example of a sigmoidal function. Specifically, we will say that a function $g(\cdot)$ is a *sigmoidal function* if $g\colon \Re \to (-1,1)$ [i.e., g maps $\Re = (-\infty, \infty)$ into $(-1,1)$], if $g(0) = 0$, if $g(\cdot)$ is smooth [i.e., $g(\cdot)$ is continuously differentiable], if $dg(\sigma)/d\sigma \stackrel{\triangle}{=} g'(\sigma) > 0$ for all $\sigma \in \Re$, if $\lim_{\sigma \to \infty} g(\sigma) = 1$, and if $\lim_{\sigma \to -\infty} g(\sigma) = -1$.

2.2. ANALOG HOPFIELD MODEL

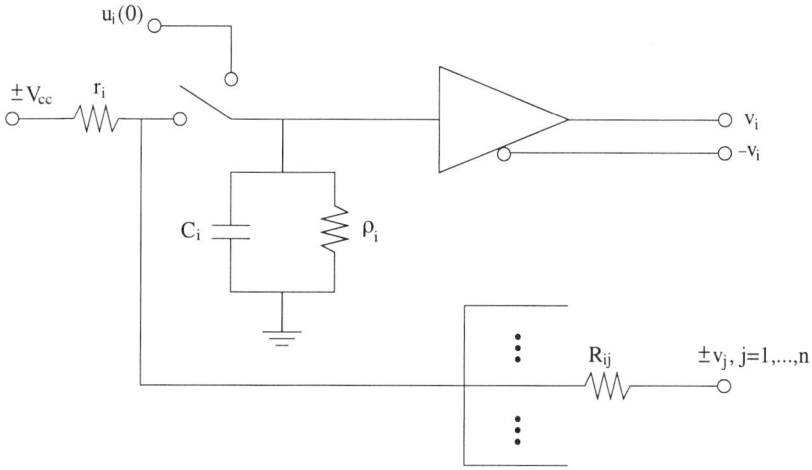

Figure 2.2.2: Implementation of the analog Hopfield neural network model.

In the circuit of Fig. 2.2.2, the neurons (represented by amplifiers) are connected to each other, as shown, where $\pm V_{cc}/r_i$ is the input current to the ith neuron, $u_i(0)$ is the initial condition (initial current) for the ith neuron, and R_{ij} denotes the resistor connecting the output of the jth neuron to the input of the ith neuron.

Invoking Kirchhoff's current law at the node of each amplifier input results in the following set of differential equations,

$$\frac{du_i}{dt} = \frac{1}{C_i}\left[\sum_{j=1}^{n}\frac{1}{R_{ij}}(\pm v_j) - \left(\frac{1}{\rho_i} + \frac{1}{r_i} + \sum_{j=1}^{n}\frac{1}{R_{ij}}\right)u_i \right.$$
$$\left. + \frac{\pm V_{cc}}{r_i}\right], \quad i = 1, \cdots, n. \qquad (2.2.2)$$

If in the above circuit we let

$$t_{ij} = \begin{cases} +1/R_{ij}, & \text{if } R_{ij} \text{ is connected to } v_j \\ -1/R_{ij}, & \text{if } R_{ij} \text{ is connected to } -v_j, \end{cases}$$

$$\frac{1}{R_i} = \frac{1}{\rho_i} + \frac{1}{r_i} + \sum_{j=1}^{n}\frac{1}{R_{ij}},$$

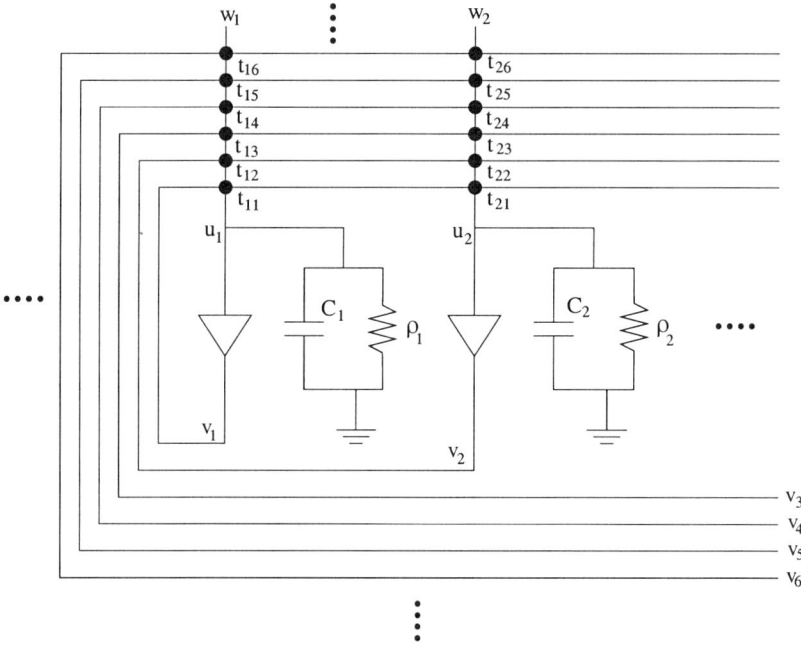

Figure 2.2.3: Symbolic representation of the analog Hopfield neural network model.

and
$$w_i = \frac{\pm V_{cc}}{r_i},$$
then (2.2.2) assumes the form
$$\begin{cases} C_i \, (du_i/dt) = -u_i/R_i + \sum_{j=1}^{n} t_{ij} v_j + w_i \\ v_i = g(\lambda u_i), \quad i = 1, \cdots, n \end{cases} \quad (2.2.3)$$

where $g(\cdot)$ is given in (2.2.1). This is the equation given by Hopfield in [16]. We note in passing that the usual symbolic representation of neural networks is as shown in Fig. 2.2.3, where the dots indicate neuron interconnections.

Compared to other models, the Hopfield analog neural network model is easily implemented by electronic circuits and has been used

2.2. ANALOG HOPFIELD MODEL

in various applications (see, e.g., [16], [18], and [47]). However, this model suffers also from deficiencies, some of which are noted below:

a) *Concerning the implementation of (2.2.3):* Since the variable $u = (u_1, \cdots, u_n)^T$ may assume values over all of $\Re^n$, the components of u may assume very large values and scaling may pose problems in implementations. Furthermore, whenever the value of R_{ij} is altered to adjust the corresponding value of t_{ij} in (2.2.3), the value of R_i in (2.2.3) changes also.

b) *Concerning the analysis of system (2.2.3):* As will be seen in Chapter 3, the set of equilibrium points of (2.2.3) corresponds to the set of solutions of the equations

$$\sum_{j=1}^{n} t_{ij} g(\lambda u_j) - \frac{u_i}{R_i} + w_i = 0, \quad i = 1, \cdots, n.$$

Since it is difficult to solve this set of equations, it may be difficult to verify the performance of system (2.2.3).

c) *Concerning the synthesis of system (2.2.3):* In Chapter 8, an energy function of the form

$$E(v) = -\frac{1}{2} v^T \tilde{T} v - v^T w + \frac{1}{\lambda} \sum_{i=1}^{n} \int_0^{v_i} \frac{1}{R_i} g_i^{-1}(\sigma) d\sigma$$

is employed, where $v = (v_1, \cdots, v_n)^T$, $\tilde{T} = [t_{ij}]$, $w = (w_1, \cdots, w_n)^T$ and $g_i^{-1}(\cdot)$ denotes the inverse of $g_i(\cdot)$. In the synthesis procedure for system (2.2.3) (presented in Chapter 8) the third term in the energy function is neglected, with the consequence that the location of the equilibrium points cannot be precisely synthesized.

The effects of the integration terms in the energy function $E(v)$ can be reduced by increasing the gain λ of the nonlinear amplifiers. Thus, λ is usually taken to be very large. However, as will be discussed in Chapter 3, large values of λ may result in periodic motions for system (2.2.3). In particular, this may happen when the diagonal elements of $\tilde{T} = [t_{ij}]$ have negative values. On the other hand, if we want to reduce the number of spurious equilibrium points (i.e., undesirable asymptotically stable equilibria) of system (2.2.3), we need to choose large negative eigenvalues for $\tilde{T} = [t_{ij}]$ and the matrix $\tilde{T}$ synthesized in this way will have negative diagonal elements.

Returning now to the representation of the Hopfield neural network given in (2.2.3), if we let $u = (u_1, \cdots, u_n)^T = (x_1, \cdots, x_n)^T = x$, $a_i = 1/(R_i C_i)$, $A = \text{diag}[a_1, \cdots, a_n]$, $I_i = w_i/C_i$, $I = (I_1, \cdots, I_n)^T$, $T_{ij} = t_{ij}/C_i$, $T = [T_{ij}]$, $y_i = g_i(\lambda u_i)/C_i = s_i(x_i)$, $y = (y_1, \cdots, y_n)^T$, and $S(x) = (s_1(x_1), \cdots, s_n(x_n))^T$, we can represent (2.2.3) equivalently by

$$\begin{cases} \dot{x} = -Ax + Ty + I \\ y = S(x). \end{cases} \qquad (2.2.4)$$

This expression, or very similar ones, are very frequently used in the literature in representing the analog Hopfield neural network model.

Next, we would like to point to a variant of the model given in (2.2.4), frequently used in the case of cellular neural networks and other applications. In this case, the sigmoidal functions $s_i(\cdot)$ are replaced by the saturation function given by

$$\text{sat}(x) = (\text{sat}(x_1), \cdots, \text{sat}(x_n))^T,$$

where (see Fig. 2.1.1b),

$$\text{sat}(x_i) = \begin{cases} 1, & x_i > 1 \\ x_i, & -1 \leq x_i \leq 1 \\ -1, & x_i < -1. \end{cases} \qquad (2.2.5)$$

In this case, (2.2.4) assumes the form

$$\begin{cases} \dot{x} = -Ax + Ty + I \\ y = \text{sat}(x). \end{cases} \qquad (2.2.6)$$

We will address the analysis and synthesis of system (2.2.6) in Chapters 5, 8, and 9.

2.3 Discrete Hopfield Neural Network Model

In [15] and [16] Hopfield presents, respectively, models for continuous (i.e., analog) and discontinuous neural networks. As mentioned ear-

2.3. DISCRETE HOPFIELD MODEL

lier, associated with each of these models is an energy function which the trajectories of the system seek to minimize. The network is considered to have n neurons whose inputs and outputs are represented, respectively, by the vectors $u = (u_1, \cdots, u_n)^T$ and $v = (v_1, \cdots, v_n)^T$.

As pointed out in Section 2.1, the dynamics of the discontinuous model are described in the following manner: each neuron computes its output according to the formula

$$\begin{cases} u_i(k) = \sum_{j=1}^{n} T_{ij} v_j(k) + I_i \\ v_i(k+1) = \text{sgn}(u_i(k)), \quad i = 1, \cdots, n \end{cases} \quad (2.3.1)$$

where $T_{ij} \in \Re$ denotes the strength of connection from neuron j to neuron i and I_i represents an external input to the ith neuron. The order in which neurons change states is completely *random* and *asynchronous*, but the mean rate of change of the state, w, is fixed. In the above, the function sgn is the sign function defined as

$$\text{sgn}(\sigma) = \begin{cases} 1, & \sigma > 0 \\ -1, & \sigma < 0. \end{cases}$$

In the case where $\sigma = 0$, $v_i(k+1)$ retains its previous value $v_i(k)$.

On the other hand, as shown in the preceding section, the equation that describes the dynamics of Hopfield's continuous (resp., analog) model can be simplified to

$$\begin{cases} \dot{u}_i = \sum_{j=1}^{n} T_{ij} v_j - b_i u_i + I_i \\ v_i = g_i(u_i), \quad i = 1, \cdots, n \end{cases} \quad (2.3.2)$$

where $\dot{u}_i = du_i/dt$, $T_{ij} \in \Re$, $b_i \in \Re$, $I_i \in \Re$, and $g_i(\cdot)$ is a sigmoidal function.

The design (resp., synthesis) of associative memories for the discontinuous model has been considered in numerous papers (see, e.g., [5], [22], [38] and [39]). A difficulty in designing these networks is due to the discontinuous nature of the input-output relationships. Frequently, it is possible to store desired patterns as stable states of (2.3.1); however, the discrete nature of the model's dynamical

46   CHAPTER 2. SOME NEURAL NETWORK MODELS

equation makes it difficult to guarantee that a pattern (stored as an equilibrium point) will attract neighboring states. This model is difficult to implement in hardware due to the requirement of a large number of interconnections and the inherent capacitances and delays. Accordingly, this model is often implemented on a digital computer where the requirement of random asynchronous switching times is approximated by a pseudo random switching sequence. Synchronous models have also been considered (see, e.g., [11] and [30]).

As pointed out earlier, associative memories can of course also be implemented by Hopfield's continuous-time (resp., analog) model, as discussed, e.g., in [16], [21], [23], [32], and [33], and as will be demonstrated in Chapter 8. In particular the design method of [15] is applicable in the high gain limit where system (2.3.2) approaches system (2.3.1). (For a detailed discussion of the high gain limit model of the analog Hopfield neural network, refer to Section 2.5). However, this technique does not guarantee to store each of the desired patterns (as asymptotically stable equilibrium points). On the other hand (see Chapter 8), the methods discussed in [7], [21], [23], [32], and [33] guarantee to store each desired pattern. These methods are compared in [7] (see also Chapter 8). Here again, problems may arise in implementing this circuit in hardware because of inherent parasitic dynamics, parameter inaccuracies, and the amount of space required to implement a large number of resistors. For a study of implementation questions, refer, e.g., to [44]–[46]. Also, some questions concerning qualitative limitations incurred in the implementation process of such networks are addressed in Chapters 6, 7, and 9 of the present book.

Most applications to date of the Hopfield neural network models have been implemented by special purpose software. Thus, either (2.3.2) has been simulated by numerical routines on digital computers or (2.3.1) has been implemented in a synchronous or pseudo-synchronous manner. To avoid problems that arise in the simulations of both models, in the design of the discontinuous model (2.3.1), and the implementation of the continuous model (2.3.2), a discrete-time *synchronous* model that approximates the continuous model (2.3.2)

2.3. DISCRETE HOPFIELD MODEL

has been employed, as described in the following.

By Euler's method, (2.3.2) can be approximated in discrete-time by replacing

$$\dot{u}(t) \approx \frac{u((k+1)\Delta T) - u(k\Delta T)}{\Delta T} \quad \text{for } k\Delta T \leq t \leq (k+1)\Delta T. \quad (2.3.3)$$

In the above equation, ΔT denotes the sampling period, and as $\Delta T \to 0$, the accuracy of the approximation increases. Applying (2.3.3) to (2.3.2) yields

$$\frac{u_i((k+1)\Delta T) - u_i(k\Delta T)}{\Delta T} = \sum_{j=1}^{n} T_{ij} v_j(k\Delta T) - b_i u_i(k\Delta T) + I_i,$$

$$i = 1, \cdots, n.$$

From the above expression it follows that

$$\begin{aligned} u_i(k+1) &= \sum_{j=1}^{n} T_{ij} v_j(k) + (1 - \Delta T b_i) u_i(k) + I_i \\ &= \sum_{j=1}^{n} T_{ij} v_j(k) - a_i u_i(k) + I_i, \quad i = 1, \cdots, n, \end{aligned} \quad (2.3.4)$$

where $a_i = \Delta T b_i - 1$, and where by a slight abuse in notation, we let $u_i(k) = (1/\Delta T) u_i(k\Delta T)$ and $v_i(k) = v_i(k\Delta T)$. The equations describing (2.3.4) and (2.3.1) are very similar. For both systems, the input to each neuron is a weighted sum of the outputs of all neurons. The features that distinguish model (2.3.4) from model (2.3.1) include the *synchronous mode* operation of (2.3.4) and the use of a sigmoidal input-output function to represent the neurons in (2.3.4). These features give the model (2.3.4) two advantages over the model (2.3.1): first, (2.3.4) allows direct implementation in software or special purpose hardware, and second, as will be seen later, model (2.3.4) allows design techniques that guarantee both the stability of stored patterns and the attractivity to stored patterns. We will present a detailed analysis of the dynamics of the discrete time, synchronous model described by (2.3.4) in the next chapter.

2.4 Generalizations of the Hopfield Model

A generalization to the analog Hopfield neural network model that we will address in the subsequent chapters is described by equations of the form

$$\dot{x} = -H(x)(-Tx + S(x) - I) \qquad (2.4.1)$$

where $x = (x_1, \cdots, x_n)^T \in (-1,1)^n \triangleq (-1,1) \times \cdots \times (-1,1)$ (n times), $\dot{x} = dx/dt$, H is a function from $(-1,1)^n$ into $\Re^{n \times n}$ (i.e., for each $x \in (-1,1)^n$, $H(x)$ is an $n \times n$ matrix), $T = [T_{ij}]$ is an $n \times n$ constant matrix, $S(x) = (s_1(x_1), \cdots, s_n(x_n))^T$ where $s_i : (-1,1) \to \Re$ and $I = (I_1, \cdots, I_n)^T$ is a constant real n-vector. In (2.4.1), x_i denotes the state variable associated with the ith neuron, the matrix T represents neuron interconnections, $s_i(\cdot)$ represents the ith neuron, I_i represents an external input for the ith neuron, and $H(x)$ represents an "amplification function." In subsequent chapters, we will impose additional restrictions on $H(x)$, $S(x)$, and T, as needed.

We now show that in particular, the Hopfield model,

$$\begin{cases} C_i\,(du_i/dt) = \sum_{j=1}^{n} T_{ij}v_j - u_i/R_i + I_i \\ v_i = g_i(\lambda u_i), \quad i = 1, \cdots, n, \end{cases} \qquad (2.4.2)$$

is a special case of system (2.4.1). As in Section 2.2, we assume in (2.4.2) that for each i, $C_i > 0$, $R_i > 0$ and I_i are constants, $T = [T_{ij}]$ is a constant matrix, $u_i \in \Re$, $v_i \in (-1,1)$, and $v_i = g_i(\lambda u_i)$, where $\lambda > 0$ is a constant. The function $g_i(\cdot)$ is assumed to be a sigmoidal function, i.e., $g_i(\cdot)$ is assumed to have the following properties: $g_i : \Re \to (-1,1)$ is monotone-increasing, $g_i(0) = 0$, $g_i(\sigma) = -g_i(-\sigma)$, the inverse $g_i^{-1} : (-1,1) \to \Re$ exists, and g_i and g_i^{-1} are C^1-functions (i.e., g_i and g_i^{-1} are continuously differentiable).

Now, when we represent system (2.4.2) in terms of the variables v_i, $i = 1, \cdots, n$, we have

$$\frac{dv_i}{dt} = \frac{dv_i}{du_i}\frac{du_i}{dt} = \left(\frac{du_i}{dv_i}\right)^{-1}\frac{1}{C_i}\left(\sum_{j=1}^{n} T_{ij}v_j - \frac{u_i}{R_i} + I_i\right)$$

2.4. GENERALIZED HOPFIELD MODEL

$$= -\lambda \left(\frac{dg_i^{-1}(v_i)}{dv_i} \right)^{-1} \frac{1}{C_i} \left(-\sum_{j=1}^{n} T_{ij} v_j + \frac{g^{-1}(v_i)}{\lambda R_i} - I_i \right), \quad (2.4.3)$$

$$i = 1, \cdots, n.$$

If in (2.4.3), we let $(v_1, \cdots, v_n)^T = x$,

$$\operatorname{diag}\left[\lambda \left(C_1 \frac{dg_1^{-1}(v_1)}{dv_1} \right)^{-1}, \cdots, \lambda \left(C_n \frac{dg_n^{-1}(v_n)}{dv_n} \right)^{-1} \right] = H(x),$$

$$\left(\frac{g^{-1}(v_1)}{\lambda R_1}, \cdots, \frac{g^{-1}(v_n)}{\lambda R_n} \right)^T = S(x)$$

$[T_{ij}] = T$, and $(I_1, \cdots, I_n)^T = I$, then system (2.4.3) assumes the form of equation (2.4.1). Thus, system (2.4.3), or equivalently, system (2.4.2), is a special case of system (2.4.1).

Another generalization of the Hopfield neural network model that we will address (in Chapter 7) is the Cohen-Grossberg neural network model [4] described by equations of the form

$$\dot{x}_i = -a_i(x_i) \left(b_i(x_i) - \sum_{j=1}^{n} t_{ij} s_j(x_j) \right), \quad i = 1, \cdots, n \quad (2.4.4)$$

where the function $a_i(\cdot)$ is bounded, positive, and continuous, the function $b_i(\cdot)$ is continuous, $T = [t_{ij}]$ is a symmetric matrix, $s_i(\cdot)$ is a sigmoidal function, $\lim_{x_i \to \infty} b_i(x_i) = \infty$, and $\lim_{x_i \to -\infty} b_i(x_i) = -\infty$. We will make additional assumptions for (2.4.4), as needed. In (2.4.4), x_i denotes the state variable associated with the ith neuron, the function $a_i(\cdot)$ represents an "amplification function," the matrix T represents neuron interconnections and the sigmoidal function $s_i(\cdot)$ represents the ith neuron. Now, as pointed out in [1], if in (2.4.2) we let $1/C_i = a_i(u_i)$, $u_i/R_i - I_i = b_i(u_i)$, $T_{ij} = t_{ij}$, and $g_j(\lambda u_j) = s_j(u_j)$, then system (2.4.2) is also a special case of system (2.4.4), i.e., the Hopfield neural network is *under the above assumptions* a special case of the Cohen-Grossberg model.

2.5 Analog Hopfield Neural Networks with Infinite Gain Amplifiers

We will also address neural networks described by discontinuous differential equations of the form

$$\frac{dx}{dt} = F(x) \tag{2.5.1}$$

with

$$F(x) = -Ax + TS(x) + I \tag{2.5.2}$$

where $x = (x_1, \cdots, x_n)^T \in \Re^n$, $F: \Re^n \to \Re^n$ is a measurable function (in the Lebesgue sense), $A = \mathrm{diag}[a_1, \cdots, a_n]$ is an $n \times n$ constant diagonal matrix with each $a_i > 0$, $T = [T_{ij}]$ is an $n \times n$ constant matrix, $I = (I_1, \cdots, I_n)^T$ is a constant vector, and $S: \Re^n \to \Re^n$ is a measurable function defined by $S(x) = (\mathrm{sgn}(x_1), \cdots, \mathrm{sgn}(x_n))^T$, where $\mathrm{sgn}: \Re \to \Re$ is a measurable function defined by

$$\mathrm{sgn}(\sigma) = \begin{cases} 1, & \text{if } \sigma > 0 \\ \text{undefined}, & \text{if } \sigma = 0 \\ -1, & \text{if } \sigma < 0. \end{cases} \tag{2.5.3}$$

The neural network model discussed above is motivated by the analog Hopfield model

$$\begin{cases} C_i \left(du_i/dt \right) = -u_i/R_i + \sum_{j=1}^{n} T_{ij} v_j + I_i \\ v_i = g_i(\lambda u_i), \quad i = 1, \cdots, n \end{cases} \tag{2.5.4}$$

where $g_i(\lambda u_i) = (2/\pi)\tan^{-1}\big((\pi/2)\lambda u_i\big)$, $C_i > 0$, $R_i > 0$, $T_{ij} \in \Re$, and $I_i \in \Re$. As was shown in Section 2.2, this system can be realized by electronic circuits in which each nonlinear function $g_i(\cdot)$ is implemented by a nonlinear amplifier with u_i the input voltage, v_i the output voltage and λ the gain of the amplifier. In practice, λ is a very large positive number. We want to know what will happen if λ becomes arbitrarily large. In this case, the nonlinear amplifiers may be viewed as hard threshold switches. To understand the behavior of

2.5. INFINITE GAIN ANALOG HOPFIELD MODEL

this kind of circuit, we need to study an ideal mathematical model described by the set of equations

$$\begin{cases} C_i(du_i/dt) = -u_i/R_i + \sum_{j=1}^{n} T_{ij}v_j + I_i \\ v_i = g_i(u_i) = \text{sgn}(u_i), \quad i = 1, \cdots, n. \end{cases} \quad (2.5.5)$$

In connection with (2.5.5), we assume without loss of generality that $C_i = 1$, $i = 1, \cdots, n$. If we now let $(u_1, \cdots, u_n)^T = x$, $T = [T_{ij}]$, $A = \text{diag}[1/R_1, \cdots, 1/R_n]$, and $I = (I_1, \cdots, I_n)^T$, then system (2.5.5) assumes the form of system (2.5.1). Thus, the neural network model given by (2.5.1), (2.5.2), may be viewed as a modified analog Hopfield neural network model (2.5.4) in which the gains of the nonlinear functions (amplifiers) are high enough to be considered infinite.

Under appropriate conditions (which will be specified later in Chapter 3), the behavior of the output values of $g_i(\cdot)$ agrees with the *discrete asynchronous model* introduced by Hopfield in [15], as follows [see also the McCulloch-Pitts model, (2.1.1), in Section 2.1]:

$$v_i^+ = \begin{cases} 1, & \text{if } \sum_{j=1}^{n} T_{ij}v_j + I_i > 0 \\ -1, & \text{if } \sum_{j=1}^{n} T_{ij}v_j + I_i < 0 \end{cases} \quad (2.5.6)$$

where $v = (v_1, \cdots, v_n)^T \in \Re^n$ with $v_i = \pm 1$, $T = [T_{ij}]$ is an $n \times n$ symmetric matrix with $T_{ii} = 0$, $i = 1, \cdots, n$, and $I = (I_1, \cdots, I_n)^T$ is a constant vector. This model updates in an asynchronous manner in the sense that during each cycle, only one component of v is updated by the formula given above.

From the above discussion it is clear that in terms of the input of the nonlinear functions, the system (2.5.1), (2.5.2) behaves like the analog Hopfield model while in terms of the output of the nonlinear functions, the system (2.5.1), (2.5.2) behaves like the discrete Hopfield model. Thus, a study of system (2.5.1), (2.5.2) (which will be conducted in Chapter 3) enables one to better understand what may happen when the gains of the nonlinear functions (amplifiers) are very high. Moreover, a synthesis procedure that we will present in Chapter 8 will turn out to be applicable to both the analog and discrete Hopfield models.

2.6 Linear Systems Operating on a Closed Hypercube

We will also concern ourselves with neural networks described by equations of the form

$$\frac{dx}{dt} = Tx + I \tag{2.6.1}$$

with the constraints

$$-1 \leq x_i \leq 1, \quad i = 1, \cdots, n \tag{2.6.2}$$

where

$$x = (x_1, \cdots, x_n)^T \in D^n \triangleq \{x \in \Re^n : -1 \leq x_i \leq 1, \ i = 1, \cdots, n\},$$

$T = [T_{ij}]$ is a real $n \times n$ constant matrix, and $I = (I_1, \cdots, I_n)^T$ is a constant vector.

We note that system (2.6.1), (2.6.2) is defined on the closed subset D^n of $\Re^n$ (i.e., a *closed hypercube*) instead of an open subset of $\Re^n$, as is usually the case. The definition of solution of system (2.6.1), (2.6.2) on the boundary of D^n will be given in Chapter 3, as will questions of existence, uniqueness and continuation of solutions of this system.

One of the reasons for considering and studying system (2.6.1), (2.6.2) is that systems of this type provide remedies to several basic disadvantages in the analog Hopfield model, pointed out in Section 2.2. In the following, we discuss some of the issues concerning the implementation of neural networks described by equations (2.6.1), (2.6.2), making reference to the circuit given in Fig. 2.6.1. In this circuit there are n identical operational (i.e., linear) amplifiers, symbolized in Fig. 2.6.2. In this figure, u_i denotes the input voltage, v_i represents the output voltage, and $\pm V_{cc}$ denotes the power supply voltage. The input-output relation of the ith operational amplifier is given by

$$v_i = \begin{cases} V_{cc}, & \text{if } u_i > V_{cc}/\lambda \\ \lambda u_i, & \text{if } -V_{cc}/\lambda \leq u_i \leq V_{cc}/\lambda \\ -V_{cc}, & \text{if } u_i < -V_{cc}/\lambda \end{cases}$$

2.6. LINEAR SYSTEMS ON A HYPERCUBE

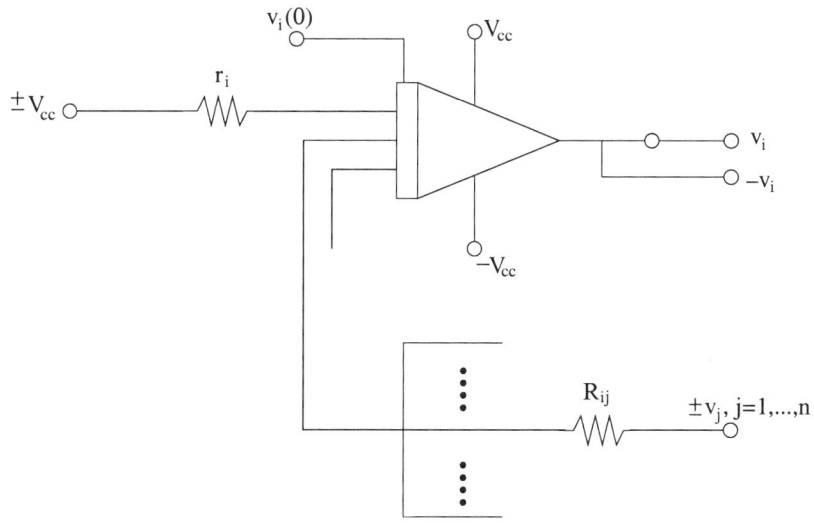

Figure 2.6.1: Implementation of the system described by (2.6.1), (2.6.2).

where λ denotes the gain of the operational amplifiers. By employing a feedback capacitor C_i, the ith operational amplifier becomes an integrator as illustrated in Fig. 2.6.3. In the circuit which implements the neural network (2.6.1), (2.6.2), these n integrators are interconnected as shown in Fig. 2.6.1. In this circuit, $\pm V_{cc}/r_i$ denotes the input current to the ith integrator, $v_i(0)$ represents the initial condition for the ith integrator, and each R_{ij} denotes the resistor connecting the output of the jth integrator to the input of the ith integrator.

If in Fig. 2.6.1 we take the voltage V_{cc} as unit, then each component v_i of v can vary from -1 to 1. When $-1 < v_i < 1$ for $i = 1, \cdots, n$, the resulting circuit can be described by a set of ordinary linear differential equations given by

$$\frac{dv_i}{dt} = \frac{1}{C_i}\left(\sum_{j=1}^{n}\frac{1}{R_{ij}}(\pm v_j) + \frac{\pm V_{cc}}{r_i}\right), \quad i = 1, \cdots, n \qquad (2.6.3)$$

54 CHAPTER 2. SOME NEURAL NETWORK MODELS

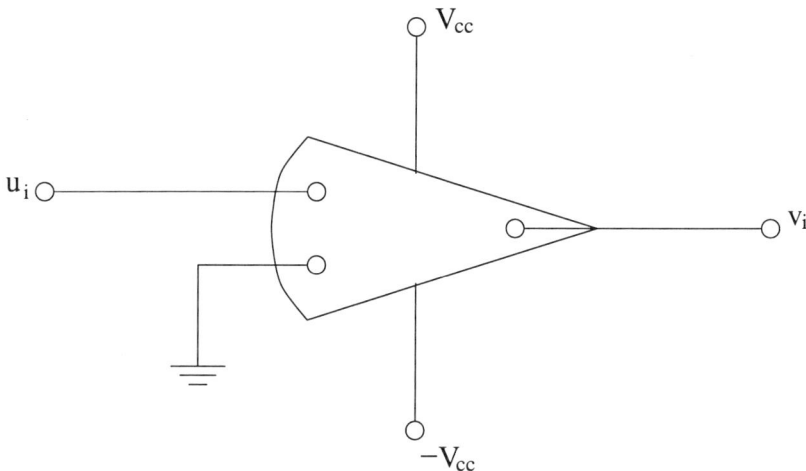

Figure 2.6.2: The ith operational amplifier of the system described by (2.6.1), (2.6.2).

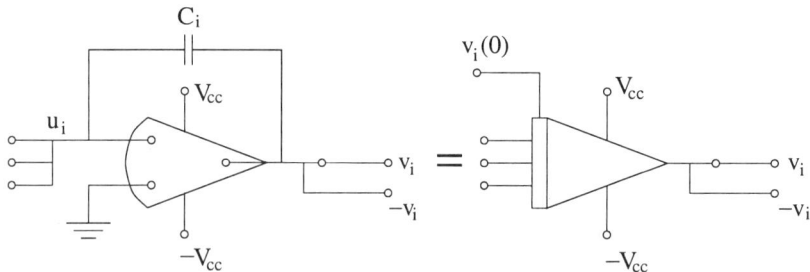

Figure 2.6.3: The ith neural cell of system (2.6.1), (2.6.2).

2.6. LINEAR SYSTEMS ON A HYPERCUBE

with the constraints

$$-1 < v_i < 1, \quad i = 1, \cdots, n.$$

If in (2.6.3) we let $C_i = 1$, $1 \leq i \leq n$, $x = (x_1, \cdots, x_n)^T = u$, $T = [T_{ij}]$, where

$$T_{ij} = \begin{cases} +1/R_{ij}, & \text{if } R_{ij} \text{ is connected to } v_j \\ -1/R_{ij}, & \text{if } R_{ij} \text{ is connected to } -v_j, \end{cases}$$

and $I = (I_1, \cdots, I_n)^T$, where

$$I_i = \frac{\pm V_{cc}}{r_i},$$

then (2.6.3) assumes the form

$$\frac{dx}{dt} = Tx + I$$

with the constraints

$$-1 \leq x_i \leq 1, \quad i = 1, \cdots, n.$$

These equations are identical to (2.6.1) and (2.6.2), respectively.

In usual applications, electronic circuits of the type depicted in Fig. 2.6.1 operate in the unsaturated (i.e., in the linear) mode and efforts are made to stay clear of saturation regions. In the next chapter, however, we will demonstrate that the circuit in Fig. 2.6.1, when operated in an extended mode, which includes saturation of the state variables, exhibits properties associated with recurrent neural networks. We will give in Chapter 4 a proper definition of solution of system (2.6.1), (2.6.2) where the variable x defined on D^n indeed describes the behavior of the circuit given in Fig. 2.6.1, including the saturation. Thus, the circuit in Fig. 2.6.1 will serve as an implementation of the neural network model (2.6.1), (2.6.2).

In Chapter 4, we will show that under reasonable assumptions, the equilibrium points of neural network (2.6.1), (2.6.2) can be determined easily and systematically. Also, by making use of the energy function

$$E(x) = -\frac{1}{2} x^T T x - x^T I,$$

a synthesis procedure developed for the Hopfield neural network [and its extension given by (2.4.1)] will be modified to apply to the neural network (2.6.1), (2.6.2) as well. Furthermore, it will be shown in Chapter 4 that operational amplifiers with large gains appear to stabilize the circuit given in Fig. 2.6.1. Moreover, it will be shown that interconnecting matrices T with large negative eigenvalues may be used to synthesize the neural network (2.6.1), (2.6.2) with a resulting reduction in the number of spurious equilibrium points.

The above observations suggest that system (2.6.1), (2.6.2) overcomes some of the disadvantages of the Hopfield analog neural network model (pointed out in Section 2.2) while maintaining the basic structure of the Hopfield neural network model.

A comparison of the Hopfield neural network model (2.2.3) and the neural network described by equations (2.6.1), (2.6.2) points to the following similarities and differences. As pointed out in Section 2.4, in terms of the variables v_i, $i = 1, \cdots, n$, we can represent the Hopfield model (2.2.3) by

$$\frac{dv}{dt} = H(v)(-S(v) + Tv + I) \qquad (2.6.4)$$

where $v = (v_1, \cdots, v_n)^T \in (-1,1)^n$,

$$H(v) = \mathrm{diag}\left[\lambda\left(C_1 \frac{dg_1^{-1}(v_1)}{dv_1}\right)^{-1}, \cdots, \lambda\left(C_n \frac{dg_n^{-1}(v_n)}{dv_n}\right)^{-1}\right],$$

$$S(v) = \left(\frac{g^{-1}(v_1)}{\lambda R_1}, \cdots, \frac{g^{-1}(v_n)}{\lambda R_n}\right)^T,$$

$T = [T_{ij}]$, and $I = (I_1, \cdots, I_n)^T$. System (2.6.4) has the identical set of equilibrium points and the identical set of asymptotically stable equilibrium points as the system described by the equations

$$\frac{dv}{dt} = -S(v) + Tv + I. \qquad (2.6.5)$$

Now system (2.6.5) can be implemented by the electronic circuit depicted in Fig. 2.6.4. In this circuit, $u_i = (1/\lambda)g^{-1}(v_i)$, $i = 1, \cdots, n$

2.6. LINEAR SYSTEMS ON A HYPERCUBE

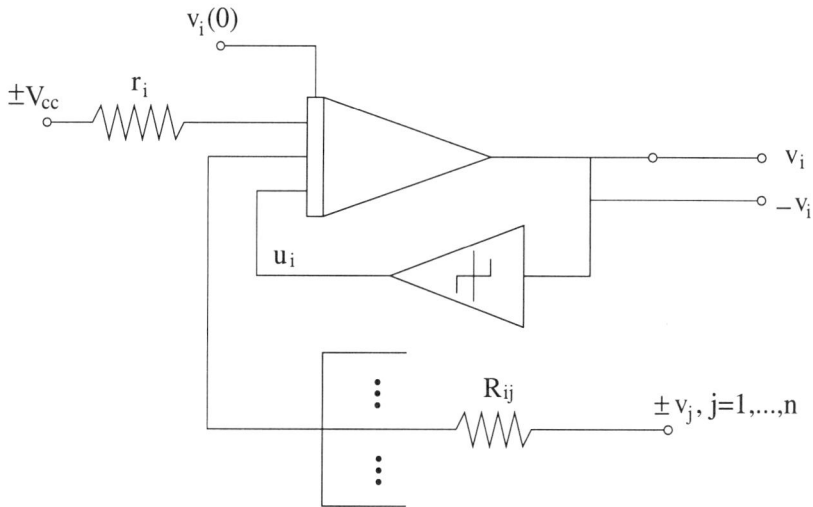

Figure 2.6.4: The implementation of system (2.6.5).

and each integrator is an ideal integrator in the sense that it *cannot* be saturated. When the parameter λ tends towards infinity, the circuit in Fig. 2.6.4 can be described by saturated integrators as in the circuit of Fig. 2.6.1. Thus, the Hopfield model (2.2.3) and the neural network model described by (2.6.1), (2.6.1), appear to be closely related.

The neural network (2.6.1), (2.6.2) is easily simulated by digital computers or by array processors, using difference equations of the form

$$x((k+1)h) = F(\Phi x(kh) + \Gamma) \qquad (2.6.6)$$

where $x(kh) \in D^n$, h is the sampling period, $F: \Re^n \to D^n$, $F(x) = (F_1(x_1), \cdots, F_n(x_n))^T$ with

$$F_i(\sigma) \triangleq \text{sat}(\sigma) = \begin{cases} 1, & \text{if } \sigma > 1 \\ \sigma, & \text{if } -1 \leq \sigma \leq 1 \\ -1, & \text{if } \sigma < -1, \end{cases}$$

$\Phi = [\Phi_{ij}] = \exp(hT)$, and

$$\Gamma = I \cdot \left(\int_0^h \exp(\eta T) d\eta \right).$$

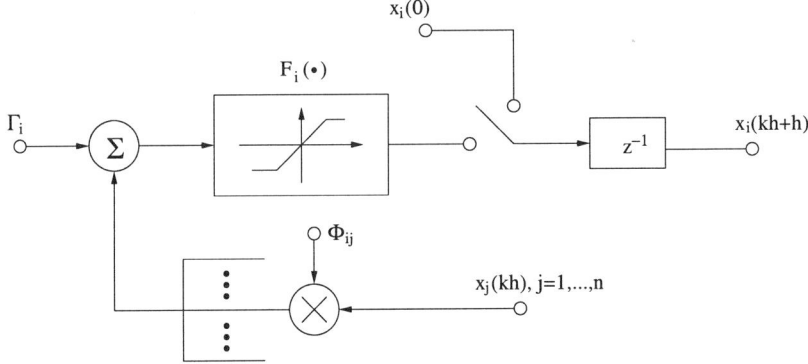

Figure 2.6.5: Block diagram of system (2.6.6).

The block diagram of system (2.6.6) is depicted in Fig. 2.6.5.

Independent of the continuous-time system (2.6.1), (2.6.2), and its discrete-time counterpart (2.6.6), we will also concern ourselves with discrete-time systems described by equations of the form

$$x(k+1) = \text{sat}(Ax(k) + I). \tag{2.6.7}$$

[Systems (2.6.6) and (2.6.7) are related by letting $A = \Phi$, $I = \Gamma$, and $h = 1$.] Such systems have been studied extensively in the literature under the names *brain-state-in-a-box* (BSB) and *linear systems operating on a closed hypercube* (see, e.g., [10], [12], [19], [36], [37]).

2.7 Summary

There are numerous models of recurrent neural networks that have been considered in the literature (refer, e.g., to [6], [13], [50]). In the present chapter we singled out several of the more important of these models, and we discussed these, when appropriate, in the context of applications to associative memories. In subsequent chapters, we will conduct qualitative analyses of these models and we will provide synthesis (resp., design) procedures for these models (concentrating on applications to associative memories).

2.7. SUMMARY

For historic reasons we first introduced the McCulloch-Pitts model given by

$$\begin{cases} v_i(k+1) = \text{sgn}(u_i(k)), & 1 \leq i \leq n \\ u_i(k) = \sum_{j=1}^{n} T_{ij} v_j(k) + I_i, & 1 \leq i \leq n \end{cases} \quad (2.7.1)$$

where each neuron is represented by the sign function, $\text{sgn}(\cdot)$, u_i denotes the input to the ith neuron, v_i represents the output of the ith neuron, T_{ij} specifies the interconnection strength between the jth and ith neurons, and I_i represents the external input to neuron i. The states in system (2.7.1) switch *asynchronously*.

Closely related to (2.7.1) is the discrete neural network described by equations of the form

$$\begin{cases} v_i(k+1) = g(u_i(k)), & 1 \leq i \leq n \\ u_i(k) = \sum_{j=1}^{n} T_{ij} v_j(k) + I_i, & 1 \leq i \leq n \end{cases}$$

where $g(\cdot)$ denotes a sigmoidal function and where the switching amongst states takes place in a *synchronous* manner.

Next, we addressed in some detail the analog Hopfield neural network (and its implementation), described by equations of the form

$$\begin{cases} C_i (du_i/dt) = -1/R_i + \sum_{j=1}^{n} t_{ij} v_j + w_i \\ v_i = g_i(\lambda u_i), \quad i = 1, \cdots, n \end{cases} \quad (2.7.2)$$

where, as before, u_i and v_i denote neuron inputs and outputs, respectively, w_i denotes the external input to the ith neuron, $C_i > 0$ and $R_i > 0$ are capacitances and resistances, respectively, and $t_{ij} \in \Re$ represent neuron interconnection weights determined by resistors (see Fig. 2.2.2 and the discussion in Section 2.2). Each neuron in (2.7.2) is modeled by an amplifier with gain given, e.g., by

$$v_i = g_i(\lambda u_i) = \frac{2}{\pi} \tan^{-1}\left(\frac{\pi}{2} \lambda u_i\right). \quad (2.7.3)$$

Using appropriate definitions, equation (2.7.2) can be written in vector form as

$$\begin{cases} \dot{x} = -Ax + Ty + I \\ y = S(x) \end{cases} \quad (2.7.4)$$

CHAPTER 2. SOME NEURAL NETWORK MODELS

where $S(x) = (s_1(x_1), \cdots, s_n(x_n))^T$ and $s_i(x_i) = g_i(\lambda u_i)/C_i$.

A variant of (2.7.4) that we considered are neural networks described by equations of the form

$$\begin{cases} \dot{x} = -Ax + Ty + I \\ y = \text{sat}(x) \end{cases} \quad (2.7.5)$$

where $\text{sat}(x) = (\text{sat}(x_1), \cdots, \text{sat}(x_n))^T$ and where $\text{sat}(\cdot)$ denotes the saturation function [refer to (2.2.5)]. This model is frequently used in cellular neural network applications (see, e.g., [3], [26], [27]).

To approximate the analog Hopfield neural network by digital computer simulations or by means of specialized digital hardware, we introduced the discrete-time model described by equations of the form

$$u_i(k+1) = \sum_{j=1}^{n} T_{ij} v_j(k) - a_i u_i(k) + I_i, \quad i = 1, \cdots, n \quad (2.7.6)$$

where all symbols are defined in (2.3.4).

We next considered two generalizations to the analog Hopfield neural network model. The first of these is described by equations of the form

$$\dot{x} = -H(x)(-Tx + S(x) - I) \quad (2.7.7)$$

where all symbols are defined in (2.4.1). The second of these, known as the Cohen-Grossberg model, is described by equations of the form

$$\dot{x}_i = -a_i(x_i) \left(b_i(x_i) - \sum_{j=1}^{n} t_{ij} s_j(x_j) \right), \quad i = 1, \cdots, n \quad (2.7.8)$$

where all symbols are defined in (2.4.4).

Some of the synthesis procedures for the analog Hopfield neural network work best for very large amplifier gains. When in (2.7.3), λ_i is arbitrarily large, the analog Hopfield neural network assumes the form of the variable structure system given by

$$\frac{dx}{dt} = F(x) \quad (2.7.9)$$

2.7. SUMMARY

with
$$F(x) = -Ax + TS(x) + I \qquad (2.7.10)$$

where $S(x) = (s_1(x_1), \cdots, s_n(x_n))^T$ and each $s_i(\cdot)$ denotes the sign function, and where the remaining symbols are defined as in equation (2.5.2). It turns out that under appropriate assumptions, the output values of the neurons in the above model agree with the discrete asynchronous model introduced by Hopfield, given by

$$v_i^+ = \begin{cases} 1, & \text{if } \sum_{j=1}^{n} T_{ij}v_j + I_i > 0 \\ -1, & \text{if } \sum_{j=1}^{n} T_{ij}v_j + I_i < 0 \end{cases} \qquad (2.7.11)$$

where all symbols are defined in (2.5.6).

The preceding neural network models are concerned with the analog Hopfield neural network, variants to this network, generalizations of this network, and synchronous and asynchronous digital networks which are counterparts to the analog Hopfield neural networks. The last class of neural networks that we considered has a structure which differs significantly from the networks described thus far. The continuous-time networks of this class are described by equations of the form

$$\frac{dx}{dt} = Tx + I \qquad (2.7.12)$$

with the constraints

$$-1 \leq x_i \leq 1, \quad i = 1, \cdots, n \qquad (2.7.13)$$

while the discrete counterpart of these networks are described by equations of the form

$$x(k+1) = \text{sat}(Ax(k) + I) \qquad (2.7.14)$$

where $\text{sat}(x) = (\text{sat}(x_1), \cdots, \text{sat}(x_n))^T$ denotes the saturation function, and where the remaining symbols in (2.7.12)–(2.7.14) are defined as in Section 2.6. We discussed in some detail implementation issues of the above networks.

2.8 Notes and References

Section 2.1 is based on material presented in [32]. For additional recurrent neural network models and applications to associative memories, refer to the references cited at the end of this chapter (e.g., [6], [13], [50]).

Section 2.2 is based primarily on material presented in [21] and [23] while Section 2.3 is based on [34]. For a good general exposition on VLSI design and implementation issues, refer to the monograph [31].

Our presentation in Section 2.4 relies on material given in [21]. Refer to [4] for a detailed presentation of the Cohen-Grossberg model.

The material of Section 2.5 is based on [22]. For other aspects and applications of variable structure systems (notably control systems), refer, e.g., to [48].

Finally, the material in Section 2.6 relies on [23] and [36]. In addition to neural network applications, systems with state saturation constraints arise also in several other areas, including digital signal processing and control systems (see, e.g., [27]).

Bibliography

[1] GA Carpenter, MA Cohen, S Grossberg. Computing with neural networks. Science 235:1226–1227, 1987.

[2] HH Chen. High order correlation model for associative memory. In: JS Denker. Ed. Neural Networks for Computing, AIP Conference Proceedings, no 151, Snowbird, UT, 1986, pp 86–99.

[3] LO Chua, L Yang. Cellular neural networks: Theory. IEEE Transactions on Circuits and Systems 35:1257–1272, 1988.

[4] M Cohen, S Grossberg. Absolute stability of global pattern formation and parallel memory storage by competitive neural networks. IEEE Transactions on Systems, Man, and Cybernetics 13:815–826, 1983.

BIBLIOGRAPHY

[5] LN Cooper, F Liberman, E Oja. Theory for the acquisition and loss of neuron specificity in visual cortex. Biological Cybernetics 33:9–28, 1979.

[6] JS Denker. Ed. Neural Networks for Computing, AIP Conference Proceedings, no 151, Snowbird, UT, 1986.

[7] JA Farrell, AN Michel. A synthesis procedure for Hopfield's continuous time associative memory. IEEE Transactions on Circuits and Systems 37:877–884, 1990.

[8] NR Franks. Army ants: A collective intelligence. American Scientist 77:139–145, 1989.

[9] B Gold. Hopfield model applied to vowel and consonant discrimination. In: JS Denker. Ed. Neural Networks for Computing, AIP Conference Proceedings, no 151, Snowbird, UT, 1986, pp 158–164.

[10] RM Golden. The 'brain-state-in-a-box' neural model is a gradient descent algorithm. Mathematical Psychology 30:73–80, 1986.

[11] EG Goles, G Vichniac. Lyapunov functions for parallel neural networks. IEEE Transactions on Circuits and Systems 36:165–181, 1989.

[12] HJ Greenberg. Equilibria of the brain-state-in-a-box (BSB) neural model. Neural Networks 1:323–324, 1988.

[13] S Haykin. Neural Networks: A Comprehensive Foundation. Upper Saddle River, NJ: Prentice-Hall, 1999.

[14] GE Hinton, JA Anderson. Eds. Parallel Models of Associative Memory. New Jersey: Lawrence Erlbaum, 1981.

[15] JJ Hopfield. Neural networks and physical systems with emergent collective computational abilities. Proceedings of the National Academy of Sciences USA 79:2554–2558, 1982.

[16] JJ Hopfield. Neurons with graded response have collective computational properties like those of two-state neurons. Proceedings of the National Academy of Sciences USA 81:3088–3092, 1984.

[17] JJ Hopfield, DI Feinstein, RE Palmer. 'Unlearning' has a stabilizing effect in collective memories. Nature 304:158–159, 1983.

[18] JJ Hopfield, DW Tank. 'Neural' computation of decisions in optimization problems. Biological Cybernetics 52:141–152, 1985.

[19] S Hui, SH Żak. Dynamical analysis of the brain-state-in-a-box (BSB) neural models. IEEE Transactions on Neural Networks 3:86–94, 1992.

[20] T Kohonen. Self-Organization and Associative Memory. Berlin: Springer-Verlag, 1988.

[21] JH Li, AN Michel, W Porod. Qualitative analysis and synthesis of a class of neural networks. IEEE Transactions on Circuits and Systems 35:976–987, 1988

[22] JH Li, AN Michel, W Porod. Analysis and synthesis of a class of neural networks: Variable structure systems with infinite gains. IEEE Transactions on Circuits and Systems 36:713–731, 1989.

[23] JH Li, AN Michel, W Porod. Analysis and synthesis of a class of neural networks: Linear systems operating on a closed hypercube. IEEE Transactions on Circuits and Systems 36:1405–1422, 1989.

[24] WA Little. The existence of persistent states in the brain. Mathematical Biosciences 19:101–120, 1974.

[25] WA Little, GL Shaw. Analytic study of the memory storage capacity of a neural network. Mathematical Biosciences 39:281–290, 1978.

[26] D Liu, AN Michel. Sparsely interconnected neural networks for associative memories with applications to cellular neural networks. IEEE Transactions on Circuits and Systems-II: Analog and Digital Signal Processing 41:295–307, 1994.

[27] D Liu, AN Michel. Dynamical Systems with Saturation Nonlinearities: Analysis and Design. Lecture Notes in Control and Information Sciences, vol 195. Berlin, Germany: Springer-Verlag, 1994.

BIBLIOGRAPHY

[28] T Maxwell. Nonlinear dynamics of artificial neural systems. In: JS Denker. Ed. Neural Networks for Computing, AIP Conference Proceedings, no 151, Snowbird, UT, 1986, pp 299–304.

[29] WS McCulloch, W Pitts. A logical calculus of the ideas immanent in nervous activity. Bulletin of Mathematical Biophysics 5:115–133, 1943.

[30] RJ McEliece, EC Posner, ER Rodemich, SS Venkatesh. The capacity of the Hopfield associative memory. IEEE Transactions on Information Theory 33:461–482, 1987.

[31] C Mead. Analog VLSI and Neural Systems. Reading, MA: Addison Wesley, 1989.

[32] AN Michel, JA Farrell. Associative memories via neural networks. IEEE Control Systems Magazine 10:6–17, 1990.

[33] AN Michel, JA Farrell, W Porod. Qualitative analysis of neural networks. IEEE Transactions on Circuits and Systems 36:229–243, 1989.

[34] AN Michel, JA Farrell, HF Sun. Analysis and synthesis techniques for Hopfield type synchronous discrete time neural networks with application to associative memory. IEEE Transactions on Circuits and Systems 37:1356–1366, 1990.

[35] AN Michel, D Liu. Theory and applications of sparsely interconnected neural networks. Neural, Parallel and Scientific Computations 4:305–324, 1996.

[36] AN Michel, J Si, G Yen. Analysis and synthesis of a class of discrete-time neural networks described on hypercubes. IEEE Transactions on Neural Networks 2:32–46, 1991.

[37] R Perfetti. A synthesis procedure for brain-state-in-a-box neural networks. IEEE Transactions on Neural Networks 6:1071–1080, 1995.

[38] L Personnaz, I Guyon, G Dreyfus. Information storage and retrieval in spin-glass like neural networks. Journal de Physique Lettres 46:L359–L365, 1985.

[39] L Personnaz, I Guyon, G Dreyfus. Collective computational properties of neural networks: New learning mechanism. Physical Review A 34:4217–4228, 1986.

[40] D Psaltis, CH Park. Nonlinear discriminant functions and associative memories. In: JS Denker. Ed. Neural Networks for Computing, AIP Conference Proceedings, no 151, Snowbird, UT, 1986, pp 370–375.

[41] FR Rosenblatt. Two theorems of statistical separability in the perception mechanization of thought processes. Proceedings of the Symposium Held at the National Physics Laboratory, H. M. Stationary Office, London, 1958, vol 1, pp 421–456.

[42] FR Rosenblatt. Principles of Neurodynamics. New York, NY: Spartan, 1962.

[43] DE Rumelhart, KL McClelland. Eds. Parallel Distributed Processing, vol 1. Cambridge, MA: MIT Press, 1986.

[44] FMA Salam. A model of neural circuits for programmable VLSI implementation. Proceedings of the 1989 IEEE International Symposium on Circuits and Systems, Portland, OR, 1989, pp 849–851.

[45] FMA Salam. New artificial neural net models: Basic theory and characteristics. Proceedings of the 1990 IEEE International Symposium on Circuits and Systems, New Orleans, LA, 1990, pp 200–205.

[46] DB Schwarz. Dynamics of microfabricated electronic neural networks. Applied Physics Letters 50:1110–1112, 1987.

[47] DW Tank, JJ Hopfield. Simple 'neural' optimization networks: An A/D converter, signal decision circuit, and a linear programming circuit. IEEE Transactions on Circuits and Systems 33:533–541, 1986.

[48] VI Utkin. Variable structure systems with sliding modes. IEEE Transactions on Automatic Control 22:212–222, 1977.

[49] B Widrow, R Winter. Neural nets for adaptive filtering and adaptive pattern recognition. Computer 18:25–39, 1988.

[50] JM Zurada. Introduction to Artificial Neural Systems. St. Paul, MN: West Publishing Company, 1992.

Chapter 3

Qualitative Analysis of Analog Hopfield-Type Neural Networks: Global Results

In the present chapter we first conduct a qualitative analysis of the generalized analog Hopfield neural network model, (2.4.1), presented in Section 2.4. Since the conventional analog Hopfield neural network model is a special case of this class of networks, the results of the present chapter pertain to the conventional Hopfield neural network, presented in Section 2.2, as well. Next, we conduct a qualitative analysis of the analog Hopfield neural network model with infinite gain amplifiers, (2.5.1), developed in Section 2.5.

We are primarily concerned with *global results* in this chapter. In Chapter 5, we will address local stability results of the two Hopfield neural network models developed in Sections 2.2 and 2.3.

Questions that we will address in the present chapter include existence, uniqueness and continuation of solutions of the equations describing the networks; existence and determination of the locations of the equilibria of a network; estimates of the total number of equilibria of a network; estimates of the total number of asymptotically stable equilibria of a network; and the global stability properties of a network.

3.1 Generalized Analog Hopfield Neural Network Model: System (L)

In the present chapter we consider a class of nonlinear, autonomous, ordinary differential equations of the form

$$\dot{x} = -H(x)(-Tx + S(x) - I). \tag{L}$$

We will define all symbols in (L) at a later point. Here it suffices to state that x is an n-vector, $\dot{x}$ denotes the derivative of x with respect to time t, $H(x)$ is a matrix-valued function, T is a matrix, $S(x)$ is a vector-valued function, and I denotes an input vector.

This system of equations can be used to model neural networks. With an appropriate set of assumptions, which we will give later, the system (L) will constitute a slight generalization of the Hopfield model (see Sections 2.2 and 2.4).

We will establish the following results for system (L):

1) We show that system (L) possesses unique solutions which exists for all $t \geq 0$.

2) We associate with system (L) an energy function E and we show that E decreases monotonically along nonequilibrium solutions of (L), as t increases and that each nonequilibrium solution of (L) tends to an equilibrium of (L) as t becomes large.

3) We show that for (L) there are only a finite number of equilibrium points.

4) We show that if $\tilde{x}$ is a stable equilibrium for (L), then it is also asymptotically stable.

5) We show that an (asymptotically) stable equilibrium $\tilde{x}$ is a local minimum of E.

For the special case of the conventional analog Hopfield neural network model with infinite gain amplifiers we will later in the chapter identify 2^n regions in n-space and we will show that in each of these regions there is at most one asymptotically stable equilibrium of the network. This in turn will enable us to establish an upper bound for the number of asymptotically stable equilibrium points of a network, provided that some reasonable restrictions are met.

3.2 Notation and Some Preliminaries

The present section consists of three parts. First, we establish some of the notation used throughout this chapter. Next, we provide some essential preliminary results on differential equations and stability theory.

A. Notation

Let V and W be arbitrary sets. Then $V \cup W$, $V \cap W$, $V - W$, and $V \times W$ denote the union, intersection, difference and Cartesian product of V and W, respectively. If V is a subset of W, we write $V \subset W$ and if x is an element of V, we write $x \in V$. If f is a function from V into W, we write $f: V \to W$ and we let $f(U) = \{f(x) \in W : x \in U\}$ for $U \subset V$, and $f^{-1}(y) = \{x \in V : f(x) = y\}$ for $y \in W$. Let $\emptyset$ denote the empty set, let $\Re$ denote the set of real numbers, and let $\Re^+ = [0, \infty)$. If $V_1, \cdots, V_n$ are n arbitrary sets, their Cartesian product is denoted by $\prod_{i=1}^{n} V_i = V_1 \times \cdots \times V_n$. If in particular, $V = V_1 = \cdots = V_n$, we write $\prod_{i=1}^{n} V_i = V^n$. Let $\Re^n$ be real n-space. If $x \in \Re^n$, then $x^T = (x_1, \cdots, x_n)$ denotes the transpose of x. When using a norm for $x \in \Re^n$, $|x|$, we will at first (through Section 3.5) have in mind $|x| = \max_{1 \leq i \leq n} \{|x_i|\}$. If $x \in \Re^n$ and $Y \subset \Re^n$, then $x \perp Y$ will mean that $x^T \cdot y = 0$ for all $y \in Y$. If $V \subset \Re^n$, then $\overline{V}$, V°, and ∂V represent the closure, interior, and boundary of V in $\Re^n$, respectively. Also, we let $B(\tilde{x}, r) = \{x \in \Re^n : |x - \tilde{x}| < r\}$ for $\tilde{x} \in \Re^n$

and $r > 0$. If $A = [a_{ij}]$ is an arbitrary matrix, then A^T denotes the transpose of A and the norm of A is defined as $\|A\| = \sup_{|x|<1}\{|Ax|\}$ (cf. [11], Chapter 10, §2). If A is a symmetric matrix, by $A > 0$ we mean that A is positive definite and by $A \geq 0$ we mean that A is positive semidefinite. If $E_1, \cdots, E_n$ are n vector spaces over $\Re$, $L(E_1, \cdots, E_n; \Re)$ denotes the set of continuous multilinear maps from $\prod_{i=1}^{n} E_i$ to $\Re$ (cf. [1], Appendix A). If in particular, $E_1 = \cdots = E_n = E$, we write $L(E_1, \cdots, E_n; \Re) = L^n(E; \Re)$. For a function $f : V \to W$, where $V \subset \Re^n$, $W \subset \Re$, the kth-order derivative (cf. [1], Chapter 4) is denoted by $D^k f : V \to L^k(\Re^n; \Re)$, if it exists. A function $F : V \to W$, where $V \subset \Re^n$, $W \subset \Re^m$, is said to be a class C^k or a C^k-function if for each component of F, the kth-order derivative exists and is continuous.

Given a C^2-function $g : V \to \Re$ where $V \subset \Re^n$, we denote the gradient of g by $\nabla g(x) = (\partial g_1(x), \cdots, \partial g_n(x))^T = Dg(x, \cdot)$ and we denote the $n \times n$ Jacobian matrix of g by $J_g(x) = [\partial^2 g(x)/\partial x_i \partial x_j] = D^2 g(x, \cdot, \cdot)$. An element $\tilde{x} \in V$ is called a critical point of g if $\nabla g(\tilde{x}) = 0$. Also, $\tilde{x} \in V$ is said to be a local minimum of g if there is an open neighborhood U of $\tilde{x}$ such that for all $x \in U$, $g(x) \geq g(\tilde{x})$.

B. Systems of Ordinary Differential Equations

We will consider systems of first order, autonomous ordinary differential equations of the form

$$\dot{x} = f(x) \tag{E}$$

where $x = (x_1, \cdots, x_n)^T \in G$, G is a non-empty connected open subset in $\Re^n$, $t \in \Re$, $\dot{x} = dx/dt$ and f is a C^1-function from G into $\Re^n$. We will have occasion to utilize the properties of (E) enumerated below (cf. [10], Chapter 2).

Lemma 3.2.1 For each $\tilde{x} \in G$, there is a unique non-continuable solution of (E), given by

$$\varphi(\cdot, 0, \tilde{x}) : [0, \tilde{t}) \to G$$

3.2. NOTATION AND SOME PRELIMINARIES 73

with $\varphi(0, 0, \tilde{x}) = \tilde{x}$. This solution is non-continuable in the sense that if there is another solution of (E)

$$\varphi_1(\cdot, 0, \tilde{x}) : [0, \tilde{t}_1) \to G$$

with $\varphi_1(0, 0, \tilde{x}) = \tilde{x}$, we have $\tilde{t}_1 \leq \tilde{t}$ and $\varphi_1 = \varphi$ on $[0, \tilde{t}_1)$. We call the function $\varphi(\cdot, 0, \tilde{x})$ the *solution* of (E) starting at $\tilde{x}$. For purposes of brevity, we frequently write $\varphi(t, \tilde{x})$ or $\varphi(t)$ in place of $\varphi(t, 0, \tilde{x})$, when the initial conditions $(0, \tilde{x})$ are understood. ∎

Lemma 3.2.2 ([10], Chapter 2, Corollary 3.2) Assume that G is bounded. Then for any solution $\varphi(\cdot, \tilde{x}) : [0, \tilde{t}) \to G$, either $\varphi(t) \to \partial G$ as $t \to \tilde{t}$ or $\tilde{t} = +\infty$. ∎

A constant solution $\varphi(t, \tilde{x}) \equiv \tilde{x}$ is said to be an *equilibrium of* (E). Equivalently, any point $\tilde{x} \in G$ such that $f(\tilde{x}) = 0$ is an equilibrium of (E).

Lemma 3.2.3 For a nonequilibrium solution $\varphi(\cdot, \tilde{x}) : [0, \tilde{t}) \to G$, $f(\varphi(t, \tilde{x})) \neq 0$, for any $0 \leq t < \tilde{t}$. ∎

The proof of this lemma is a direct consequence of the uniqueness of the solutions of (E).

C. Stability of an Equilibrium

We now summarize a few concepts and results from the Lyapunov stability theory.

An equilibrium $\varphi(t) \equiv \tilde{x}$ of (E) is said to be *isolated* if there is an $r > 0$ such that for any $x \in B(\tilde{x}, r) - \{x\}$, $f(x) \neq 0$.

Let $\tilde{x}$ be an isolated equilibrium of (E). For the following definitions, we assume that solutions $\varphi(\cdot, 0, x)$ for (E) exist for all $t \geq 0$ when $|x - \tilde{x}| < h$ for some $h > 0$.

a) $\tilde{x}$ is said to be *stable* if for any $\varepsilon > 0$ ($\varepsilon < h$), there is a $\delta = \delta(\varepsilon) > 0$ such that $|\varphi(t, 0, x) - \tilde{x}| < \varepsilon$, for all $t \in [0, +\infty)$ whenever $|x - \tilde{x}| < \delta$;

b) $\tilde{x}$ is said to be *asymptotically stable* if it is stable and if there is an $\eta > 0$ ($\eta < h$) such that $\lim_{t \to +\infty} |\varphi(t,0,x) - \tilde{x}| = 0$ whenever $|x - \tilde{x}| < \eta$;

c) $\tilde{x}$ is said to be *unstable* if it is not stable.

Given a C^1-function $g\colon G \to \Re$, we define the function $D_{(\mathrm{E})}g\colon G \to \Re$ by $D_{(\mathrm{E})}g(x) = \nabla g(x)^T f(x)$ and we call $D_{(\mathrm{E})}g$ the *derivative of g with respect to t along the solutions of* (E).

A continuous function $\psi\colon \Re^+ \to \Re^+$ is said to belong to class $\mathcal{K}$ (i.e., $\psi \in \mathcal{K}$) if $\psi(0) = 0$ and $\psi(s)$ is monotonically increasing in s.

In the following, we assume without loss of generality that the origin is an isolated equilibrium of (E), so that $f(0) = 0$. We let $B(0,r) \stackrel{\triangle}{=} B(r)$. We have (cf. [10], Chapter 5, §9):

Lemma 3.2.4 *The equilibrium $x = 0$ of* (E) *is asymptotically stable if there exists a C^1-function $v\colon B(r) \to \Re$ for some $r > 0$ ($r < h$) and functions $\psi_1, \psi_2 \in \mathcal{K}$ such that $v(0) = 0$,*

$$v(x) \geq \psi_1(|x|),$$

and

$$D_{(\mathrm{E})}v(x) \leq -\psi_2(|x|)$$

for all $x \in B(r)$. ∎

The above result states that the equilibrium $x = 0$ of (E) is asymptotically stable if there exists a positive definite function v whose time derivative, evaluated along the solutions of (E), is negative definite.

Next, we present two results from the *invariance theory* for differential equations. In doing so, we require the following notion: A point $a \in \Re^n$ is said to lie in the *limit set* $\Omega(\varphi)$ of a solution φ of (E) if there exists a sequence $\{t_m\} \to \infty$ as $m \to \infty$ such that $\lim_{m \to \infty} \varphi(t_m) = a$. For proofs of the next two results, refer to Lemmas 11.9 and 11.10 in [10], Chapter 5.

Lemma 3.2.5 If a solution $\varphi(t, x_0)$ of (E) remains in a compact set for $0 \leq t < \infty$, then its limit set $\Omega(\varphi)$ is a nonempty, compact and invariant set with respect to (E). Moreover, $\varphi(t, x_0)$ approaches the set $\Omega(\varphi)$ as $t \to \infty$ [i.e., for every $\varepsilon > 0$ there exists a t' such that for every $t > t'$ there exists a point $a \in \Omega(\varphi)$ (possibly depending on t) such that $|\varphi(t, x_0) - a)| < \varepsilon$]. ∎

Lemma 3.2.6 Let v be a continuously differentiable function defined on a domain $G \subset \Re^n$ containing the origin and let $D_{(E)}v(x) \leq 0$ for all $x \in G$. Let $x_0 \in G$ and let $\varphi(t, x_0)$ be a bounded solution of (E) whose trajectory lies in G for all $t \geq 0$ and let the limit set $\Omega(\varphi)$ of $\varphi(t, x_0)$ lie in G. Then $D_{(E)}v = 0$ at all points of $\Omega(\varphi)$. [Recall that the *trajectory* of a solution φ of (E) is the projection of the locus of points in the t-x space determined by $\varphi(t)$ for all $t \geq 0$ onto the x-space.] ∎

3.3 Assumptions for the Generalized Hopfield Model

We will consider neural networks described by differential equations of the form

$$\dot{x} = -H(x)(-Tx + S(x) - I) \qquad (L)$$

where $x = (x_1, \cdots, x_n)^T \in (-1, 1)^n$, $\dot{x} = dx/dt$, H is a function from $(-1, 1)^n$ into $R^{n \times n}$ [i.e., for each $x \in (-1, 1)^n$, $H(x)$ is an $n \times n$ matrix], $T = [T_{ij}]$ is an $n \times n$ constant matrix, $S(x) = (s_1(x_1), \cdots, s_n(x_n))^T$ where $s_i \colon (-1, 1) \to \Re$ and $I = (I_1, \cdots, I_n)^T$ is a constant real vector. In the present section, we will impose realistic restrictions on the functions $H(x)$ and $S(x)$ and on the matrix T, and we will discuss some of the consequences of these restrictions.

Assumption (A) For system (L) assume the following:
a) For every fixed $x \in (-1, 1)^n$, $H(x)$ is symmetric and positive definite.
b) T is symmetric.

c) For each i, $1 \leq i \leq n$, $s_i: (-1,1) \to \Re$ is monotone-increasing, $s_i(0) = 0$, $s_i(x_i) = -s_i(-x_i)$, the inverse $s_i^{-1}: \Re \to (-1,1)$ exists, s_i and s_i^{-1} are C^1-functions,

$$\int_0^{x_i} s_i(\sigma) d\sigma \to +\infty \text{ as } x_i \to 1,$$

and furthermore, $s_i''(x_i) = d^2 s_i(x_i)/dx_i^2$ exists. [From these assumptions, it is clear that $x_i s_i(x_i) > 0$ for $x_i \neq 0$, $\lim_{\rho \to 1} s_i(\rho) = +\infty$, $\lim_{\rho \to -1} s_i(\rho) = -\infty$ and for any $x_i \in (-1,1)$, $s_i'(x_i) = ds_i(x_i)/dx_i > 0$ and $s_i'(x_i) = s_i'(-x_i)$.] ∎

Remark 3.3.1 The hypothesis concerning $H(x)$ in Assumption (A) for system (L) is weaker than the corresponding hypothesis made in [4] for the Hopfield model. The hypotheses concerning matrix T and the functions s_i, $1 \leq i \leq n$, enumerated in Assumption (A) for system (L) are identical to corresponding ones made in [4] for the Hopfield model, save that in Assumption (A) it is assumed that s_i'' exists for each i. ∎

As in [3] and [4], we associate with system (L) an energy function $E: (-1,1)^n \to \Re$, given by

$$E(x) = -\frac{1}{2} x^T T x + \sum_{i=1}^n \int_0^{x_i} s_i(\rho) d\rho - x^T I. \quad (3.3.1)$$

The first-order derivative of E, $DE: (-1,1)^n \to L(\Re^n; \Re)$ is given by

$$DE(x,y) = \nabla E(x)^T y$$

where $\nabla E(x)$ is the gradient of E and

$$\nabla E(x) = \left(\frac{\partial E(x)}{\partial x_1}, \cdots, \frac{\partial E(x)}{\partial x_n} \right)^T = -Tx + S(x) - I.$$

The second-order derivative of E, $D^2 E: (-1,1)^n \to L^2(\Re^n; \Re)$ is given by

$$D^2 E(x,y,z) = y^T J_E(x) z$$

3.3. ASSUMPTIONS FOR THE HOPFIELD MODEL

where $J_E(x)$ is the Jacobian matrix of E and

$$J_E(x) = \left[\frac{\partial^2 E(x)}{\partial x_i \partial x_j}\right] = -T + \text{diag}[s_1'(x_1), \cdots, s_n'(x_n)].$$

Also, the third-order derivative of E, $D^3 E: (-1,1)^n \to L^3(\Re^n; \Re)$ is given by

$$D^3 E(x, y, z, u) = \sum_{i=1}^{n} s_i''(x_i) y_i z_i u_i$$

where $s_i''(x_i) = d^2 s_i(x_i)/dx_i^2$. Finally. the derivative of E along solutions of (L) with respect to time t is given by

$$\begin{aligned} D_{(\text{L})} E(x) &= \nabla E(x)^T (-H(x)(-Tx + S(x) - I)) \\ &= -\nabla E(x)^T H(x) \nabla E(x). \end{aligned}$$

Lemma 3.3.1 If system (L) satisfies Assumption (A) and the energy function E is defined as above, then for any $\{x_m\} \subset (-1,1)^n$ such that $x_m \to \partial(-1,1)^n$ as $m \to +\infty$, we have $E(x_m) \to +\infty$ as $m \to +\infty$.

Proof: Let $a = \sup\{|-x^T T x - x^T I| : x \in (-1,1)^n\}$. We have $a \leq \|T\| + |I| < +\infty$. Let

$$f_i(\xi) = \int_0^{\xi} s_i(\rho) d\rho$$

$\xi \in (-1,1)$, $i = 1, \cdots, n$. By Assumption (A), for each i, $f_i(\xi) \geq 0$ and $\lim_{\xi \to 1} f_i(\xi) = +\infty$ and $\lim_{\xi \to -1} f_i(\xi) = +\infty$. Let $f(x) = \max_{1 \leq i \leq n} \{f_i(x_i)\}$. We have $E(x) \geq f(x) - a$. The lemma now follows, since $f(x_m) \to +\infty$ as $x_m \to \partial(-1,1)^n$. ∎

Lemma 3.3.2 If (L) satisfies Assumption (A), then $x \in (-1,1)^n$ is an equilibrium of (L) if and only if $\nabla E(x) = 0$. Thus the set of critical points of E is identical to the set of equilibrium points of system (L).

Proof: Since x is a critical point of E if and only if $\nabla E(x) = -Tx + S(x) - I = 0$ and since x is an equilibrium of (L) if and only if $-H(x)(-Tx + S(x) - I) = 0$, the lemma follows since $H(x)$ is non-singular. ∎

Assumption (B) Given Assumption (A), we assume the following:

a) There is no $x \in (-1,1)^n$ satisfying the relations:

(1) $\nabla E(x) = 0$,

(2) $\det(J_E(x)) = 0$,

(3) $J_E(x) \geq 0$,

(4) $(s_1''(x_1), \cdots, s_n''(x_n))^T \perp N$, where

$$N = \{z = (y_1^3, \cdots, y_n^3)^T \in \Re^n :$$

$$J_E(x)(y_1, \cdots, y_n)^T = 0\},$$

simultaneously.

b) The set of equilibrium points of (L) is discrete [i.e., each equilibrium of (L) is isolated]. ∎

Assumption (C) Given Assumption (A), we assume that there is no $x \in (-1,1)^n$ satisfying the equations

(1) $\nabla E(x) = 0$,

(2) $\det(J_E(x)) = 0$,

simultaneously. ∎

Remark 3.3.2 Clearly, Assumption (C) implies the first part of Assumption (B). By the Inverse Function Theorem (cf. [1], Chapter 3), Assumption (C) implies that each zero of $\nabla E(\cdot)$ is isolated, and thus, by Lemma 3.3.2, each equilibrium of (L) is isolated. It follows that Assumption (C) implies Assumption (B). Note, however, that Assumption (C) may be easier to apply than (B). ∎

3.3. ASSUMPTIONS FOR THE HOPFIELD MODEL

Lemma 3.3.3 If Assumption (A) is true for system (L) with T fixed, then Assumption (C) [and hence, Assumption (B)] will be true for almost all $I \in \Re^n$ in the sense of the Lebesgue measure.

Proof: For fixed T, we define a C^1-function $K\colon (-1,1)^n \to \Re^n$ by
$$K(x) = \nabla E(x) + I = -Tx + S(x).$$
By Sard's Theorem (cf. [1], Theorem 2.8), there exists $Q \subset \Re^n$ with measure 0 such that if $K(x) \in \Re^n - Q$, $\det(DK(x)) \neq 0$. Thus, when $I \in \Re^n - Q$, if $\nabla E(x) = 0$, then $K(x) = 0 + I = I \in \Re^n - Q$ and $\det(J_E(x)) = \det(DK(x)) \neq 0$. ∎

Remark 3.3.3 By this lemma, any given Hopfield model (see Section 2.2) can be altered to satisfy Assumption (B) by changing the external input I by an arbitrarily small amount. ∎

Assumption (D) Given Assumption (A), we assume that for each i, $s_i\colon (-1,1) \to \Re$ is a C^2-function and $s_i''(\rho) > 0$ for $\rho \in (0,1)$. ∎

Remark 3.3.4 Again, the above is not a strong assumption. For example, let us consider the specific case treated in [4],
$$s_i(\rho) = \frac{2}{\lambda \pi R_i} \tan\left(\frac{\rho \pi}{2}\right).$$
We have that
$$s_i'(\rho) = \frac{1}{\lambda R_i \cos^2(\rho \pi / 2)}$$
and
$$s_i''(\rho) = \frac{\pi \sin(\rho \pi / 2)}{\lambda R_i \cos^3(\rho \pi / 2)}$$
which is continuous and $s_i''(\rho) > 0$ for $\rho \in (0,1)$. So s_i satisfies the Assumption (D). ∎

3.4 Main Results (Generalized Hopfield Model)

In this section we present several results which characterize the qualitative behavior of system (L). The results presented in this section for system (L) make use of Assumption (B). Since Assumption (C) implies Assumption (B), these results hold under Assumption (C) as well.

Theorem 3.4.1 If system (L) satisfies (A) and (B), then
1) for any $x \in (-1,1)^n$, there is a unique solution $\varphi(\cdot, 0, x)$ for (L);
2) along a nonequilibrium solution of system (L), energy function E given in (3.3.1) decreases monotonically. Thus, no non-constant periodic solution exists;
3) each solution of (L) exists on $[0, +\infty)$;
4) each nonequilibrium solution of (L) converges to an equilibrium of (L) as $t \to +\infty$;
5) there are only finitely many equilibrium points for (L).

Proof: a) Part 1) follows from Lemma 3.2.1.

b) The derivative of E with respect to t along the nonequilibrium solution $\varphi: [0, \tilde{t}) \to (-1, 1)^n$ is given by

$$D_{(L)}E(\varphi(t)) = -\nabla E(\varphi(t))^T \cdot H(\varphi(t)) \cdot \nabla E(\varphi(t)), \quad t \in [0, \tilde{t}).$$

By lemma 3.2.3, for any $t \in [0, \tilde{t})$, we have

$$H(\varphi(t)) \cdot \nabla E(\varphi(t)) \neq 0$$

and $\nabla E(\varphi(t)) \neq 0$. Since $H(\varphi(t))$ is positive definite,

$$\nabla E(\varphi(t))^T \cdot H(\varphi(t)) \cdot \nabla E(\varphi(t)) > 0.$$

Therefore, $D_{(L)}E(\varphi(t)) < 0$. Hence, for $0 \leq t_1 < t_2 < \tilde{t}$, we have

$$E(\varphi(t_2)) - E(\varphi(t_1)) = \int_{t_1}^{t_2} D_{(L)}E(\varphi(t))dt < 0.$$

3.4. MAIN RESULTS

c) Suppose that Part 3) of the theorem is false, i.e., φ exists only on $[0, \tilde{t})$, $\tilde{t} > 0$. By Lemma 3.2.2, $\varphi(t) \to \partial(-1,1)^n$ as $t \to \tilde{t}$. By Lemma 3.3.1, there exists a t, $0 < t < \tilde{t}$ such that $E(\varphi(0)) < E(\varphi(t))$. But this contradicts Part 2) of the theorem.

d) By Part 2) of the present theorem and by Lemma 3.3.1, for any nonequilibrium solution $\varphi(\cdot, \tilde{x}) : [0, +\infty) \to (-1,1)^n$ of system (L), there exists a $\sigma > 0$ such that $\varphi([0, +\infty)) \subset C$ where $C = (-1+\sigma, 1-\sigma)^n$. Let $\Omega(\varphi) = \{x \in (-1,1)^n : \text{there exists } \{t_m\} \subset [0,+\infty), t_m \to +\infty, x = \lim_{m\to\infty} \varphi(t_m)\}$. Each element in $\Omega(\varphi)$ is said to be an Ω-*limit point of* φ (cf. [10], Chapter 5; see also Section 3.2C of the present chapter). We have $\Omega(\varphi) \subset \varphi(\overline{[0,+\infty)}) \subset \overline{C} \subset (-1,1)^n$. Since $\overline{C}$ is compact and $\varphi([0,+\infty))$ contains infinitely many points, we know that $\Omega(\varphi) \neq \emptyset$ (by the Bolzano-Weierstrass Property, cf. [8]). By an invariance theorem for ordinary differential equations (see Lemmas 3.2.5 and 3.2.6; or [10], Chapter 5, lemmas 11.9 and 11.10), $\varphi(t)$ approaches $\Omega(\varphi)$ [in the sense that for any $\varepsilon > 0$, there exists $\hat{t} > 0$ such that for any $t > \hat{t}$, there exists $x_t \in \Omega(\varphi)$ such that $|\varphi(t) - x_t| < \varepsilon$] and for every $x \in \Omega(\varphi)$,

$$D_{(\text{L})}E(x) = -\nabla E(x)^T H(x) \nabla E(x) = 0.$$

Since $H(x)$ is positive definite, this implies $\nabla E(x) = 0$. Therefore, every Ω-limit point of φ is an equilibrium of system (L). By Assumption (B), the set of equilibrium points of (L) is discrete. So is $\Omega(\varphi)$. Since $\Omega(\varphi) \subset \overline{C}$ and since $\overline{C}$ is compact, it follows that $\Omega(\varphi)$ is finite. We claim that $\Omega(\varphi)$ contains only one point. If otherwise, take $\hat{x} \in \Omega(\varphi)$, and let $\varepsilon > 0$ be the minimal distance from x to the nearest point in $\Omega(\varphi) - \{x\}$. As discussed above, there exists $\hat{t} > 0$ such that for every $t > \hat{t}$, there exists $x_t \in \Omega(\varphi)$ having the property that $|\varphi(t) - x_t| < \varepsilon/3$. Let $B_1 = B(\hat{x}, \varepsilon/3)$ and $B_2 = B(x, \varepsilon/3)$ where $x \in \Omega(\varphi) - \{\hat{x}\}$. B_1 and B_2 are disconnected. We have $\varphi((\hat{t}, +\infty)) \subset B_1 \cup B_2$ and by the definition of $\Omega(\varphi)$, $\varphi((\hat{t},+\infty)) \cap B_1 \neq \emptyset$ and $\varphi((\hat{t},+\infty)) \cap B_2 \neq \emptyset$. But this contradicts the connectedness of $\varphi((\hat{t},+\infty))$. We have thus shown that each solution of system (L) converges to an Ω-limit set which is a singleton, containing an equilibrium of (L).

e) Let $b = \sup\{|-Tx - I|: x \in (-1,1)^n\}$. We have $b \leq \|T\| + |I| < +\infty$. By Assumption (A), for each i, we have $s_i(\rho) \to \pm\infty$ as $\rho \to \pm 1$. Therefore, $|\nabla E(x)| \geq |S(x)| - b \to +\infty$ as $x \to \partial(-1,1)^n$. Hence, there exists δ, $0 < \delta < 1/2$ such that $\nabla E(x) \neq 0$ outside of $C(-1+\delta, 1-\delta)^n$. By Lemma 3.3.2, all equilibrium points of (L) are in $\overline{C}$ which is compact. By the compactness of $\overline{C}$ and Part b) of Assumption (B), the set of equilibrium points of (L) is finite. ∎

Theorem 3.4.2 Suppose that system (L) satisfies Assumptions (A) and (B). If $\tilde{x}$ is an equilibrium of (L), then the following statements are equivalent:

(1) $\tilde{x}$ is stable;

(2) $\tilde{x}$ is a local minimum of function E;

(3) $J_E(\tilde{x}) > 0$;

(4) $\tilde{x}$ is asymptotically stable.

The above result states that if an equilibrium of (L) is stable then it is also asymptotically stable. Furthermore, only asymptotically stable equilibrium points of (L) correspond to local minima of the energy function E.

Proof of Theorem 3.4.2:

a) (1) $\Longrightarrow$ (2) Assume that $\tilde{x}$ is a stable equilibrium of (L). For purposes of contradiction, assume that $\tilde{x}$ is not a local minimum of E. Then there exists a sequence $\{x_m\} \subset (-1,1)^n$ such that $0 < |x_m - \tilde{x}| < 1/m$ and $E(x_m) < E(\tilde{x})$. By Assumption (B), there exists an $\varepsilon > 0$ such that there are no equilibrium points in $B(\tilde{x}, \varepsilon) - \{\tilde{x}\}$. Then for any δ, $\varepsilon > \delta > 0$, choose m such that $1/m < \delta$. In this case we have $x_m \in B(\tilde{x}, \delta) - \{\tilde{x}\} \subset B(\tilde{x}, \varepsilon) - \{\tilde{x}\}$ and x_m is not an equilibrium. From Part 4) of Theorem 3.4.1, it follows that the solution $\varphi(\cdot, x_m)$ converges to an equilibrium of (L), say $\hat{x}$. By Part 2) of Theorem 3.4.1, $E(\hat{x}) < E(x_m) < E(\tilde{x})$, $\hat{x} \neq \tilde{x}$. Hence $\hat{x}$ is not contained in $B(\tilde{x}, \varepsilon)$ and $\varphi(t, x_m)$ will leave $B(\tilde{x}, \varepsilon)$ as $t \to \infty$. Therefore, $\tilde{x}$ is unstable. We have arrived at a contradiction. Hence, $\tilde{x}$ must be a local minimum of E.

3.4. MAIN RESULTS

b) (2) $\Longrightarrow$ (3) Assume that $\tilde{x}$ is a local minimum of the energy function E. The proof is again by contradiction. We distinguish between two cases: (i) $J_E(\tilde{x})$ is not positive definite but it is positive semidefinite, and (ii) $J_E(\tilde{x})$ is not positive semidefinite.

In case (i), we have $\nabla E(\tilde{x}) = 0$ and $\det(J_E(\tilde{x})) = 0$. By Part a) of Assumption (B), there exists $y \in \Re^n$, $y \neq 0$ such that $J_E(\tilde{x})y = 0$, $D^3 E(\tilde{x}, y, y, y) = (s_1''(\tilde{x}_1), \cdots, s_n''(\tilde{x}_n)) \cdot (y_1^3, \cdots, y_n^3)^T \neq 0$. From the Taylor expansion of E at $\tilde{x}$ (cf. [1], Chapter 4), we obtain

$$E(\tilde{x}+ty) = E(\tilde{x}) + t\nabla E(\tilde{x})y + \frac{t^2}{2}y^T J_E(\tilde{x})y + \frac{t^3}{6}D^3(\tilde{x},y,y,y) + o(t^3),$$

$$t \in [-1, 1]$$

where $\lim_{t \to 0} o(t^3)/t^3 = 0$. Since $\nabla E(\tilde{x}) = 0$ and $J_E(\tilde{x})y = 0$, we have

$$E(\tilde{x}+ty) = E(\tilde{x}) + \frac{t^3}{6}D^3(\tilde{x},y,y,y) + o(t^3), \quad t \in [-1,1].$$

Since $D^3(\tilde{x}, y, y, y) \neq 0$, there exists $\delta > 0$ such that

$$E(\tilde{x}+ty) - E(\tilde{x}) = \frac{t^3}{6}D^3(\tilde{x},y,y,y) + o(t^3) < 0, \quad t \in (-\delta, 0),$$

$$\text{if } D^3(\tilde{x},y,y,y) > 0$$

and

$$E(\tilde{x}+ty) - E(\tilde{x}) = \frac{t^3}{6}D^3(\tilde{x},y,y,y) + o(t^3) < 0, \quad t \in (0, \delta),$$

$$\text{if } D^3(\tilde{x},y,y,y) < 0.$$

Therefore, $\tilde{x}$ is not a local minimum of E.

In case (ii), $J_E(\tilde{x})$ is not positive semidefinite. Then there exists $y \in \Re^n$ such that $y \neq 0$, $y^T J_E(\tilde{x})y < 0$. A Taylor expansion of E at $\tilde{x}$ yields

$$E(\tilde{x}+ty) = E(\tilde{x}) + t\nabla E(\tilde{x})y + \frac{t^2}{2}y^T J_E(\tilde{x})y + o(t^2), \quad t \in [0,1]$$

where $\lim_{t \to 0} o(t^2)/t^2 = 0$. Since $\nabla E(\tilde{x}) = 0$, we have

$$E(\tilde{x} + ty) = E(\tilde{x}) + \frac{t^2}{2} y^T J_E(\tilde{x}) y + o(t^2), \quad t \in [0, 1].$$

Since $y^T J_E(\tilde{x}) y < 0$, there exists a $\delta > 0$ such that

$$E(\tilde{x} + ty) - E(\tilde{x}) = \frac{t^2}{2} y^T J_E(\tilde{x}) y + o(t^2) < 0, \quad t \in (0, \delta).$$

Once more, $\tilde{x}$ is not a local minimum of E.

From the contradictions generated in cases (i) and (ii), we have $J_E(\tilde{x}) > 0$.

c) (3) $\implies$ (4) Assume that $J_E(\tilde{x})$ is positive definite. Then there exists an open neighborhood U of $\tilde{x}$ such that on U, the function defined by $v(x) = E(x) - E(\tilde{x})$ is positive definite with respect to $\tilde{x}$ [i.e., $v(\tilde{x}) = 0$ and $v(x) > 0$, $x \neq \tilde{x}$] and $D_{(L)}v(x) = -\nabla v(x)^T H(x) \nabla v(x) < 0$ for $x \neq \tilde{x}$. It follows from the fundamental stability theory of Lyapunov (cf. [10], Chapter 5, §9; also Section 3.2C) that $\tilde{x}$ is asymptotically stable.

d) (4) $\implies$ (1) Assume that $\tilde{x}$ is asymptotically stable. Then $\tilde{x}$ is clearly stable, by definition. ∎

We conclude with a note concerning the locations and estimates of the largest number of asymptotically stable equilibria for the network (L). Through faulty use of the mean value theorem, it was erroneously concluded in [6] (refer to footnote 1 in [7]) that for system (L) there is at most one asymptotically stable equilibrium point within each of the 2^n regions (quadrants) of the state space given by

$$\Lambda(\xi_1, \cdots, \xi_n) = \{x \in (-1, 1)^n : \xi_i x_i > 0, \ 1 \leq i \leq n\},$$

where $\xi_i = 1$ or -1, $1 \leq i \leq n$. In [12], a specific example of an analog Hopfield neural network [which is a special case of (L)] with more than one asymptotically stable equilibrium within a single quadrant is given. It turns out, however, that in the case of the analog Hopfield neural network with infinite gain amplifiers, the difficulties described

3.5. INFINITE GAIN ANALOG HOPFIELD MODEL (N)

above can be circumvented. In the remainder of the present chapter we will conduct a qualitative analysis of the analog Hopfield neural network model with infinite gain amplifiers. For such systems, we will obtain results which are in the spirit of the results established above for system (L), along with results concerning the location and estimates of the largest number of asymptotically stable equilibria for such networks.

3.5 Analog Hopfield Neural Network Model with Infinite Gain Amplifiers: System (N)

In the present chapter we also consider neural networks described by discontinuous differential equations of the form

$$\frac{dx}{dt} = F(x) \tag{N}$$

with

$$F(x) = -Ax + TS(x) + I \tag{3.5.1}$$

where $x = (x_1, \cdots, x_n)^T \in \Re^n$, $F \colon \Re^n \to \Re^n$ is a measurable function, $A = \text{diag}[\rho_1, \cdots, \rho_n]$ is an $n \times n$ constant matrix with each $\rho_i > 0$, $T = [T_{ij}]$ is an $n \times n$ constant matrix, $I = (I_1, \cdots, I_n)^T$ is a constant vector, and $S \colon \Re^n \to \Re^n$ is a measurable function defined by $S(x) = (\text{sgn}(x_1), \cdots, \text{sgn}(x_n))^T$ where

$$\text{sgn}(\sigma) = \begin{cases} 1, & \text{if } \sigma > 0 \\ \text{undefined}, & \text{if } \sigma = 0 \\ -1, & \text{if } \sigma < 0. \end{cases}$$

The function F is not defined on the set $M = \{x \in \Re^n \colon \text{there is at least one } i, 1 \leq i \leq n, \text{ such that } x_i = 0\}$. The set M is said to make up the discontinuous surfaces of system (N).

This class of neural networks corresponds to the analog Hopfield model with the gains of the nonlinear functions infinite, as discussed in Section 2.5.

In the remainder of this chapter, we establish results for system (N) along the following lines:

a) Since the function $F(x)$ is not continuous, a definition of solution of system (N) is developed. On the surfaces M where $F(\cdot)$ is discontinuous, solutions in the sliding mode are considered. Making use of this definition of solutions for system (N), we show that for any initial condition, there is a solution of (N), and all such solutions can be extended to the infinite time interval.

b) The concept of equilibrium point for system (N) is made precise. We show that in each of 2^n regions which are separated by M, there exists at most one asymptotically stable equilibrium point.

c) If in one of the above regions, say G, there is an equilibrium point, say x_0, then G is contained in the domain of attraction of x_0.

d) We call the elements in the range of the function S the *output vectors* of (N). We show that there is a one to one correspondence between stable output vectors and asymptotically stable equilibrium points in $\Re^n - M$. (The term "stable output vector" will be defined precisely in Section 3.7.)

Under the assumptions that T is symmetric and the main diagonal elements, T_{ii}, $1 \leq i \leq n$, of T are nonnegative, we associate with system (N) an energy function, and we show that:

e) The set of local minimum points of E is contained in the set of stable output vectors of (N). These two sets are equal if $T_{ii} = 0$, $i \leq i \leq n$. This is quite different from the analog Hopfield model.

f) Solutions of (N) will not be in a sliding mode.

g) If T is positive semidefinite, along each output sequence [i.e., along each sequence of output vectors of (N)], the energy function decreases monotonically, and system (N) will not exhibit periodic solutions.

h) If T is not positive semidefinite, g) is true with respect to asynchronous solutions of (N). (The term "asynchronous solution" will be defined precisely in Section 3.7.)

3.6 Definition and Properties of the Solutions of System (N)

When using a norm for $x \in \Re^n$, $|x|$, we will have in mind in the remainder of this chapter the Euclidean norm, i.e.,

$$|x| = \left(\sum_{i=1}^{n} x_i^2\right)^{\frac{1}{2}}.$$

We let

$$B^n = \{x \in \Re^n : x_i = 1 \text{ or } -1, \ i = 1, \cdots, n\}.$$

Also, we let Sym(n) denote the symmetric group of order n (cf. [5]).

Since the right hand side of system (N) is not continuous on $\Re^n$, we first have to generalize the usual definition of solution for ordinary differential equations with continuous right hand side (see, e.g., [10]).

For each i, $i = 1, \cdots, n$, let

$$M_i = \left\{x = (x_1, \cdots, x_n)^T \in \Re^n : x_i = 0\right\} \tag{3.6.1}$$

$$M = \cup M_i, \ 1 \leq i \leq n. \tag{3.6.2}$$

Then each M_i is a subspace of $\Re^n$ of dimension $(n-1)$. The right hand side function $F(x)$ of the system (N) is defined only on $\Re^n - M$ and M is said to be the set of discontinuous surfaces of system (N). Note that M separates $\Re^n$ into 2^n nonintersecting regions defined by

$$\begin{aligned}G(\xi) &= G(\xi_1, \cdots, \xi_n) \\ &= \{x \in \Re^n : \xi_i x_i > 0, \ 1 \leq i \leq n\}, \ \xi \in B^n.\end{aligned} \tag{3.6.3}$$

Note that for any $z \in G(\xi)$, we have that $\xi_i = \text{sgn}(z_i)$, $i = 1, \cdots, n$. On each $G(\xi)$, the right hand side function $F(x)$ is well defined and continuous. Thus the properties of the system (N), when confined to each $G(\xi)$, can be studied in the usual way. On each $G(\xi)$, the function $S(x) = \xi$ is a constant and $F(x)$ is a linear function which can be extended on $\Re^n$ as

$$F_\xi : \Re^n \to \Re^n, \ F_\xi(x) = -Ax + (T\xi + I) = -A(x - x_\xi) \tag{3.6.4}$$

where
$$x_\xi = A^{-1}(T\xi + I). \tag{3.6.5}$$

For each $\xi \in B^n$, we define a linear differential equation as follows:

$$\frac{dx}{dt} = F_\xi(x) \tag{N_ξ}$$

where $x \in \Re^n$. Since $F(x) \equiv F_\xi(x)$ on $G(\xi)$, the behavior of system (N) is the same as the behavior of system (N_ξ) on each region $G(\xi)$.

Since $A = \text{diag}(\rho_1, \cdots, \rho_n)$ is diagonal, the ith components of (N_ξ) can be described as

$$\frac{dx_i}{dt} = F_{\xi i}(x) = -\rho_i(x_i - x_{\xi i}). \tag{$N_{\xi i}$}$$

Thus the components of a solution $x = x(t)$ of (N_ξ) are independent of each other. From the basic theory of ordinary differential equations (cf. [10]), we have the following result.

Lemma 3.6.1 For a linear system (N_ξ),

1) (N_ξ) has a unique equilibrium point

$$x_\xi = A^{-1}(T\xi + I)$$

which is asymptotically stable in the large.

2) For any M_i, $\Re^n$ is divided by M_i into 2 parts

$$\Re_i^+ = \left\{ x = (x_1, \cdots, x_n)^T \in \Re^n : \xi_i x_i > 0 \right\}$$

and

$$\Re_i^- = \left\{ x = (x_1, \cdots, x_n)^T \in \Re^n : \xi_i x_i < 0 \right\}.$$

If x_ξ is in $\Re_i^+$, then all of the solutions of (N_ξ) starting in M_i tend towards and into $\Re_i^+$. If x_ξ is in $\Re_i^-$, then all of the solutions of (N_ξ) starting in M_i tend towards and into $\Re_i^-$. If x_ξ is in M_i, then all of the solutions of (N_ξ) starting in M_i remain in M_i.

3.6. SOLUTIONS OF SYSTEM (N)

3) If $\xi \in G(\xi)$, all solutions of (N_ξ) starting in $\partial G(\xi)$ tend towards and into $G(\xi)$.

Proof: 1) Part 1 follows since $F_\xi(x_\xi) = 0$ and the eigenvalues of A are real and negative.

2) To prove Part 2, without loss of generality, we assume that $\xi_i = 1$, $i = 1, \cdots, n$. If $\tilde{x} \in M_j$, then from the equation $(N_{\xi j})$, the jth component of the tangent of the solution of (N_ξ) at $\tilde{x}$ is

$$F_{\xi j}(\tilde{x}) = -\rho_j(\tilde{x}_j - x_{\xi j}) = \rho_j x_{\xi j}.$$

Hence at $\tilde{x}$, x_j increases as t increases and so the solution of (N) will pass through M_j into $G(\xi)$ from the outside.

3) Part 3 follows from Part 2. ∎

To study the properties of system (N) on all $\Re^n$, we first have to give a proper definition of the solutions for (N). We require the notation given below. Let

$$\Lambda = \left\{\xi = (\xi_1, \cdots, \xi_n)^T : \xi_i = \pm 1 \text{ or } 0,\ 1 \le i \le n\right\} \quad (3.6.6)$$

and

$$\Lambda_m = \Big\{\xi = (\xi_1, \cdots, \xi_n)^T \in \Lambda : \xi_{\sigma(i)} = 0,\ 1 \le i \le m \text{ and } \xi_{\sigma(i)} = \pm 1,$$
$$m < i \le n,\ \sigma \in \text{Sym}(n)\Big\},\ 0 \le m \le n. \quad (3.6.7)$$

The number of elements in Λ_m is equal to

$$\frac{n!\, 2^{n-m}}{m!(n-m)!},$$

and the number of elements in $\Lambda = \bigcup_{0 \le m \le n} \Lambda_m$ is 3^n. For each $\xi \in \Lambda$, let

$$C(\xi) = \Big\{x = (x_1, \cdots, x_n)^T \in \Re^n : x_i = 0 \text{ if } \xi_i = 0, \\ x_i \xi_i > 0 \text{ if } \xi_i \ne 0\Big\}. \quad (3.6.8)$$

From the notation given above, we have the following result.

Lemma 3.6.2

1) $\Lambda_0 = B^n$ and $C(\xi) = G(\xi)$, for any $\xi \in \Lambda_0$.
2) For any $\xi, \eta \in \Lambda$, $\xi \neq \eta$, $C(\xi) \cap C(\eta) = \emptyset$.
3) $M = \cup C(\xi)$, $\xi \in \cup \Lambda_m$, $1 \leq m \leq n$.
4) For any $\xi \in \Lambda_0$ and for any $\eta \in \Lambda$, $C(\eta) \cap \partial G(\xi) \neq 0$ implies $C(\eta) \subset \partial G(\xi)$.
5) For any $\eta = (\eta_1, \cdots, \eta_n)^T \in \Lambda_m$ and $\sigma \in \text{Sym}(n)$ such that $\eta_{\sigma(i)} = 0$, $1 \leq i \leq m$, let $\tilde{\Lambda}$ be the set $\{\xi \in \Lambda_0 : C(\eta) \subset \partial G(\xi)\}$. Then $\tilde{\Lambda} = \{\xi \in \Lambda_0 : \xi_{\sigma(i)} = \eta_{\sigma(i)}, \text{ for } m < i \leq n\}$.
6) For any $\eta = (\eta_1, \cdots, \eta_n)^T \in \Lambda_m$ and $\sigma \in \text{Sym}(n)$ such that $\eta_{\sigma(i)} = 0$, $1 \leq i \leq m$, $M_{\sigma(1)} \cap \cdots \cap M_{\sigma(m)}$ is an $(n-m)$-dimensional subspace of $\Re^n$. $C(\eta)$ is an open subset of $M_{\sigma(1)} \cap \cdots \cap M_{\sigma(m)}$, and $C(\eta)$ is a connected component of

$$\left(M_{\sigma(1)} \cap \cdots \cap M_{\sigma(m)}\right) - \left(M_{\sigma(m+1)} \cap \cdots \cap M_{\sigma(n)}\right).$$

The projection map

$$P: \Re^n \to M_{\sigma(1)} \cap \cdots \cap M_{\sigma(m)}$$

turns out to be

$$P_{\sigma(i)}(x) = 0 \text{ for } 1 \leq i \leq m \qquad (3.6.9)$$

and

$$P_{\sigma(i)}(x) = x_{\sigma(i)} \text{ for } m < i \leq n. \qquad \blacksquare \qquad (3.6.10)$$

Claim 3.6.1 For each m, $0 \leq m \leq n$, we can define by induction S_m, W_m and D_m with the properties that S_m, W_m are sets of functions from a subinterval of $[0, \infty)$ to $\Re^n$, and $D_m \subset \Re^n$ such that

i) $D_i \cap D_m = \emptyset$, for $0 \leq i < m$,

ii) $D_0 \cup \cdots \cup D_m \supset C(\eta)$, for any $C(\eta)$, $\eta \in \Lambda_m$, and

3.6. SOLUTIONS OF SYSTEM (N)

iii) either $D_m \supset C(\gamma)$ or $D_m \cap C(\gamma) = \emptyset$, for any $C(\gamma)$, $\gamma \in \Lambda_j$, $m < j \leq n$.

Proof: We prove Claim 3.6.1 in two steps.

Step 1): For $m = 0$, let S_0 be the set of functions

$$\varphi = \varphi(\cdot): (0, \tilde{t}\,) \to C(\xi)$$

with properties as follows:

a) $\xi \in \Lambda_0 = B^n$,

b) φ is a C^1-function and

$$\frac{d\varphi}{dt} = F_\xi(\varphi(t)) \text{ on } (0, \tilde{t}\,). \tag{3.6.11}$$

Let $D_0 = \{\tilde{x} \in \Re^n : \text{there is } \varphi \in S_0 \text{ such that } \varphi(0+) = \lim_{t \to 0+} \varphi(t) = \tilde{x}\}$. Let $W_0 = \{\psi = \psi(\cdot, \tilde{x}): [0, \tilde{t}\,) \to \overline{C}(\eta): \tilde{x} \in D_0, \eta \in \Lambda_0, \psi(0, \tilde{x}) = \tilde{x}, \psi \text{ is continuous and there is } \varphi \in S_0 \text{ such that on } (0, \tilde{t}\,), \psi \equiv \varphi\}$.

According to these definitions, S_0 is the set of solutions of (N_ξ) on $G(\xi) = C(\xi)$, where $\xi \in \Lambda_0$. W_0 is the set of functions obtained by continuously extending the solutions in S_0 to $t = 0$. In other words, W_0 is the set of solutions of (N_ξ) in $G(\xi)$ with the starting points in $G(\xi) \cup \partial G(\xi)$, where $\xi \in \Lambda_0$. D_0 is the set of starting points of the solutions in W_0. It follows from the Existence Theorem of differential equations (cf. [10]) that for any $\xi \in \Lambda_0$, and for any $\tilde{x} \in G(\xi)$, there is a solution in W_0 with starting point $\tilde{x}$. This means that $D_0 \supset C(\xi)$ for any $\xi \in \Lambda_0$. For any $C(\gamma)$, $\gamma \in \Lambda_j$, $0 < j \leq n$, if $C(\gamma) \cap D_0 \neq \emptyset$, then there is $\psi \in W_0$ such that $\psi = \psi(\cdot, \tilde{x}): [0, \tilde{t}\,) \to G(\xi) \cup \partial G(\xi)$ where $\xi \in \Lambda_0$, $\tilde{x} \in C(\gamma) \cap \partial G(\xi)$, and the ψ is a solution of (N_ξ) starting at $\tilde{x}$ towards and into $G(\xi)$. Then by Lemma 3.6.1, $x_\xi \in G(\xi)$ and for any $x \in \partial G(\xi)$, the solution of (N_ξ) starting at x will also tend towards and into $G(\xi)$, that is, $D_0 \supset \partial G(\xi)$. By Lemma 3.6.2, $C(\gamma) \cap \partial G(\xi) \neq \emptyset$ implies $\partial G(\xi) \supset C(\gamma)$. Thus $D_0 \supset C(\gamma)$. We have proved that for any j, $0 < j \leq n$, and for any $C(\gamma)$, $\gamma \in \Lambda_j$, if $C(\gamma) \cap D_0 \neq \emptyset$, then $D_0 \supset C(\gamma)$.

Step 2): For $0 < m \leq n$, suppose that for each k, $0 \leq k < m$, S_k, D_k, and W_k have been defined with the properties that S_k, W_k

are sets of functions from a subinterval of $[0, \infty)$ to $\Re^n$, and $D_k \subset \Re^n$ such that

i) $D_i \cap D_k = \emptyset$, for $0 \leq i < k$,

ii) $D_0 \cup \cdots \cup D_k \supset C(\eta)$, for any $C(\eta)$, $\eta \in \Lambda_k$, and

iii) either $D_k \supset C(\gamma)$ or $D_k \cap C(\gamma) = \emptyset$, for any $C(\gamma)$, $\gamma \in \Lambda_j$, $k < j \leq n$.

Let S_m be the set of functions $\varphi = \varphi(\cdot): (0, \tilde{t}) \to C(\eta)$, with properties as follows:

a) $\eta \in \Lambda_m$, $C(\eta) \cap D_0 \cup \cdots \cup D_{m-1} = \emptyset$. (By the definition of Λ_m, there is $\sigma \in \mathrm{Sym}(n)$ with $\eta_{\sigma(i)} = 0$ for $1 \leq i \leq m$, $\eta_{\sigma(i)} \neq 0$ for $m < i \leq n$ such that $C(\eta) = \{x = (x_1, \cdots, x_n)^T : x_{\sigma(i)} = 0$ for $1 \leq i \leq m$ and $x_{\sigma(i)} \eta_{\sigma(i)} > 0$ for $m < i \leq n\}$. Then $C(\eta)$ is in the $(n-m)$-dimensional subspace $M_{\sigma(1)} \cap \cdots \cap M_{\sigma(m)}$ of $\Re^n$.)

b) φ is an absolutely continuous function with

$$\frac{d\varphi(t)}{dt} = \sum_{\xi \in \tilde{\Lambda}} \lambda_\xi(t) P\big(F_\xi(\varphi(t))\big), \quad m < i \leq n, \text{ a.e. on } (0, \tilde{t}) \quad (3.6.12)$$

where P is the projection from $\Re^n$ to $M_{\sigma(1)} \cap \cdots \cap M_{\sigma(m)}$,

$$\tilde{\Lambda} = \{\xi \in \Lambda_0 : C(\eta) \subset \partial G(\xi)\}$$
$$= \{\xi \in \Lambda_0 : \xi_{\sigma(i)} = \eta_{\sigma(i)}, \text{ for } m < i \leq n\},$$

and for each $\xi \in \tilde{\Lambda}$, $\lambda_\xi : (0, \tilde{t}) \to [0, \infty)$ is a measurable parameter function such that

$$\sum_{\xi \in \tilde{\Lambda}} \lambda_\xi(t) = 1 \text{ on } (0, \tilde{t}) \quad (3.6.13)$$

and

$$0 \leq \lambda_\xi(t) \leq 1, \text{ for any } \xi \in \tilde{\Lambda} \text{ on } (0, \tilde{t}). \quad (3.6.14)$$

Let

$$D_m = \Big\{\tilde{x} \in \Re^n - D_0 \cup \cdots \cup D_{m-1} :$$
$$\varphi(0+) = \lim_{t \to 0+} \varphi(t) = \tilde{x}, \, \varphi \in S_m\Big\}.$$

3.6. SOLUTIONS OF SYSTEM (N)

Let

$$W_m = \{\psi = \psi(\cdot, \tilde{x}) : [0, \tilde{t}) \to \overline{C}(\eta) : \tilde{x} \in D_m, \ \eta \in \Lambda_m, \ \psi(0, \tilde{x}) = \tilde{x},$$
$$\psi \text{ is continuous and there is } \varphi \in S_m \text{ such that on } (0, \tilde{t}), \ \psi \equiv \varphi\}.$$

First, we have that $D_i \cap D_m = \emptyset$ for $0 \leq i < m$. Next, for any $C(\eta)$, $\eta \in \Lambda_m$ such that $C(\eta) \cap D_0 \cup \cdots \cup D_{m-1} = \emptyset$, we need to show that $C(\eta)$ is contained in D_m. Without loss of generality, assume that for $\eta = (\eta_1, \cdots, \eta_n)^T$, $\eta_i = 0$ for $1 \leq i \leq m$ and $\eta_i = 1$ for $m < i \leq n$. Let $\tilde{\Lambda} = \{\xi \in \Lambda_0 : C(\eta) \subset \partial G(\xi)\}$. Then $\tilde{\Lambda} = \{\xi \in \Lambda_0 : \xi_i = 1$ for $m < i \leq n\}$, and the projection map $P : \Re^n \to M_1 \cap \cdots \cap M_m$ has value $P_i(x) = 0$ for $1 \leq i \leq m$ and $P_i(x) = x_i$ for $m < i \leq n$. Take $\xi \in \tilde{\Lambda}$. Since F_ξ is continuous on an open neighborhood U of $\tilde{x}$ in $\Re^n$, then $P(F_\xi(\cdot))$ is continuous on the open neighborhood $U \cap C(\eta)$ of $\tilde{x}$ in $C(\eta)$. It follows from the Existence Theorem of differential equations that there is a C^1-function $\varphi = \varphi(\cdot) : (0, \tilde{t}) \to C(\eta) \cap U$ such that

$$\frac{d\varphi(t)}{dt} = P\big(F_\xi(\varphi(t))\big) \text{ on } (0, \tilde{t})$$

and $\varphi(0+) = \tilde{x}$. The function φ satisfies (3.6.12) with the parameter functions defined as $\lambda_\xi \equiv 1$ and $\lambda_\beta \equiv 0$, for $\beta \in \tilde{\Lambda}$, $\beta \neq \xi$, on $(0, \tilde{t})$. Thus, $\varphi \in S_m(t)$ and $\tilde{x} = \varphi(0+) \in D_m$. We have proved that for any $C(\eta)$, $\eta \in \Lambda_m$, $D_0 \cup \cdots \cup D_m \supset C(\eta)$. Finally, for any $C(\gamma) \in \Lambda_j$, $m < j \leq n$, such that $C(\gamma) \cap D_m \neq \emptyset$, we need to show that $C(\gamma)$ is contained in D_m. Without loss of generality, we assume that for $\gamma = (\gamma_1, \cdots, \gamma_n)^T$, $\gamma_i = 0$ for $1 \leq i \leq j$ and $\gamma_i = 1$ for $j < i \leq n$. Also we assume that there is a function $\varphi : (0, \tilde{t}) \to C(\eta)$ in S_m such that $\eta_i = 0$ for $1 \leq i \leq m$ and $\eta_i = 1$ for $m < i \leq n$. Furthermore, we assume that φ is an absolutely continuous function which satisfies

$$\frac{d\varphi(t)}{dt} = \sum_{\xi \in \tilde{\Lambda}} \tilde{\lambda}_\xi(t) P\big(F_\xi(\varphi(t))\big), \ m < i \leq n, \text{ a.e. on } (0, \tilde{t}). \quad (3.6.15)$$

Here P is the projection of $\Re^n \to M_1 \cap \cdots \cap M_m$ with $P_i(x) = 0$ for $1 \leq i \leq m$ and $P_i(x) = x_i$ for $m < i \leq n$, and $\tilde{\Lambda} = \{\xi \in \Lambda_0 : C(\eta) \subset \partial G(\xi)\} = \{\xi \in \Lambda_0 : \xi_i = 1, \text{ for } m < i \leq n\}$, and for each $\xi \in \tilde{\Lambda}$,

$\tilde{\lambda}_\xi : (0, \tilde{t}) \to [0, \infty)$ is a measurable parameter function such that

$$\sum_{\xi \in \tilde{\Lambda}} \tilde{\lambda}_\xi(t) = 1 \text{ on } (0, \tilde{t}), \qquad (3.6.16)$$

$$0 \leq \tilde{\lambda}_\xi(t) \leq 1, \text{ for any } \xi \in \tilde{\Lambda} \text{ on } (0, \tilde{t}), \qquad (3.6.17)$$

and

$$\varphi(0+) = \tilde{x}, \qquad (3.6.18)$$

where $\tilde{x} \in C(\gamma) \cap D_m$.

Fact There are constants $\hat{\lambda}_\xi$, $\xi \in \tilde{\Lambda}$ such that

$$\sum_{\xi \in \tilde{\Lambda}} \hat{\lambda}_\xi = 1 \text{ on } (0, \tilde{t}), \qquad (3.6.19)$$

$$0 \leq \tilde{\lambda}_\xi \leq 1, \text{ for any } \xi \in \tilde{\Lambda} \text{ on } (0, \tilde{t}), \qquad (3.6.20)$$

and

$$\sum_{\xi \in \tilde{\Lambda}} \hat{\lambda}_\xi x_{\xi_i} > 0, \quad m < i \leq j. \qquad (3.6.21)$$

Proof of the Fact: Let $A_1 = \left\{ y = (y_1, \cdots, y_k)^T \in \Re^k : y_i = \sum_{\xi \in \tilde{\Lambda}} \hat{\lambda}_\xi x_{\xi_{m+i}} > 0, 1 \leq i \leq j - m, \text{ where } \sum_{\xi \in \tilde{\Lambda}} \hat{\lambda}_\xi = 1 \text{ and } 0 \leq \hat{\lambda}_\xi \leq 1, \right.$ for any $\left. \xi \in \hat{\Lambda} \right\}$ and let $A_2 = \{ y = (y_1, \cdots, y_k)^T \in \Re^k : y_i > 0 \}$ where $k = j - m$. Then A_1 and A_2 are convex sets in $\Re^k$. Suppose the fact is not true. Then $A_1 \cap A_2 = \emptyset$ and there is a k-dimensional subspace P of $\Re^k$ which separates A_1 and A_2 (cf. Hahn-Banach Theorem [8]). Take a vector z_0 which is normal to P and which points into the direction of set A_2. Since $\varphi(t) \in C(\eta)$ for $t \in (0, \tilde{t})$, we have that $\varphi_i(t) > 0$ for $m < i \leq j$ and $(\varphi_{m+1}(t), \cdots, \varphi_j(t))^T \cdot z_0 > 0$, for any

3.6. SOLUTIONS OF SYSTEM (N)

$t \in (0, \tilde{t})$. On the other hand, from (3.6.15)–(3.6.18), we have that

$$\begin{aligned} d\varphi_i(t)/dt &= \sum_{\xi \in \tilde{\Lambda}} \tilde{\lambda}_\xi(t) P_i\Big(F_\xi(\varphi(t))\Big) \\ &= \sum_{\xi \in \tilde{\Lambda}} \tilde{\lambda}_\xi(t) \Big(F_\xi(\varphi(t))\Big)_i \\ &= \sum_{\xi \in \tilde{\Lambda}} \tilde{\lambda}_\xi(t) \Big(-\rho_i(\varphi_i(t) - x_{\xi i})\Big) \\ &= -\rho_i \left(\varphi_i(t) - \sum_{\xi \in \tilde{\Lambda}} \tilde{\lambda}_\xi(t) x_{\xi i}\right) \end{aligned}$$

and that $(\varphi_{m+1}(t), \cdots, \varphi_j(t))^T \cdot z_0 \leq 0$, for any $t \in (0, \tilde{t})$. This contradiction shows that the fact is true.

Next, take a set of constants $\hat{\lambda}_\xi$, $\xi \in \tilde{\Lambda}$, which satisfy (3.6.19)–(3.6.21). Then for any $\hat{x} \in C(\gamma)$, there is an open neighborhood U of $\hat{x}$ in $\Re^n$ such that on the reduced open subset $U \cap C(\eta)$ in $C(\eta)$, we have that for any $x \in U \cap C(\eta)$, $x_i > 0$, $j < i \leq n$, and

$$\sum_{\xi \in \tilde{\Lambda}} \hat{\lambda}_\xi P_i\Big(F_\xi(x)\Big) = \sum_{\xi \in \tilde{\Lambda}} \hat{\lambda}_\xi F_{\xi i}(x) = \sum_{\xi \in \tilde{\Lambda}} \hat{\lambda}_\xi \Big(-\rho_i(x_i - x_{\xi i})\Big) > 0,$$

$$m < i \leq j.$$

By the Existence Theorem of differential equations, the system

$$\frac{dx(t)}{dt} = \sum_{\xi \in \tilde{\Lambda}} \hat{\lambda}_\xi P\Big(F_\xi(x)\Big)$$

has a solution $\chi: (0, t_1) \to C(\eta)$, with

$$\chi(0+) = (0, \cdots, 0, \hat{x}_{j+1}, \cdots, \hat{x}_n)^T = \hat{x}.$$

Thus we have proved that for any $C(\gamma) \subset \Lambda_j$, $m < j$, such that $C(\gamma) \cap D_m \neq \emptyset$, $C(\gamma)$ is contained in D_m.

By Steps 1 and 2, we can define, by induction, the sets S_m, W_m, D_m, $0 \leq m \leq n$, with the desired properties. ∎

Definition 3.6.1 *A function φ in $S = \cup S_i$ is said to be a (local) solution of* (N). *A function $\psi = \psi(\cdot, \tilde{x})$ in $W = \cup W_i$ is said to be* a (local) *solution of* (N) *starting at* $\tilde{x}$. In particular, solutions in S_0 or W_0 are said to be *in the usual sense*, while solutions in S_j or W_j, $j > 0$, are said to be *in a sliding mode*. ∎

Remark 3.6.1 For each $G(\xi)$, $\xi \in B^n$, a function with its image in $G(\xi)$ is a solution of system (N) in the sense of Definition 3.6.1 if and only if it is a solution of (N_ξ) in the usual sense. The definition of solutions of system (N) in the sliding mode with their images in the discontinuous surfaces M constitutes a generalized definition of solutions of discontinuous systems in the sense of Filippov (cf. [9] and [13]). ∎

Lemma 3.6.3

1) $D_0 \cup \cdots \cup D_n = \Re^n$.
2) For any $\tilde{x} \in \Re^n$, there is a (local) solution of system (N) starting at $\tilde{x}$.

Proof: Part 1) follows since for each $C(\xi)$, $\xi \in \Lambda$, $C(\xi) \subset D_0 \cup \cdots \cup D_n$, and $\Re^n \subset \cup C(\xi)$.

Part 2) follows since for any $\tilde{x} \in D_m$, $0 \leq m \leq n$, there is a (local) solution of (N) starting at $\tilde{x}$ because of Claim 3.6.1. ∎

Definition 3.6.2

1) For $\tilde{x} \in \Re^n$, a function $\psi = \psi(\cdot, \tilde{x}) : [0, \tilde{t}) \to \Re^n$ is said to be a *solution of* (N) *starting at* $\tilde{x}$ if
   a) $\psi(0, \tilde{x}) = \tilde{x}$,
   b) for any $t \in [0, \tilde{t})$, there is $\delta > 0$ such that $t + \delta < \tilde{t}$ and ψ restricted to $(t, t + \delta)$ is a (local) solution as defined in Definition 3.6.1.

2) The function ψ is said to be *in a sliding mode* during the period $(t, t + \delta)$ if we have $\psi((t, t + \delta)) \subset M$. Also, ψ is said to have *no sliding mode* if ψ is not in a sliding mode on any interval. ∎

3.7. EQUILIBRIA AND OUTPUT VECTORS OF (N)

Theorem 3.6.1

1) Every solution of system (N), $\psi = \psi(\cdot, \tilde{x}): [0, \tilde{t}\,) \to \Re^n$, can be extended to the interval $[0, \infty)$ in the sense that there is a solution of system (N), $\psi_1 = \psi_1(\cdot, \tilde{x}): [0, \infty) \to \Re^n$, such that $\psi_1 \equiv \psi$ on $[0, \tilde{t}\,)$.

2) For any $\tilde{x} \in \Re^n$, there is a solution of (N) starting at $\tilde{x}$ which is defined on the interval $[0, \infty)$.

Proof: If Part 1) is not true, there is a solution of (N), $\psi = \psi(\cdot, \tilde{x}): [0, \tilde{t}\,) \to \Re^n$, such that for any solution of (N),

$$\psi_1 = \psi_1(\cdot, \tilde{x}): [0, t_2) \to \Re^n$$

we have that if $\psi_1 = \psi$ on $[0, \tilde{t}\,)$, then $\tilde{t} = t_2$. This is contradictory to Part 2) of Lemma 3.6.3.

Part 2) follows from Lemma 3.6.3 and from Part 1). ∎

In the remainder of this chapter, we only consider solutions of (N) defined on the infinite interval $[0, \infty)$.

3.7 Qualitative Properties of the Equilibrium Points and of the Output Vectors of System (N)

We are at last in a position to conduct a careful study of the qualitative properties of the neural network (N). Similarly as in Section 3.2C, we make the following definitions for system (N).

Definition 3.7.1 A vector $\tilde{x} \in R^n$ is said to be an *equilibrium (point) of* (N) if the function $\psi(\cdot, \tilde{x}): [0, \infty) \to \Re^n$ defined by $\psi(t, \tilde{x}) \equiv \tilde{x}$, is a solution of (N). In particular, an equilibrium point of (N) in $R^n - M$ is said to be an *equilibrium point in the usual sense*. ∎

Definition 3.7.2 Let $\tilde{x}$ be an equilibrium point of (N).

1) $\tilde{x}$ is said to be *stable* if for every $\varepsilon > 0$, there is a $\delta = \delta(\varepsilon) > 0$ such that $|\psi(t, 0, x) - \tilde{x}| < \varepsilon$ for all $t \in [0, +\infty)$ whenever $|x - \tilde{x}| < \delta$.

2) $\tilde{x}$ is said to be *asymptotically stable* if it is stable and if there is an $\eta > 0$ such that $\lim\limits_{t \to +\infty} |\psi(t, 0, x) - \tilde{x}| = 0$ whenever $|x - \tilde{x}| < \eta$.

3) $\tilde{x}$ is said to be *unstable* if it is not stable. ∎

Theorem 3.7.1 For $\xi \in \Lambda_0$, consider $G(\xi)$ and x_ξ as defined in (3.6.3)–(3.6.5). The following is true.
1) If $x_\xi \notin G(\xi)$, there is no equilibrium point of (N) in the region $G(\xi)$.
2) If $x_\xi \in G(\xi)$, x_ξ is the unique equilibrium point of (N) in the region $G(\xi)$, and x_ξ is also asymptotically stable and $G(\xi)$ is contained in the domain of attraction of x_ξ.

Proof: Under our definitions, on $G(\xi)$ the concepts of the solutions, equilibrium points and their stability properties [for (N)] are identical to those of (N_ξ). Therefore, the theorem follows from Lemma 3.6.1. ∎

Theorem 3.7.2 Let $\tilde{x} \in M$. If $x_\xi = \tilde{x}$ for any $\xi \in \tilde{\Lambda}$, where $\tilde{\Lambda} = \{\xi \in \Lambda_0 : \tilde{x} \in \partial G(\xi)\}$, then $\tilde{x}$ is an asymptotically stable equilibrium point of (N) and $U = (\cup G(\xi) \cup \partial G(\xi))^0$ is contained in the domain of attraction of $\tilde{x}$.

Proof: Without loss of generality, assume there is an m, $1 \leq m \leq n$, such that $\tilde{x} = (\tilde{x}_1, \cdots, \tilde{x}_n)^T$ with $\tilde{x}_j = 0$, $1 \leq j \leq m$, and $\tilde{x}_j > 0$, $m < j \leq n$. Then $\tilde{\Lambda} = \{\xi \in \Lambda_0 : \xi_j > 0, m < j \leq n\}$. On each $\partial G(\xi) \cup G(\xi)$, $\xi \in \tilde{\Lambda}$, $F_\xi(x) = -A(x - x_\xi) = -A(x - \tilde{x})$. According to Definition 3.6.1, we can easily check that on the open neighborhood $U = (\cup G(\xi) \cup \partial G(\xi))^0 = \{x \in \Re^n : x_j > 0, m < j \leq n\}$, the set of solutions of (N) is identical to the set of solutions of the continuous system

$$\frac{dx}{dt} = -A(x - \tilde{x}) \tag{N_c}$$

3.7. EQUILIBRIA AND OUTPUT VECTORS OF (N)

in the usual sense. Therefore, it follows from the theory of linear systems that $\tilde{x}$ is asymptotically stable with U contained in the domain of attraction. ∎

Remark 3.7.1 Consider the case $m = n = 2$ in Theorem 3.7.2. We have $\tilde{x} = (0,0)^T$, and $\pm T_{i1} \pm T_{i2} - I_i = 0$, $i = 1, 2$. So $T_{ij} = 0$, $1 \leq i, j \leq 2$, and $I_1 = I_2 = 0$. The system (N) is reduced to

$$\begin{cases} dx_1/dt = -a_1 x_1 \\ dx_2/dt = -a_2 x_2. \end{cases} \quad (\text{N}_c)$$

Now the right-hand side of the system (N_c) is continuous and defined on all of $\Re^2$. Theorem 3.7.2 tells us that the solutions and qualitative properties of the equilibrium points of (N_c) will be the same whether we study (N_c) as a continuous system in the usual sense or whether we study (N_c) as a discontinuous system with the right-hand side function defined only on $\Re^2 - M$, where $M = \{x = (x_1, x_2,)^T : x_1 = 0 \text{ and/or } x_2 = 0\}$, under the concepts of Definitions 3.6.2, 3.7.1 and 3.7.2. ∎

Remark 3.7.2 When the system reaches an equilibrium point $\tilde{x}$, two possibilities exist:
1) if $\tilde{x} \in \Re^n - M$, the output of the function $S(\cdot)$ is unchanged, or
2) if $\tilde{x} \in M$, components of the output of the functions $S(\cdot)$ may be oscillating between 1 and -1. ∎

In some cases we are interested in the behavior of the output of system (N) rather than in the behavior of the variable $x \in \Re^n$. Under the output of the system (N) we have in mind the variable $S(x)$ which resides in the set B^n. For given $x \in \Re^n$, we call $\xi = S(x)$ an *output vector* of system (N).

Definition 3.7.3 $\tilde{\xi} \in B^n$ is said to be a *stable output vector* of system (N) if there is a solution $\psi = \psi(\cdot, \tilde{x}) : [0, +\infty) \to \Re^n$ of system (N) and $\tilde{t} \in [0, +\infty)$ such that $\psi((\tilde{t}, +\infty)) \subset G(\tilde{\xi})$. $\tilde{\xi} \in B^n$ is said to be an *unstable output vector* of system (N) if $\tilde{\xi}$ is not a stable output vector. ∎

The next result follows readily from Theorem 3.7.1.

Theorem 3.7.3

1) For any $\xi \in B^n$, ξ is a stable output vector of system (N) if and only if $x_\xi \in G(\xi)$.

2) As t increases, if the output vector of system (N) reaches a stable output vector ξ, then the corresponding solution of system (N) will converge to the stable equilibrium point x_ξ as $t \to +\infty$.

3) If no component of x_ξ is 0, then for any $\xi \in B^n$, the map $\xi \to x_\xi$ determines a one-to-one correspondence between the set of stable output vectors of system (N) and the set of stable equilibrium points of system (N) in $\Re^n - M$. ∎

3.8 Qualitative Analysis of System (N) in Terms of an Energy Function

Similarly as in Section 3.4, where we studied the generalized analog Hopfield neural network model using an energy function, we employ in the present section an energy function in studying some of the qualitative properties of neural network (N). We begin by making the following assumptions for system (N).

Assumption 3.8.1 For system (N), we will assume:

1) $T = [T_{ij}]$ is symmetric,

2) $T_{ii} \geq 0$, $1 \leq i \leq n$, and

3) no component of x_ξ is 0 for any $\xi \in B^n$. ∎

Remark 3.8.1 For system (N), consider a fixed $n \times n$ matrix T. Then for almost all vectors $I \in \Re^n$, Part 3) of Assumption 3.8.1 is true.

3.8. ENERGY FUNCTION ANALYSIS OF (N)

Proof: There are a finite number of elements in B^n, and for each $\xi \in B^n$, there are only a finite number of different values of I with components of $x_\xi = A^{-1}(T\xi + I)$ equal to zero. ∎

Definition 3.8.1 If system (N) satisfies Assumption 3.8.1, then
1) the *energy function* $E: B^n \to \Re$ of system (N) is defined as

$$E(\xi) = -\frac{1}{2}\xi^T T\xi - \xi^T I + c \quad (3.8.1)$$

where c is a constant, and

2) $\xi \in B^n$ is said to be a *(local) minimum* of the energy function E if $E(\xi) \leq E(\eta)$, for $\eta \in J(\xi)$, where

$$J(\xi) = \{\eta \in B^n: \text{there is a } k \text{ such that } \eta_k \xi_k < 0, \text{ and}$$

$$\eta_i \xi_i > 0, \ i \neq k\}. \quad (3.8.2)$$

Also for any $\eta \in J(\xi)$, η is said to be an *adjacent* vector of ξ in B^n. ∎

Lemma 3.8.1 Assume that system (N) satisfies Assumption 3.8.1. Let ξ and $\eta \in B^n$ be two adjacent vectors. Assume that there is an integer k such that $\eta_k \xi_k < 0$, and $\eta_i \xi_i > 0$, $i \neq k$. Then the following is true:

1)
$$E(\eta) - E(\xi) = 2\rho_k \xi_k x_{\xi k} - 2T_{kk} \quad (3.8.3)$$

where $x_{\xi k}$ is the kth component of x_ξ.

2) If $E(\eta) < E(\xi)$ and $T_{kk} = 0$, then $\xi_k x_{\xi k} < 0$.

3) If $E(\eta) \geq E(\xi)$, then $\xi_k x_{\xi k} > 0$.

Proof: 1) By Definition 3.8.1 and from $\rho_k x_{\xi k} = \sum\limits_{j=1}^{n} T_{kj}\xi_j + I_k$, we have

$$E(\eta) - E(\xi) = 2\xi_k \left(\sum_{j \neq k} T_{kj}\xi_j + I_k \right)$$
$$= 2\rho_k \xi_k x_{\xi k} - 2T_{kk}\xi_k^2$$
$$= 2\rho_k \xi_k x_{\xi k} - 2T_{kk}.$$

2) If $E(\eta) < E(\xi)$ and $T_{kk} = 0$, we have that

$$\xi_k x_{\xi k} = \frac{1}{\rho_k}(\rho_k \xi_k x_{\xi k} - T_{kk}) < 0.$$

3) If $E(\eta) \geq E(\xi)$, then $2\rho_k \xi_k x_{\xi k} - 2T_{kk} \geq 0$. Since $T_{kk} \geq 0$, $\rho_k > 0$ and $\xi_k x_{\xi k} \neq 0$, we have that $\xi_k x_{\xi k} > 0$. ∎

Theorem 3.8.1 Assume that system (N) satisfies Assumption 3.8.1. Then the following is true:

1) A local minimum of the energy function E is a stable output vector of system (N).

2) If $T_{ii} = 0$, $1 \leq i \leq n$, then a stable output vector of system (N) is a local minimum of the energy function E.

Proof: 1) If $\xi \in B^n$ is a local minimum of E, by Lemma 3.8.1, Part 3, $\xi_k x_{\xi k} > 0$, for $1 \leq k \leq n$, and thus $x_\xi \in G(\xi)$. By Theorem 3.7.3, ξ is a stable output vector of (N).

2) If $T_{ii} = 0$, $1 \leq i \leq n$, and $\xi \in B^n$ is a stable output vector of system (N), then by Theorem 3.7.3 $\xi_k x_{\xi k} \geq 0$, for $1 \leq k \leq n$. If ξ is not a local minimum of E, then by Lemma 3.8.1, Part 2, there is a k such that $\xi_k x_{\xi k} < 0$. This contradiction establishes the proof. ∎

Remark 3.8.2 1) Theorem 3.8.1 shows that there is a one-to-one correspondence between the set of local minima of E and the set of stable output vectors of system (N) under the condition $T_{ii} = 0$, $1 \leq i \leq n$. Without this condition, the output of system (N) may get stuck at some vector which is not a local minimum of the energy function E. The reason for this can be seen clearly from formula (3.8.3). Therefore, when using the energy function to synthesize system (N), we will want T_{ii} as small as possible, provided that $T_{ii} \geq 0$.

2) When there is a negative T_{ii}, the energy function E for system (N), given in (3.8.1), need not necessarily decrease monotonically with increasing time. This is quite different from the behavior of the analog Hopfield model (c.f. [4] and [6]; see also Theorem 3.4.1). ∎

3.8. ENERGY FUNCTION ANALYSIS OF (N)

Theorem 3.8.2 If system (N) satisfies Assumption 3.8.1, no solution of system (N) will be in the sliding mode during any time period, i.e., $D_0 = \Re^n$.

Proof: If the theorem is not true, there is a solution of system (N) $\varphi: [0, +\infty) \to \Re^n$ and an interval $(t_0, t_0 + \varepsilon)$ such that φ is in the sliding mode on $(t_0, t_0 + \varepsilon)$. Without loss of generality, assume that there are integers k and m, $1 \leq k \leq m \leq n$, such that

$$x_0 = \varphi(t_0) \in (M_1 \cap \cdots \cap M_m) - (M_{m+1} \cap \cdots \cap M_n)$$

and

$$\varphi((t_0, t_0 + \varepsilon)) \subset (M_1 \cap \cdots \cap M_k) - (M_{k+1} \cap \cdots \cap M_n).$$

By Claim 3.6.1 and Lemma 3.6.2, $x_0 \in D_k$. Let

$$\tilde{\Lambda} = \{\xi = (\xi_1, \cdots, \xi_n)^T \in B^n : \xi_i = \text{sgn}(x_{0i}),\ k < i \leq n\}$$

and take $\tilde{\xi} \in \tilde{\Lambda}$ such that $E(\tilde{\xi}) \leq E(\xi)$, for any $\xi \in \tilde{\Lambda}$. In view of Lemma 3.8.1, $\xi_i x_{\xi i} > 0$, $1 \leq i \leq k$. Consider the solution $\chi = \chi(\cdot, x_0): [0, +\infty) \to \Re^n$ of the system (N_ξ) with the initial condition x_0. Since $\xi_i x_{\xi i} > 0$, for $1 \leq i \leq k$, and $x_{0i} \neq 0$, for $k < i \leq n$, there is a $\delta > 0$ such that $\chi((0, \delta)) \subset G(\xi)$. So $x_0 \in D_0 \cap D_k \neq \emptyset$, a contradiction. This proves the theorem. ∎

Corollary 3.8.1 If system (N) satisfies Assumption 3.8.1, no equilibrium of (N) is in M.

Proof: If $x \in M$ is an equilibrium of (N) then by Definition 3.6.1, $x \in D_k$ for some $k > 0$. By Theorem 3.8.2, $x \in D_k \cap D_0 \neq \emptyset$. This is a contradiction. Thus we have proved the corollary. ∎

Definition 3.8.2 Assume that system (N) satisfies Assumption 3.8.1. According to Theorem 3.8.2, for any solution of system (N), $\varphi = \varphi(, x_0): [0, +\infty) \to \Re^n$, we can define a constant k_φ and two associated sequences $T_\varphi = \{t_i \in (0, +\infty) : 1 \leq i \leq k_\varphi\}$ and $B_\varphi = \{\xi_i \in B^n : 1 \leq i \leq k_\varphi\}$ by induction as follows:

i) For $k = 1$, by Theorem 3.8.2, there is $\varepsilon > 0$ and $\xi \in B^n$ such that $\varphi((0, \varepsilon)) \subset G(\xi)$. Let $\xi_1 = \xi$ and let $t_1 = \sup\{t \in (0, +\infty) : \varphi((0, t)) \subset G(\xi_1)\}$. If $t_1 = +\infty$, let $k_\varphi = 1$.

ii) For $k > 1$, suppose that t_i and ξ_i, $1 \leq i \leq k - 1$, have been defined and $t_{k-1} \neq +\infty$. By Theorem 3.8.2, there is $\varepsilon > 0$ and $\xi \in B^n$ such that $\varphi((t_{k-1}, t_{k-1} + \varepsilon)) \subset G(\xi)$. Let $\xi_k = \xi$ and let $t_k = \sup\{t \in t_{k-1}, +\infty) : \varphi((t_{k-1}, t)) \subset G(\xi_k)\}$. If $t_k = +\infty$ or $k = 2^n$, let $k_\varphi = k$.

iii) If for any finite integer k, $t_k \neq +\infty$, let $k_\varphi = +\infty$.

B_φ is said to be the *output sequence* of system (N) associated with the solution φ, k_φ is said to be the *length* of B_φ, and T_φ is said to be the *time sequence* associated with solution φ. ∎

From Definition 3.8.2 and Lemma 3.6.1, we have:

Lemma 3.8.2 Suppose that system (N) satisfies Assumption 3.8.1. If $T_\varphi = \{t_i \in (0, +\infty) : 1 \leq i \leq k_\varphi\}$ and $B_\varphi = \{\xi_i \in B^n : 1 \leq i \leq k_\varphi\}$ are the two associated sequences of a solution φ of system (N), then

1) $0 < t_1 < \cdots t_k < t_{k+1} < \cdots$,

2) for any k, $\xi_k \neq \xi_{k+1}$ and $\varphi(t) = \xi_k$, for $t \in (t_{k-1}, t_k)$. ∎

Lemma 3.8.3

1) With the same assumptions and notation as in Lemma 3.8.2, for an integer k, $1 \leq k < k_\varphi$, let $\eta = \xi_k$, $\eta^+ = \xi_{k+1}$, and $\Delta \eta = (\Delta \eta_1, \cdots, \Delta \eta_n)^T = \eta^+ - \eta$. Suppose η^+ and η differ in m components. We can find a permutation $\sigma \in \text{Sym}(n)$ such that $\sigma(1) < \cdots < \sigma(m)$, $\Delta \eta_{\sigma(i)} = -2\eta_{\sigma(i)}$ for $1 \leq i \leq m$, and $\Delta \eta_{\sigma(i)} = 0$ for $m < i \leq n$. Then we have

$$\begin{aligned} \Delta E &= E(\eta^+) - E(\eta) \\ &= 2(\eta_\sigma)^T (T\eta + I)_\sigma - 2(\eta_\sigma)^T T_\sigma \eta_\sigma \\ &< -2(\eta_\sigma)^T T_\sigma \eta_\sigma \end{aligned} \quad (3.8.4)$$

where η_σ is the m-dimensional vector consisting of $\sigma(1), \cdots, \sigma(m)$ components of η, $(T\eta + I)_\sigma$ is the m-dimensional vector

3.8. ENERGY FUNCTION ANALYSIS OF (N)

consisting of $\sigma(1), \cdots, \sigma(m)$ components of $T\eta + I$, and T_σ is the $m \times m$ matrix consisting of $\sigma(1), \cdots, \sigma(m)$ columns and rows of T.

2) $E(\eta^+) < E(\eta)$ if $T_\sigma \geq 0$. In particular, when $m = 1$, we have $\Delta E < -2(\eta_{\sigma(1)})^T T_{\sigma(1)\sigma(1)}\eta_{\sigma(1)} = -2T_{\sigma(1)\sigma(1)} < 0$. (This is similar to what we have shown in Lemma 3.8.1.)

Proof: 1) In the notation of the lemma, we have

$$\Delta E = E(\eta^+) - E(\eta)$$
$$= \left[-(1/2)(\eta + \Delta\eta)^T T(\eta + \Delta\eta) - (\eta + \Delta\eta)^T I + c\right]$$
$$- \left[-(1/2)\eta^T T\eta - \eta^T I + c\right]$$
$$= -(\Delta\eta)^T(T\eta + I) - (1/2)(\Delta\eta)^T T(\Delta\eta)$$
$$= 2(\eta_\sigma)^T (T\eta + I)_\sigma - 2(\eta_\sigma)^T T_\sigma \eta_\sigma.$$

Also, by Lemma 3.6.1, for $1 \leq i \leq m$, the ith components of η_σ and $(T\eta + I)_\sigma$ differ in their signs. We obtain $2(\eta_\sigma)^T (T\eta + I)_\sigma < 0$ and $\Delta E < -2(\eta_\sigma)^T T_\sigma \eta_\sigma$.

2) Part 2) follows from Part 1). ∎

Theorem 3.8.3 Suppose that system (N) satisfies Assumption 3.8.1, and $T_\varphi = \{t_i \in (0, +\infty) : 1 \leq i \leq k_\varphi\}$ and $B_\varphi = \{\xi_i \in B^n : 1 \leq i \leq k_\varphi\}$ are the two associated sequences of a solution φ of system (N). If $T \geq 0$, i.e., T is positive semidefinite, then

1) $E(\xi_{i+1}) < E(\xi_i)$, $1 \leq i < k_\varphi$,

2) $k_\varphi \leq 2^n$ and $t_{k_\varphi} = +\infty$, and

3) ξ_{k_φ} is a stable output vector of (N).

Proof: Part 1) follows from Lemma 3.8.3 and from the fact that if $T \geq 0$, then so are all of its principal complimentary minors.

2) Suppose $k_\varphi > 2^n$. Since B^n contains only 2^n elements, there must be i and j, $1 \leq i < j \leq k_\varphi$, such that $E(\xi_i) = E(\xi_j)$. This contradicts Part 1). Therefore, $k_\varphi \leq 2^n$. By Definition 3.8.2, $t_{k_\varphi} = +\infty$.

3) Since $\varphi((t_{k_\varphi-1}, +\infty)) \subset G(\xi_{k_\varphi})$, by Definition 3.7.3, ξ_{k_φ} is a stable output vector of (N). ∎

Remark 3.8.3 In Theorem 3.8.3, Part 1) states that the energy function decreases monotonically along the output sequence. Parts 2) and 3) state that the output sequences do not oscillate and they will converge to stable output vectors of (N) during a finite number of steps. ∎

Corollary 3.8.2 Suppose that system (N) satisfies Assumption 3.8.1 and $T \geq 0$. Then each solution of (N) converges to an (asymptotically) stable equilibrium point of (N) as $t \to +\infty$. In particular, if the output sequence of a solution φ of system (N) converges to ξ_0, then φ converges to $x_{\xi_0} = T\xi_0 + I$ as $t \to +\infty$.

Proof: For a solution φ of (N), by Theorem 3.8.3, there is a $t_0 \in (0, +\infty)$ and a $\xi_0 \in B^n$ such that $\varphi((t_0, +\infty)) \subset G(\xi_0)$. It follows from Lemma 3.6.1 and Theorem 3.7.3 that φ converges to $x_{\xi_0} = T\xi_0 + I$ as $t \to +\infty$, and x_{ξ_0} is an asymptotically stable equilibrium point of (N). ∎

When T is not positive semidefinite, we may consider a special kind of solution of (N) for which the results of Theorem 3.8.3 still hold.

Definition 3.8.3 1) For $\xi, \eta \in B^n$, η is said to be *reachable* from ξ if there is a sequence $\{\beta_0, \cdots, \beta_m\} \subset B^n$ such that $\xi = \beta_0$, $\eta = \beta_m$ and for each i, $1 \leq i < m$, β_i and β_{i+1} are adjacent. Furthermore, if β_i and β_{i+1} differ at the lth component, then $\beta_{i,l} \cdot x_{\beta i,l} < 0$, where $x_{\beta i} = T\beta_i + I$, and $\beta_{i,l}$, $x_{\beta i,l}$ are the lth components of β_i and $x_{\beta i}$, respectively.

2) A solution $\varphi = \varphi(\cdot, x_0): [0, +\infty) \to \Re^n$ of system (N) is said to be an *asynchronous solution* of system (N), if for each i, $1 < i \leq k_\varphi$, ξ_{k+1} is reachable from ξ_k. ∎

Remark 3.8.4 Apparently, the set of initial conditions for which solutions of (N) are not asynchronous is of measure zero. This statement is reinforced in physical implementations as well: the probability of two amplifiers with infinite gain switching simultaneously at the same precise instant is zero. ∎

3.8. ENERGY FUNCTION ANALYSIS OF (N)

Theorem 3.8.4 Suppose that system (N) satisfies Assumption 3.8.1. For any asynchronous solution φ of system (N) with the two associated sequences $T_\varphi = \{t_i \in (0, +\infty): 1 \leq i \leq k_\varphi\}$ and $B_\varphi = \{\xi_i \in B^n: 1 \leq i \leq k_\varphi\}$, we have

1) $E(\xi_{i+1}) < E(\xi_i)$, $1 \leq i < k_\varphi$,
2) $k_\varphi \leq 2^n$ and $t_{k_\varphi} = +\infty$,
3) ξ_{k_φ} is a stable output vector of (N), and
4) $\{\xi_i \in B^n: 1 \leq i \leq k_\varphi\}$ is a subsequence of a solution of the asynchronous discrete system

$$v_i^+ = \begin{cases} 1, & \text{if } \sum_{j=1}^{n} T_{ij}v_j + I_i > 0 \\ -1, & \text{if } \sum_{j=1}^{n} T_{ij}v_j + I_i < 0 \end{cases} \quad (N_d)$$

where $v = (v_1, \cdots, v_n)^T \in B^n$, $[T_{ij}] = T$, $(I_1, \cdots, I_n)^T = I$.

Proof: Part 1) follows from the definition of asynchronous solutions and Lemma 3.8.1. Parts 2) and 3) can be proved in the same way as Theorem 3.8.3. Part 4) also follows directly from the definition of asynchronous solutions. ∎

Corollary 3.8.3 Suppose that system (N) satisfies Assumption 3.8.1. Then each asynchronous solution of (N) converges to an asymptotically stable equilibrium point of (N) as $t \to +\infty$. In particular, if the output sequence of an asynchronous solution φ of system (N) converges to ξ_0, then φ converges to $x_{\xi_0} = T\xi_0 + I$ as $t \to +\infty$.

Proof: The corollary can be proved in the same way as Corollary 3.8.2. ∎

Remark 3.8.5 In Theorem 3.8.4, Part 1) states that the energy function decreases monotonically along the output sequence. Parts 2) and 3) state that the output sequences do not oscillate and they will converge to stable output vectors of (N) during a finite number of steps. Part 4) establishes a relationship between system (N) and the discrete Hopfield neural network model, provided that T_{ii} may also be positive. ∎

Definition 3.8.4 Suppose that (N) satisfies Assumption 3.8.1. A *directed graph* (V, A) associated with system (N) is defined as follows:

1) $V = B^n$, and

2) $A = \{(\xi, \eta) \in V \times V : \eta$ is adjacent to ξ and if ξ and η differ in the kth component then $x_{\xi k}\xi_k < 0$ where $x_\xi = T\xi + I\}$.

The elements in V are the *vertices* of (V, A) and the elements in A are the *arcs* of (V, A) (cf. [2]). For ξ, $\eta \in V$, η is said to be a *descendant* of ξ if there is a path from ξ to η. For $\xi \in V$, ξ is said to be a *leaf* of graph (V, A) if ξ has no descendants other than itself. ∎

Lemma 3.8.4 Suppose that system (N) satisfies Assumption 3.8.1, and (V, A) is the directed graph associated with system (N) defined above. The following is true:

1) (V, A) is a DAG (i.e., a directed acyclic graph, cf. [2]).

2) The set of leaves of (V, A) is identical to the set of stable output vectors of system (N).

3) For any $\xi \in V$, there is at least one leaf of (V, A) which is a descendant of ξ.

Proof: 1) Part 1) follows since by Theorem 3.8.4, system (N) has no oscillatory output sequences.

2) Part 2) follows from Theorem 3.7.3, Part 1).

3) Part 3) of the lemma follows since (V, A) is a DAG and for $\xi \in V$, the vertex at the end of an unextendable path starting from ξ is a leaf of (V, A). ∎

Definition 3.8.5 Suppose the system (N) satisfies Assumption 3.8.1, and $\xi \in B^n$ is a stable output vector of (N). $\eta \in B^n$ is said to be in the *domain of attraction* of ξ if η is the only leaf of (V, A) which is a descendant of ξ, where (V, A) is the directed graph associated with system (N) as defined in Definition 3.8.4. ∎

Theorem 3.8.5 Suppose that system (N) satisfies Assumption 3.8.1. If $\xi \in B^n$ is a stable output vector of (N) and $\eta \in B^n$ is in the domain of attraction of ξ, then $G(\eta)$ is contained in the domain of attraction of x_ξ, where $x_\xi = T\xi + I$.

Proof: The theorem follows from Corollary 3.8.3. ∎

3.9 Summary

In the present chapter we first investigated global qualitative properties of generalized analog Hopfield neural networks described by equations of the form

$$\dot{x} = -H(x)(-Tx + S(x) - I). \tag{L}$$

Using an energy function of the form

$$E(x) = -\frac{1}{2}x^T T x + \sum_{i=1}^{n} \int_0^{x_i} s_i(\rho)d\rho - x^T I$$

we showed that under reasonable assumptions, the following results are true:

a) for any $x \in (-1,1)^n$, there is a unique solution $\varphi(\cdot, 0, x)$ for (L);

b) along a nonequilibrium solution of (L), the energy function E decreases monotonically, and therefore, no non-constant periodic solutions exist for (L);

c) each solution of (L) exists on $[0, +\infty)$;

d) each nonequilibrium solution of (L) converges to an equilibrium of (L) as $t \to +\infty$, i.e., (L) is *globally stable*;

e) there are only finitely many equilibrium points for (L).

We further showed that under mild assumptions, the following statements are equivalent:

i) $\tilde{x}$ is a stable equilibrium of (L);

ii) $\tilde{x}$ is a local minimum of the energy function E;

iii) $J_E(\tilde{x}) > 0$, i.e., the Jacobian matrix for system (L) evaluated at $x = \tilde{x}$ is positive definite; and

iv) $\tilde{x}$ is asymptotically stable.

Results of the type given above can be used in a variety of applications. For example, the global stability property of system (L) [refer to item d) above] enables us to partition the state space of (L), using the domains of attraction of the asymptotically stable equilibria of (L). Such a partition in turn determines an equivalence relation for system (L), which in turn can be used in classification problems, including applications to associative memories. This will be demonstrated in Chapters 8 and 9.

Next, we investigated global (and some local) qualitative properties of a class of neural networks described by variable structure systems given by

$$\frac{dx}{dt} = F(x) \qquad (N)$$

with

$$F(x) = -Ax + TS(x) + I$$

where the components of the vector $S(x)$ consist of sign functions.

For system (N) we established results along the following lines:

a) We introduced an appropriate notion of solution for system (N) (including the concept of *sliding mode*) and we showed that for any initial condition, there is such a solution of (N), and that all solutions can be extended to the infinite time interval.

b) We made precise the notion of equilibrium point for system (N) and we showed that in each of 2^n regions [which are separated by the surfaces of discontinuity, M, of the right hand side of (N)], there exists at most one asymptotically stable equilibrium point.

c) If in one of the above regions, call it G, there is an equilibrium point, say x_0, then G is contained in the domain of attraction of x_0.

d) We showed that there is a one-to-one correspondence between the asymptotically stable equilibrium points in $\Re^n - M$ and the stable output vectors of (N) [the range of the function S makes up the output rectors of (N)].

Furthermore, under the assumptions that T is symmetric and the diagonal elements of T are non-negative, we used an energy function of the form

$$E(\xi) = -\frac{1}{2}\xi^T T \xi - \xi^T I + c$$

to establish the following properties of (N):

i) The set of local minima of E is contained in the set of stable output vectors of (N). These two sets are equal if $T_{ii} = 0$, $1 \leq i \leq n$.

ii) Solutions of (N) will not be in a sliding mode.

iii) If T is positive semidefinite, then along each output sequence [i.e., along each sequence of output vectors of (N)], the energy function decreases monotonically, and system (N) will not exhibit periodic solutions.

iv) If T is not positive semidefinite, then statement iii) is true with respect to asynchronous solutions of (N).

3.10 Notes and References

The results presented in Sections 3.1 through and including 3.4 are based on material established in [6]. Some of these results are in the same spirit as results developed in [3] for the Cohen-Grossberg model.

The results presented in Sections 3.5 through and including 3.8 rely on material given in [7]. We note here that variable structure systems arise in several disciplines, especially control theory. However, whereas in variable structure neural networks the objective is usually to *avoid* sliding modes, in variable structure control systems the objective is to design the controller in a manner to steer the system along sliding motions to some desired target set in the state space.

In Chapter 7 we will conduct a qualitative analysis of the Cohen-Grossberg model endowed with time delays. In the special case when the delays are zero, these results are along similar lines as some of the results that we established in Sections 3.1 through 3.4 for system (L).

Bibliography

[1] A Avez. Differential Calculus. New York, NY: Wiley, 1986.

[2] AV Aho, JE Hopcroft, JD Ullman. Data Structure and Algorithms. Reading, MA: Addison-Wesley, 1987.

[3] M Cohen, S Grossberg. Absolute stability of global pattern formation and parallel memory storage by competitive neural networks. IEEE Transactions on Systems, Man, and Cybernetics 13:815–826, 1983.

[4] JJ Hopfield. Neurons with graded response have collective computational properties like those of two-state neurons. Proceedings of the National Academy of Sciences USA 81:3088–3092, 1984.

[5] N Jacobson. Basic Algebra I. San Francisco, CA: Freeman, 1974.

[6] JH Li, AN Michel, W Porod. Qualitative analysis and synthesis of a class of neural networks. IEEE Transactions on Circuits and Systems 35:976–987, 1988.

[7] JH Li, AN Michel, W Porod. Analysis and synthesis of a class of neural networks: Variable structure systems with infinite

gains. IEEE Transactions on Circuits and Systems 36:713–731, 1989.

[8] AN Michel, CJ Herget. Applied Algebra and Functional Analysis. New York, NY: Dover Publications, 1993.

[9] AN Michel, DW Porter. Practical stability and finite-time stability of discontinuous systems. IEEE Transactions on Circuit Theory 19:123–129, 1972.

[10] RK Miller, AN Michel. Ordinary Differential Equations. New York, NY: Academic Press, 1982.

[11] HL Royden. Real Analysis. Second Edition. New York, NY: MacMillan, 1963.

[12] FMA Salam, Y Wang. Some properties of dynamic feedback neural nets. Proceedings of the 26th IEEE Conference on Decision and Control, Austin, TX, 1988, pp 337–342.

[13] VI Utkin. Variable structure systems with sliding modes. IEEE Transactions on Automatic Control 22:212–222, 1977.

Chapter 4

Stability Analysis of Linear Systems Operating on a Closed Hypercube: System (M)

In the present chapter we conduct a qualitative analysis of analog and discrete-time neural networks which constitute linear systems operating on a closed hypercube in real n-space. Such networks, which were developed in Section 2.6, are described by linear differential equations, or by linear difference equations, defined on a closed hypercube. In implementations of such systems, all the state variables are constrained by saturation nonlinearities.

We are concerned with both global and local results. Questions that we will address in the present chapter include existence, uniqueness and continuation of solutions of the equations describing the networks; determination of the locations of the equilibria of a network; estimates of the total number of the equilibria of a network; estimates of the total number of asymptotically stable equilibria of a network; local stability properties of an equilibrium; and global stability properties of a network.

4.1 Linear Continuous-Time Systems Operating on a Closed Hypercube: System (M)

In the present chapter we consider the class of neural networks addressed in Section 2.6, described by a system of first-order linear ordinary differential equations defined on a hypercube. Specifically, we will consider neural networks described by equations of the form

$$\frac{dx}{dt} = Tx + I \qquad \text{(M)}$$

with the constraints

$$-1 \leq x_i \leq 1, \quad i = 1, \cdots, n$$

where $x = (x_1, \cdots, x_n)^T \in D^n = \{x \in \Re^n : -1 \leq x_i \leq 1, i = 1, \cdots, n\}$, $T = [T_{ij}]$ is a real $n \times n$ constant matrix, and $I = (I_1, \cdots, I_n)^T$ is a constant vector. The main difference between system (M) and the usual linear systems is that the latter are defined on open subsets of $\Re^n$ while the former is defined on the closed subset D^n of $\Re^n$. For system (M), we will introduce a new concept of solution, called solution in the "saturated" mode.

We showed in Section 2.6 that system (M) can easily be implemented by analog VLSI circuits. Also, we showed in Section 2.6 that the present class of neural networks is closely related to the analog Hopfield model [4]. Thus, some of the results obtained in the present chapter can also be applied in synthesis procedures for the analog Hopfield model, provided that the amplifier gains are sufficiently high.

Under appropriate assumptions, which we will give later, we will establish for system (M) results along the following lines.

a) First, a definition of solution of system (M) is introduced. On the boundary ∂D^n, this type of solution of (M) involves the notion of "solution in a saturated mode." Making use of this concept of solution, we show that for any initial condition, there is a unique

4.2. NOTATION

solution of (M), and all such solutions can be extended to the infinite time interval.

b) The concept of equilibrium point for (M) is made precise. An efficient algorithm is then developed to determine the location of each equilibrium point of (M) and to determine whether it is asymptotically stable or unstable.

c) It is shown that system (M) has at most 3^n equilibrium points and at most 2^n asymptotically stable equilibrium points. The distribution of the equilibrium points is also addressed.

d) An energy function E for system (M) is introduced. We show that there is a one-to-one correspondence between the set of local minimum points of E and the set of asymptotically stable equilibrium points of (M).

e) We also show that along each solution of (M), the energy function E decreases monotonically, and system (M) will not exhibit periodic solutions.

Before presenting the above results, we need to establish some essential notation.

4.2 Notation

Let V and W be arbitrary sets. Then $V \cup W$, $V \cap W$, $V - W$, and $V \times W$ denote the union, intersection, difference, and Cartesian product of V and W, respectively. If V is a subset of W, we write $V \subset W$ and if x is an element of V, we write $x \in V$. If f is a function from V into W, we write $f: V \to W$ and we let $f(U) = \{f(x) \in W : x \in U\}$ for $U \subset V$, and $f^{-1}(y) = \{x \in V : f(x) = y\}$ for $y \in W$. Let $\emptyset$ denote the empty set, let $\Re$ denote the set of real numbers, and let $\Re^+ = [0, +\infty)$. Let Z denote the set of integers, and let $Z^+ = \{0, 1, 2, \cdots\}$. If $V_1, \cdots, V_n$ are n arbitrary sets, their Cartesian product is denoted by $\prod_{i=1}^{n} V_i = V_1 \times \cdots \times V_n$. If in particular, $V = V_1 = \cdots = V_n$, we write $\prod_{i=1}^{n} V_i = V^n$. Let $\Re^n$ be real n-space. If $x \in \Re^n$, then

$x^T = (x_1, \cdots, x_n)$ denotes the transpose of x. When using a norm for $x \in \Re^n$, $|x|$, we will have in mind $|x| = \sqrt{\sum_{i=1}^{n} x_i^2}$. If $x \in \Re^n$ and $Y \subset \Re^n$, then $x \perp Y$ will mean that $x^T \cdot y = 0$ for all $y \in Y$. If $V \subset \Re^n$, then $\overline{V}$, V° and ∂V represent the closure, interior and the boundary of V in $\Re^n$, respectively. Also, we let $B(\tilde{x}, r) = \{x \in \Re^n : |\tilde{x} - x| < r\}$ for $\tilde{x} \in \Re^n$ and $r > 0$. Let $B^n = \{x \in \Re^n : x_i = 1 \text{ or } -1, i = 1, \cdots, n\}$ and $D^n = \{x \in \Re^n : -1 \leq x_i \leq 1, i = 1, \cdots, n\}$. If $x, y \in \Re^n$, let $x * y = (x_1 y_1, \cdots, x_n y_n)^T$ and $\min(x) = \min\{x_i : 1 \leq i \leq n\}$. If $A = [A_{ij}]$ is an arbitrary matrix, then A^T denotes the transpose of A and the norm of A is defined as $\|A\| = \sup_{|x| \leq 1}\{|Ax|\}$. If A is a symmetric matrix, by $A > 0$ we mean that A is positive definite and by $A \geq 0$ we mean that A is positive semidefinite. $\text{Sym}(n)$ denotes the symmetric group of order n.

4.3 Definition and Properties of the Solutions of System (M)

We first give an appropriate definition of solution for system (M). This notion of solution needs to capture, e.g., the behavior of the circuit given in Fig. 2.6.1 in Chapter 2.

For each m, $0 \leq m \leq n$, let

$$\Lambda_m = \{\xi = (\xi_1, \cdots, \xi_n)^T \in \Lambda : \xi_{\sigma(i)} = 0,\ 1 \leq i \leq m \text{ and } \xi_{\sigma(i)} = \pm 1,\ m < i \leq n,\ \text{for some } \sigma \in \text{Sym}(n)\} \quad (4.3.1)$$

where

$$\Lambda = \{\xi = (\xi_1, \cdots, \xi_n)^T : \xi_i = \pm 1 \text{ or } 0,\ 1 \leq i \leq n\}. \quad (4.3.2)$$

The number of elements in Λ_m is equal to

$$\frac{n!\, 2^{n-m}}{m!(n-m)!}$$

4.3. DEFINITION AND PROPERTIES OF SOLUTIONS

and the number of elements in $\Lambda = \cup \Lambda_m$, $0 \le m \le n$, is 3^n. For each $\xi \in \Lambda$, let

$$C(\xi) = \{x = (x_1, \cdots, x_n)^T \in \Re^n : |x_i| < 1 \text{ if } \xi_i = 0, \text{ and } \\ x_i = \xi_i \text{ if } \xi_i \ne 0\}. \quad (4.3.3)$$

From the notation given above, we have:

Lemma 4.3.1

1) $\Lambda_0 = B^n$ and $C(\xi) = \{\xi\}$, for any $\xi \in \Lambda_0$.
2) $\Lambda_n = \{0\}$ and $C(0) = (D^n)^\circ = \{x \in \Re^n : -1 < x_i < 1, i = 1, \cdots, n\}$.
3) $\partial(D^n) = \cup C(\xi)$, $\xi \in \cup \Lambda_m$, $1 \le m \le n$.
4) $D^n = \cup C(\xi)$, $\xi \in \cup \Lambda_m$, $0 \le m \le n$.
5) For any $\xi, \eta \in \Lambda$, $\xi \ne \eta$, $C(\xi) \cap C(\eta) = \emptyset$. ∎

Suppose that $\xi \in \Lambda_m$ and $\sigma \in \text{Sym}(n)$ such that

$$\xi_{\sigma(i)} = 0,\ 1 \le i \le m \text{ and } \xi_{\sigma(i)} = \pm 1,\ m < i \le n. \quad (4.3.4)$$

Subsequently, we will make use of the notation

$$\begin{aligned}
T_{\text{I,I}} &= \left[T_{\sigma(i)\sigma(j)}\right]_{1 \le i,j \le m} \\
T_{\text{I,II}} &= \left[T_{\sigma(i)\sigma(j)}\right]_{1 \le i \le m, m < j \le n} \\
T_{\text{II,I}} &= \left[T_{\sigma(i)\sigma(j)}\right]_{m < i \le n, 1 \le j \le m} \\
T_{\text{II,II}} &= \left[T_{\sigma(i)\sigma(j)}\right]_{m < i,j \le n} \\
I_{\text{I}} &= \left(I_{\sigma(1)}, \cdots, I_{\sigma(m)}\right)^T \\
I_{\text{II}} &= \left(I_{\sigma(m+1)}, \cdots, I_{\sigma(n)}\right)^T \\
\xi_{\text{I}} &= \left(\xi_{\sigma(1)}, \cdots, \xi_{\sigma(m)}\right)^T \\
\xi_{\text{II}} &= \left(\xi_{\sigma(m+1)}, \cdots, \xi_{\sigma(n)}\right)^T.
\end{aligned} \quad (4.3.5)$$

Remark 4.3.1 1) For a given $\xi \in \Lambda_m$, there may exist different permutations in $\text{Sym}(n)$ for which (4.3.4) is true. For these different permutations, the notation given above will be the same up to different orders in the components. Thus, the analysis and conclusions will be identical for any of the permutations used.

2) If $m = n$, we have $T_{\text{I},\text{I}} = T$, $I_\text{I} = I$, $\xi_\text{I} = \xi$ and the $T_{\text{I},\text{II}}$, $T_{\text{II},\text{I}}$, $T_{\text{II},\text{II}}$, I_II, ξ_II do not exist. If $m = 0$, we have $T_{\text{II},\text{II}} = T$, $I_\text{II} = I$, $\xi_\text{II} = \xi$ and the $T_{\text{I},\text{I}}$, $T_{\text{I},\text{II}}$, $T_{\text{II},\text{I}}$, I_I, ξ_I do not exist. ∎

Definition 4.3.1 1) Consider $\xi \in \Lambda_m$, $0 < m \leq n$, with $\sigma \in \text{Sym}(n)$ such that $\xi_{\sigma(i)} = 0$, $1 \leq i \leq m$ and $\xi_{\sigma(i)} = \pm 1$, $m < i \leq n$. Also, consider the linear system defined by

$$\frac{dx_\text{I}}{dt} = T_{\text{I},\text{I}} x_\text{I} + T_{\text{I},\text{II}} \xi_\text{II} + I_\text{I} \quad (\text{M}_\xi)$$

where $x_\text{I} = \left(x_{\sigma(1)}, \cdots, x_{\sigma(m)}\right)^T$, $x_\text{II} = \left(x_{\sigma(m+1)}, \cdots, x_{\sigma(n)}\right)^T$ and $-1 < x_{\sigma(i)} < 1$ for $1 \leq i \leq m$.

(M_ξ) is said to be the *reduced linear system* of (M) over the region $C(\xi)$.

2) For any $\xi \in \Lambda_m$, a C^1-function $\varphi: (0, \delta) \to C(\xi)$ is said to be a *(local) solution* of system (M) if the vector function φ_I containing the $\sigma(i)$-th component of φ, $1 \leq i \leq m$, is a solution of the linear system (M_ξ), i.e.,

$$\frac{d\varphi_\text{I}(t)}{dt} = T_{\text{I},\text{I}} \varphi_\text{I}(t) + T_{\text{I},\text{II}} \xi_\text{II} + I_\text{I}, \quad t \in (0, \delta) \quad (4.3.6)$$

and

$$\min\left((T_{\text{II},\text{I}} \varphi_\text{I}(t) + T_{\text{II},\text{II}} \xi_\text{II} + I_\text{II}) * \xi_\text{II}\right) \geq 0, \quad t \in (0, \delta) \quad (4.3.7)$$

where $\varphi_\text{I} = \left(\varphi_{\sigma(1)}, \cdots, \varphi_{\sigma(m)}\right)^T$ and $\varphi_\text{II} = \left(\varphi_{\sigma(m+1)}, \cdots, \varphi_{\sigma(n)}\right)^T$.

In particular, if $\xi \in \Lambda_m$, $m < n$, the solution φ is said to be in the *saturated mode*. ∎

4.3. DEFINITION AND PROPERTIES OF SOLUTIONS

Remark 4.3.2 1) $\varphi((0,\delta)) \subset C(\xi)$ implies that

$$-1 < \varphi_{\sigma(i)}(t) < 1, \quad i = 1, \cdots, m, \ t \in (0, \delta)$$

$$\varphi_{\sigma(i)}(t) = \xi_{\sigma(i)} \quad i = m+1, \cdots, n; \ t \in (0, \delta)$$

i.e.,

$$\varphi_{\text{II}}(t) = \xi_{\text{II}} \text{ on } (0, \delta).$$

2) When $m = n$, $\Lambda_n = \{0\}$. In this case, (4.3.7) does not exist and we only need to consider (4.3.6). Furthermore, the (local) solutions in $C(0) = (D^n)^\circ = \{x \in \Re^n : -1 < x_i < 1,\ i = 1, \cdots, n\}$ defined above for system (M) will be identical to the usual solutions defined on the open subset $C(0)$ for the linear system (M_0).

3) When $m = 0$, $\Lambda_0 = B^n$ and for $\xi \in \Lambda_0$, $C(\xi) = \{\xi\}$. In this case, (4.3.6) does not exist and we only need to consider (4.3.7). Furthermore, the only function with the range in $C(\xi)$ is the constant function $\varphi(t) \equiv \xi$. ■

Definition 4.3.2 For $\tilde{x} \in D^n$, a continuous function

$$\psi = \psi(\cdot, \tilde{x}) : [0, \tilde{t}) \to D^n$$

is said to be a *solution of* (M) *starting* at $\tilde{x}$ if

a) $\psi(0, \tilde{x}) = \tilde{x}$, and

b) there are countably many non-interconnected open intervals $(t_i, t_i + \delta_i)$ such that $\overline{\cup(t_i, t_i + \delta_i)} = \overline{(0, \tilde{t})}$ and ψ restricted to each $(t_i, t_i + \delta_i)$ is a (local) solution as defined in Part 2) of Definition 4.3.1 above. ■

From the Existence Theorem of ordinary differential equations (cf. [16]), we have

Theorem 4.3.1

1) For any $x \in D^n$, there is a unique solution $\psi(\cdot, x)$ for system (M).

2) Each solution of (M) can be uniquely extended to the infinite time interval $[0, +\infty)$. ∎

Remark 4.3.3 With a little extra effort, the following information can be added to Theorem 4.3.1 [6]: Each solution of (M) is continuously differentiable with respect to time where at each t_i (see Definition 4.3.2), we mean the right derivative. ∎

4.4 Qualitative Properties of the Equilibrium Points of System (M)

In view of Theorem 4.3.1, we consider henceforth only solutions of (M) that are defined on $\Re^+ = [0, \infty)$.

Definition 4.4.1 1) A vector $\tilde{x} \in D^n$ is said to be an *equilibrium (point)* of (M) if the function $\psi(\cdot, \tilde{x}) : [0, \infty) \to D^n$ defined by $\psi(t, \tilde{x}) \equiv \tilde{x}$, is a solution of (M).

2) Let $\tilde{x}$ be an equilibrium of (M).

   i) $\tilde{x}$ is said to be *stable* if for every $\varepsilon > 0$, there is a $\delta = \delta(\varepsilon) > 0$ such that $|\psi(t, x) - \tilde{x}| < \varepsilon$ for all $t \in [0, \infty)$ whenever $|x - \tilde{x}| < \delta$.

   ii) $\tilde{x}$ is said to be *asymptotically stable* if it is stable and if there is an $\eta > 0$ such that $\lim_{t \to +\infty} |\psi(t, x) - \tilde{x}| = 0$ whenever $|x - \tilde{x}| < \eta$.

   iii) $\tilde{x}$ is said to be *unstable* if it is not stable. ∎

We now consider the following assumptions for (M).

Assumption 4.4.1

1) T is symmetric.

2) For any m, $0 \leq m \leq n$, and for any $\xi \in \Lambda_m$, the $m \times m$ matrix $T_{I,I} = [T_{\sigma(i)\sigma(j)}]_{1 \leq i,j \leq m}$, is non-singular, where $\sigma \in \text{Sym}(n)$ such that $\xi_{\sigma(i)} = 0$, $1 \leq i \leq m$ and $\xi_{\sigma(i)} = \pm 1$, $m < i \leq n$. ∎

4.4. QUALITATIVE PROPERTIES OF EQUILIBRIA

For system (M) satisfying Assumption 4.4.1, we define the following notation.

1) For $\xi = 0 \in \Lambda_n$, let

$$x_\xi = (x_{\xi 1}, \cdots, x_{\xi n})^T \in \Re^n, \quad x_\xi = -T^{-1}I. \tag{4.4.1}$$

2) For $\xi \in \Lambda_m$, $0 < m < n$, with $T_{\text{I},\text{I}}, \cdots, T_{\text{II},\text{II}}$, I_I, I_II defined in (4.3.6) and (4.3.7), let

$$x_\xi = (x_{x1}, \cdots, x_{\xi n})^T \in \Re^n \tag{4.4.2}$$

where

$$x_{\xi \text{I}} = \left(x_{\xi \sigma(1)}, \cdots, x_{\xi \sigma(m)}\right)^T = -(T_{\text{I},\text{I}})^{-1}(T_{\text{I},\text{II}}\xi_\text{II} + I_\text{I})$$

$$x_{\xi \text{II}} = \left(x_{\xi \sigma(m+1)}, \cdots, x_{\xi \sigma(n)}\right)^T = \xi_\text{II}$$

and let

$$r_\xi \in \Re, \quad r_\xi = \min\left((T_{\text{II},\text{I}}x_{\xi \text{I}} + T_{\text{II},\text{II}}\xi_\text{II} + I_\text{II}) * \xi_\text{II}\right). \tag{4.4.3}$$

3) For $\xi \in \Lambda_0 = B^n$, $C(\xi) = \{\xi\}$. Let

$$x_\xi = \xi \tag{4.4.4}$$

and

$$r_\xi \in \Re, \quad r_\xi = \min((T\xi + I) * \xi). \tag{4.4.5}$$

Assumption 4.4.2 Given Assumption 4.4.1 for system (M), we assume that for $\xi \in \Lambda_m$, $0 \leq m < n$, $x_\xi \notin \partial C(\xi)$, i.e., $x_{x\sigma(i)} \neq \pm 1$, $i = 1, \cdots, m$. ∎

Remark 4.4.1 For fixed T, Assumption 4.4.2 is true for almost all vectors I in $\Re^n$. ∎

Lemma 4.4.1 Suppose that system (M) satisfies Assumptions 4.4.1 and 4.4.2. Then for any $\xi \in \Lambda_m$, $0 \leq m < n$, $r_\xi \neq 0$.

Proof: Suppose that for some $\xi \in \Lambda_m$, $0 < m < n$, $r_\xi = 0$. Then from the notation given in (4.4.1)–(4.4.5), there is j, $1 \leq j \leq n - m$, such that the jth component of the vector $(T_{\text{II},\text{I}} x_{\xi\text{I}} + T_{\text{II},\text{II}} \xi_{\text{II}} + I_{\text{II}})$ is equal to 0. Without loss of generality, assume that $j = 1$. Take $\zeta \in \Lambda_{m+1}$, where $\zeta_{\sigma(i)} = 0$ for $1 \leq i \leq m+1$ and $\zeta_{\sigma(i)} = \xi_{\sigma(i)}$ for $m + 1 < i \leq n$. Then $r_\xi = r_\zeta \in \partial C(\xi)$ and this contradicts Assumption 4.4.2. Suppose that for some $\xi \in \Lambda_0$, $r_\xi = 0$. Then we can arrive at a contradiction in the same manner. This proves the lemma. ∎

Theorem 4.4.1 Suppose system (M) satisfies Assumptions 4.4.1 and 4.4.2. Then for any m, $0 \leq m \leq n$, and for any $\xi \in \Lambda_m$, with the notation given above, we have the following results:

Case I: $m = n$, $\xi = 0 \in \Lambda_n$.

1) If $x_\xi \notin C(\xi) = (D^n)^\circ$, there is no equilibrium point of system (M) in $(D^n)^\circ$.

2) If $x_\xi \in C(\xi) = (D^n)^\circ$, x_ξ is the unique equilibrium point of system (M) in $(D^n)^\circ$. In particular,

   i) if T is not negative definite, x_ξ is unstable, and
   ii) if $T_{\text{I},\text{I}} = T$ is negative definite, x_ξ is asymptotically stable and there are no other equilibrium points in $C(\xi) = D^n$.

Case II: $0 < m < n$, $\xi \in \Lambda_m$.

A) If $r_\xi < 0$, there is no equilibrium point of (M) in $C(\xi)$.

B) If $r_\xi > 0$, we have that

   1) If $x_\xi \notin C(\xi)$, there is no equilibrium point of system (M) in $C(\xi)$.
   2) If $x_\xi \in C(\xi)$, x_ξ is the unique equilibrium point of system (M) in $C(\xi)$. In particular,

      i) if $T_{\text{I},\text{I}}$ is not negative definite, x_ξ is unstable, and

4.4. QUALITATIVE PROPERTIES OF EQUILIBRIA   125

ii) if $T_{I,I}$ is negative definite, x_ξ is asymptotically stable, and there are no other equilibrium points in $\overline{C(\xi)}$.

Case III: $\xi \in \Lambda_0 = B^n$. (Note: $C(\xi) = \{\xi\}$.)

A) If $r_\xi < 0$, $x_\xi = \xi$ is not an equilibrium point of system (M).

B) If $r_\xi > 0$, $x_\xi = \xi$ is an asymptotically stable equilibrium point of system (M).

Proof: Case I: In this case, $\xi = 0$ and $C(\xi) = (D^n)^\circ$, and from Definition 4.4.1, solutions of (M) on $C(0)$ are identical to solutions of (M) on $C(0)$ in the usual sense. Then the conclusions of Case I of the theorem follow directly from the theory of linear differential equations (cf. [16]).

Case II: Consider $\xi \in \Lambda_m$, $0 < m < n$, and a constant function $\varphi\colon [0,+\infty) \to C(\xi)$, $\varphi(t) = \tilde{x}$. If $\tilde{x}$ is an equilibrium point of (M) in $C(\xi)$, then by Definition 4.3.1 we have that

$$T_{I,I}\tilde{x}_I + T_{I,II}\xi_{II} + I_I = 0$$

i.e., $\tilde{x}_I = x_{\xi I}$ and

$$\min\Big((T_{II,I}\tilde{x}_I + T_{II,II}\xi_{II} + I_{II}) * \xi_{II}\Big) \geq 0.$$

Since $\tilde{x} \in C(\xi)$, $\tilde{x}_{II} = \xi_{II}$, and $x_\xi = \tilde{x} \in C(\xi)$. Also, $r_\xi \geq 0$ and by Lemma 4.4.1, $r_\xi > 0$. On the other hand, if $x_\xi \in C(\xi)$ and $r_\xi > 0$, let $\rho\colon [0,+\infty) \to C(\xi)$, $\varphi(t) = x_\xi$. Then φ is a C^1-function and satisfies (4.3.6) and (4.3.7). By Definition 4.3.1, φ is a solution of (M) and by Definition 4.4.1, $\varphi \equiv x_\xi$ is an equilibrium point of (M) in $C(\xi)$.

Furthermore, suppose that x_ξ is an equilibrium point of (M). Then there is an open neighborhood U of x_ξ in $\Re^n$ such that

$$\min\Big((T_{II,I}x_I + T_{II,II}\xi_{II} + I_{II}) * \xi_{II}\Big) > 0$$

for all $x \in U \cap D^n$. If $T_{I,I} < 0$, it can be proved by induction and by the theory of linear differential equations that all solutions of

(M) starting in $U \cap D^n$ will monotonically converge to x_ξ as $t \to +\infty$. Thus x_ξ is an asymptotically stable equilibrium point of (M). On the other hand, if $T_{I,I}$ is not negative definite, then $T_{I,I}$ has a positive eigenvalue since $T_{I,I}$ is not singular. By the theory of linear differential equations, there is a $\delta_0 > 0$ such that $B(x_\xi, \delta_0) \cap D^n \subset U \cap D^n$, and for any ε, $0 < \varepsilon < \delta_0$, there is a function $\varphi\colon [0, t_0) \to C(\xi) \cap U$ such that $\varphi(0) \in C(\xi) \cap B(x_\xi, \varepsilon)$, $|\varphi(t_0) - x_\xi| > \delta_0$, and φ_I is a solution of linear system (M_ξ). Since $\varphi([0, t_0)) \subset U$, φ_{II} satisfies (4.3.7) and φ is a solution of system (M). Thus x_ξ is an unstable equilibrium point of (M) by Definition 4.4.1.

Finally, for purposes of contradiction, assume x_ξ is an asymptotically stable equilibrium point of (M) and x_ζ is another equilibrium point of (M) in $\overline{C(\xi)}$. Since x_ξ is the unique equilibrium point of (M) in $C(\xi)$, $x_\zeta \in \overline{C(\xi)} - C(\xi)$. Then there is a k, $1 \leq k \leq m$, such that $\zeta_{\sigma(k)} = 1$ or -1. By the theory of linear differential equations, the $\sigma(k)$th component of $Tx_\zeta + I$ starting at x_ζ points to x_ξ. Thus $(Tx_\zeta + I)_{\sigma(k)} \cdot \zeta_{\sigma(k)} < 0$ and $r_\zeta < 0$. This contradiction shows that x_ξ is the only equilibrium point of (M) in $\overline{C(\xi)}$.

Case III: If $r_\xi < 0$, $\varphi \equiv x_\xi$ does not satisfy (4.3.7) and x_ξ is not a solution of (M). If $r_\xi > 0$, then there is an open neighborhood U of x_ξ in $\Re^n$ such that

$$\min\left((T_{II,I}x_I + T_{II,II}\xi_{II} + I_{II}) * \xi_{II}\right) > 0$$

for all $x \in U \cap D^n$. It can be proved by induction and by the theory of linear differential equations that all solutions of (M) starting in $U \cap D^n$ will monotonically converge to x_ξ as $t \to +\infty$. Thus x_ξ is an asymptotically stable equilibrium point of (M) by Definition 4.4.1.

This concludes the proof of Theorem 4.4.1. ∎

Remark 4.4.2 1) Theorem 4.4.1 establishes an algorithm to locate all equilibrium points of (M) and to determine the stability properties of all equilibrium points.

2) In practice, due to noise, unstable equilibrium points can not be used as memory locations. However, by investigating the locations

4.4. QUALITATIVE PROPERTIES OF EQUILIBRIA

of the unstable equilibrium points of (M), the domain of attraction of each asymptotically stable equilibrium point of (M) can be approximately determined. We will illustrate this observation by means of an example in Chapter 8.

3) Since system (M) is closely related to the analog Hopfield model [refer to equations (2.6.4) and (2.6.5)], Theorem 4.4.1 may be used to determine asymptotically stable equilibrium points for the Hopfield model. This will be illustrated by means of an example in Chapter 8.

4) If for some $\xi \in \Lambda$, the corresponding $T_{I,I}$ is singular, Theorem 4.4.1 can still be applied to other vectors in Λ. If Lemma 4.4.1 is not true, we need to consider the case $r_\xi = 0$. In fact, we can study this case using the same method as was employed in Theorem 4.4.1. In this case, the conclusions might be less straightforward. ∎

Theorem 4.4.2 If system (M) satisfies Assumptions 4.4.1 and 4.4.2, we have the following results:

1) There is at most one equilibrium point of (M) in each region $C(\xi)$, $\xi \in \Lambda$.

2) There are at most 3^n equilibrium points for system (M).

3) If for $\xi \in \Lambda$ the corresponding x_ξ is an asymptotically stable equilibrium point for system (M), then

   i) x_ξ is the unique equilibrium point of system (M) in $\overline{C(\xi)}$, and

   ii) x_ξ is the unique asymptotically stable equilibrium point of system (M) in $\overline{C(\xi)} \cup C(\zeta)$, where $\zeta \in \Lambda$ such that $x_\xi \in \overline{C(\zeta)}$. In particular, if $\xi \in \Lambda_0 = B^n$ and $x_\xi = \xi$ is an asymptotically stable equilibrium point of system (M), then $x_\xi = \xi$ is the unique asymptotically stable equilibrium point of system (M) in the region $\{x \in D^n : -1 < x_i \xi_i \leq 1, 1 \leq i \leq n\}$.

4) There are at most 2^n asymptotically stable equilibrium points for system (M).

Proof: Part 1) follows from Theorem 4.4.1. Part 2) follows from the fact that D^n is separated into 3^n regions by $C(\xi)$, $\xi \in \Lambda$. Part 3) has been proved in Theorem 4.4.1. Part 4) follows from Part 3). ■

Remark 4.4.3 Theorem 4.4.2 is not only very useful to simplify the algorithm given in Theorem 4.4.1 for checking the locations of equilibrium points of system (M) but it is also useful to determine whether a given set of vectors can be synthesized as a set of asymptotically stable equilibrium points of system (M) or not [refer to the synthesis procedure for system (M) presented in Chapter 8]. ■

4.5 Qualitative Analysis of System (M) in Terms of an Energy Function

Similarly as in Sections 3.4 and 3.8, where we studied the generalized analog Hopfield neural network model (L) and the analog Hopfield neural network model with infinite gains (N), respectively, using energy functions, we employ in the present section an energy function in studying some of the qualitative properties of neural network (M). To this end, we make the following definition.

Definition 4.5.1 If T is symmetric, then

1) the *energy function* $E: D^n \to \Re$ of system (N) is defined by

$$E(x) = -\frac{1}{2}x^T T x - x^T I \qquad (4.5.1)$$

and

2) $x \in D^n$ is said to be a *(local) minimum* of the energy function E if there is an open neighborhood U of x in $\Re^n$ such that $E(x) \leq E(y)$, for any $y \in D^n \cap U$. ■

Theorem 4.5.1 Suppose system (M) satisfies Assumptions 4.4.1 and 4.4.2. Then it is true that

1) along a non-equilibrium solution of (M), the energy function E given in (4.5.1) decreases monotonically; and

4.5. ENERGY FUNCTION ANALYSIS

2) each non-equilibrium solution of (M) converges to an equilibrium of (M).

Proof: 1) It is sufficient to consider the proof for local solutions of (M) as defined in Definition 4.3.1. Consider a non-constant local solution of (M) given by $\varphi\colon (0,\delta) \to C(\xi)$, $\xi \in \Lambda_m$. With the notation given in (4.3.5), we have on $(0, \delta)$,

$$\begin{aligned}
E(\varphi(t)) &= -(1/2)\varphi(t)^T T\varphi(t) - \varphi(t)^T I \\
&= -(1/2)\left(\varphi_{\mathrm{I}}(t)^T, \varphi_{\mathrm{II}}(t)^T\right) \begin{bmatrix} T_{\mathrm{I,I}} & T_{\mathrm{I,II}} \\ T_{\mathrm{II,I}} & T_{\mathrm{II,II}} \end{bmatrix} \cdot \begin{bmatrix} \varphi_{\mathrm{I}}(t) \\ \varphi_{\mathrm{II}}(t) \end{bmatrix} \\
&\quad - \left(\varphi_{\mathrm{I}}(t)^T, \varphi_{\mathrm{II}}(t)^T\right) \begin{bmatrix} I_{\mathrm{I}} \\ I_{\mathrm{II}} \end{bmatrix} \\
&= -(1/2)\Big(\varphi_{\mathrm{I}}(t)^T T_{\mathrm{I,I}}\varphi_{\mathrm{I}}(t) + 2\varphi_{\mathrm{I}}(t)^T T_{\mathrm{I,II}}\xi_{\mathrm{II}} \\
&\quad + \xi_{\mathrm{II}}^T T_{\mathrm{II,II}}\xi_{\mathrm{II}}\Big) - (\varphi_{\mathrm{I}}(t)^T I_{\mathrm{I}} + \xi_{\mathrm{II}}^T I_{\mathrm{II}})
\end{aligned}$$

and by (4.3.6) and (4.3.7)

$$\begin{aligned}
dE(\varphi(t))/dt &= -(T_{\mathrm{I,I}}\varphi_{\mathrm{I}}(t) + T_{\mathrm{I,II}}\xi_{\mathrm{II}} + I_{\mathrm{I}})d\varphi(t)/dt \\
&= -(T_{\mathrm{I,I}}\varphi_{\mathrm{I}}(t) + T_{\mathrm{I,II}}\xi_{\mathrm{II}} + I_{\mathrm{I}})^2 \\
&< 0.
\end{aligned}$$

This proves Part 1).

2) Part 2) follows from the theory of ordinary differential equations (cf. [16]). ∎

Remark 4.5.1 1) Theorem 4.5.1 shows that system (M) has no oscillatory solutions.

2) In practice, due to noise, all solutions of system (M) will only converge to asymptotically stable equilibrium points of (M). ∎

Theorem 4.5.2 Suppose system (M) satisfies Assumptions 4.4.1 and 4.4.2. Then there is a one-to-one correspondence between the set of local minima of the energy function E and the set of asymptotically stable equilibrium points of system (M).

Proof: Suppose that $\tilde{x}$ is an asymptotically stable equilibrium point of system (M). Then there is an open neighborhood U of $\tilde{x}$ in

$\Re^n$ such that all solutions of (M) starting in $U \cap D^n$ will converge to $\tilde{x}$ as $t \to +\infty$. Since along any solution φ, the value of the energy function E decreases monotonically and the energy function E is continuous, we have that $E(\tilde{x}) < E(x)$ for $x \in U \cap D^n$. Thus $\tilde{x}$ is a local minimum of E.

On the other hand, suppose that $\tilde{x}$ is a local minimum of the energy function E. Then there is an open neighborhood U of $\tilde{x}$ in $\Re^n$ such that $E(\tilde{x}) \leq E(x)$, $x \in U \cap D^n$. By Theorem 4.5.1, Part 1, $\tilde{x}$ is an equilibrium point of system (M). If $\tilde{x}$ is not asymptotically stable, by Theorem 4.4.1, it is unstable. Thus there is a $\delta_0 > 0$ such that $B(\tilde{x}, \delta_0) \subset U$ and for any ε, $0 < \varepsilon < \delta_0$, there is a solution φ of (M) starting in $B(\tilde{x}, \varepsilon) \cap D^n$ which tends towards the exterior of $B(\tilde{x}, \delta_0) \cap D^n$. Since along solution φ, the value of the energy function E decreases monotonically and E is continuous, we have that $E(\tilde{x}) > E(x_0)$ for some point $x_0 \in (\partial B(\tilde{x}, \delta_0)) \cap D^n \subset U \cap D^n$. This contradiction shows that $\tilde{x}$ is an asymptotically stable equilibrium point of system (M).

This completes the proof of the theorem. ∎

Remark 4.5.2 1) By Theorems 4.5.1 and 4.5.2, applications developed in [5] and [17] using the Hopfield model can also be realized by use of system (M).

2) As shown in [8] (see Sections 3.1 through 3.4), for system (L), which includes the Hopfield model as a special case, there is a one-to-one correspondence between the set of asymptotically stable equilibrium points of system (L) and the set of local minima of the energy function $E_L: (-1, 1)^n \to \Re$, given by

$$E_L(x) = -\frac{1}{2}x^T T x - x^T I + \frac{1}{\lambda} \sum_{i=1}^{n} \int_0^{x_i} \frac{1}{R_i} g_i^{-1}(\rho) d\rho.$$

When $\lambda \to +\infty$, $E_L(x) \to E(x) = (1/2)x^T T x - x^T I$. From this, we may conclude that near the location of each asymptotically stable equilibrium point of system (M), there is an asymptotically stable equilibrium point of system (L) when the gain λ is large. We believe (although we have not been able to prove this yet) that this relation

4.6. DISCRETE-TIME SYSTEMS

establishes roughly a one-to-one correspondence between the sets of the asymptotically stable equilibrium points of the two systems (L) and (M). This will be illustrated by means of a specific example in Chapter 8. ∎

4.6 Linear Discrete-Time Systems Operating on a Closed Hypercube

In the present chapter we also consider the class of discrete-time neural networks addressed in Section 2.6 [see (2.6.7)], described by a system of first-order linear ordinary difference equations defined on a hypercube. Specifically, we will consider neural networks described by equations of the form

$$x_i(k+1) = \text{sat}\left(\sum_{j=1}^{n} T_{ij}x_j(k) + I_i\right), \quad k = 0,1,2,\cdots; \ i = 1,\cdots,n \quad (\text{M}_{d_i})$$

where

$$\text{sat}(\theta) = \begin{cases} 1, & \theta > 1 \\ \theta, & -1 \leq \theta \leq 1 \\ -1, & \theta < -1. \end{cases}$$

In vector form, we can express (M_{d_i}) as

$$x(k+1) = \text{sat}(Tx(k) + I), \quad k = 0,1,2,\cdots \quad (\text{M}_d)$$

where all symbols in (M_d) are defined in the obvious way.

In what follows, we will make use of the sets Λ_m, Λ, $C(\xi)$; the matrices $T_{\text{I,I}}$, $T_{\text{I,II}}$, $T_{\text{II,I}}$, $T_{\text{II,II}}$; and the vectors ξ_I, ξ_II introduced in equations (4.3.1) through (4.3.5), along with the properties of these entities summarized in Lemma 4.3.1 and Remark 4.3.1.

Definition 4.6.1 1) Consider $\xi \in \Lambda_m$, $0 < m \leq n$, with $\mu \in \text{Sym}(n)$, such that $\xi_{\mu(i)} = 0$, $1 \leq i \leq m$, and $\xi_{\mu(i)} = 1$ or -1, $m < i \leq n$. Also, consider the linear difference system defined by

$$x_\text{I}(k+1) = T_{\text{I,I}}x_\text{I}(k) + T_{\text{I,II}}\xi_\text{II} + I_\text{I} \quad (\text{M}_{d\xi})$$

where
$$x_{\mathrm{I}} = \left(x_{\mu(1)}, \cdots, x_{\mu(m)}\right)^T, \quad x_{\mathrm{II}} = \left(x_{\mu(m+1)}, \cdots, x_{\mu(n)}\right)^T$$
and
$$-1 < x_{\mu(i)} < 1, \text{ for } 1 \leq i \leq m.$$

System ($\mathrm{M_{d\xi}}$) is said to be the *reduced linear system* of system ($\mathrm{M_d}$) over the region $C(\xi)$.

2) For any $\xi \in \Lambda_m$, a function $\varphi\colon \{0, 1, \cdots, k_0\} \to C(\xi)$, is said to be a (*local*) *solution* of system ($\mathrm{M_d}$) if the vector function φ_{I} containing the $\mu(i)$-th components of φ, $1 \leq i \leq m$, is a solution of the linear system ($\mathrm{M_\xi}$), i.e.,

$$\varphi_{\mathrm{I}}(k+1) = T_{\mathrm{I,I}}\varphi_{\mathrm{I}}(k) + T_{\mathrm{I,II}}\xi_{\mathrm{II}} + I_{\mathrm{I}}, \ k \in \{0, 1, \cdots, k_0\} \quad (4.6.1)$$

and

$$\min\left((T_{\mathrm{II,I}}\varphi_{\mathrm{I}}(k) + T_{\mathrm{II,II}}\xi_{\mathrm{II}} + I_{\mathrm{II}}) * \xi_{\mathrm{II}}\right) \geq 1, \ k \in \{0, 1, \cdots, k_0\} \quad (4.6.2)$$

where
$$\varphi_{\mathrm{I}} = \left(\varphi_{\mu(1)}, \cdots, \varphi_{\mu(m)}\right)^T$$
and
$$\varphi_{\mathrm{II}} = \left(\varphi_{\mu(m+1)}, \cdots, \varphi_{\mu(n)}\right)^T.$$

In particular, if $\xi \in \Lambda_m$, $m < n$, the solution φ is said to be in a *saturated mode*. ∎

Remark 4.6.1 1) $\varphi(\{0, 1, \cdots, k_0\}) \subset C(\xi)$ implies that
$$-1 < \varphi_{\mu(i)}(k) < 1, \ i = 1, \cdots, m, \ k \in \{0, 1, \cdots, k_0\}$$
$$\varphi_{\mu(i)}(k) = \xi_{\mu(i)}, \ i = m+1, \cdots, n, \ k \in \{0, 1, \cdots, k_0\}$$
i.e.,
$$\varphi_{\mathrm{II}}(k) = \xi_{\mathrm{II}} \text{ when } k \in \{0, 1, \cdots, k_0\}.$$

2) When $m = n$, $\Lambda_n = \{0\}$. In this case, (4.6.2) has no meaning and we only need to consider (4.6.1). Furthermore, the (local)

4.6. DISCRETE-TIME SYSTEMS

solutions in $C(0) = (D^n)^\circ = \{x \in \Re^n : -1 < x_i < 1,\ i = 1, \cdots, n\}$ defined above for system (M_d) will be identical to the usual solutions defined on the open subset $C(0)$ for the linear system (M_d).

3) When $m = 0$, $\Lambda_0 = B^n$ and for $\xi \in \Lambda_0$, $C(\xi) = \{\xi\}$. In this case, (4.6.1) does not exist and we only need to consider (4.6.2). Furthermore, the only function with the range in $C(\xi)$ is the constant function $\varphi(k) \equiv \xi$. ∎

We are now in a position to make the following definition.

Definition 4.6.2 For $x_0 \in D^n$, a function $\varphi = \varphi(\cdot, x_0) \colon Z^+ \to D^n$ is said to be a *solution of* (M_d) *starting at* x_0 if

a) $\varphi(0, x_0) = x_0$, and

b) there are countably many sets $E_i = \{l_i, \cdots, l_i + k_i\}$, $l_i \in Z^+$, $k_i \in Z^+$, $l_0 = 0$ such that $E_i \cap E_j = \emptyset$ when $i \neq j$, and $\cup E_i = Z^+$, and $\varphi(k)$ restricted to each E_i is a (local) solution as defined in Definition 4.6.1. ∎

Similarly as in the case of continuous-time linear systems defined on a hypercube, we define various notions of stability of an equilibrium for system (M_d) in the following manner.

Definition 4.6.3

1) A vector $x_e \in D^n$ is said to be an *equilibrium* of system (M_d) if the function $\varphi = \varphi(\cdot, x_e) \colon Z^+ \to D^n$ defined by $\varphi(k, x_e) \equiv x_e$ is a solution of (M_d).

2) Let x_e be an equilibrium point of system (M_d). Then

   i) x_e is said to be *stable* if for every $\varepsilon > 0$, there is a $\delta = \delta(\varepsilon) > 0$ such that $|\varphi(k, x) - x_e| < \varepsilon$, for all $k \in Z^+$ whenever $|x - x_e| < \delta$;

   ii) x_e is said to be *asymptotically stable* if it is stable and if there is an $\eta > 0$ such that $\lim_{k \to \infty} |\varphi(k, x) - x_e| = 0$ whenever $|x - x_e| < \eta$; and

   iii) x_e is said to be *unstable* if it is not stable. ∎

We will have occasion to make use of the following assumptions for system (M$_d$).

Assumption 4.6.1

1) T is symmetric.
2) For any m, $0 \leq m \leq n$, and for any $\xi \in \Lambda_m$, the $m \times m$ matrix $(E_m - T_{I,I}) = (E_m - T_{\mu(i)\mu(j)})$, $1 \leq i, j \leq m$ is nonsingular, where E_m is the $m \times m$ identity matrix, and $\mu \in \text{Sym}(n)$, such that $\xi_{\mu(i)} = 0$, $1 \leq i \leq m$, and $\xi_{\mu(i)} = \pm 1$, $m < i \leq n$. ∎

For system (M$_d$) satisfying Assumption 4.6.1, we introduce the following notation.

I. For $\xi = 0 \in \Lambda_n$, let

$$x_\xi = Tx_\xi + I \in \Re^n \text{ or } x_\xi = (E_n - T)^{-1} I \quad (4.6.3)$$

where E_n denotes the $n \times n$ identity matrix.

II. For $\xi \in \Lambda_m$, $0 < m < n$ and with $T_{I,I}, \cdots, T_{II,II}$, I_I, I_{II} defined as in (4.6.1) and (4.6.2), let

$$x_\xi = (x_{\xi 1}, \cdots, x_{\xi n})^T \in \Re^n \quad (4.6.4)$$

where

$$x_{\xi I} = \left(x_{\xi \mu(1)}, \cdots, x_{\xi \mu(m)}\right)^T = (E_m - T_{I,I})^{-1}(T_{I,II}\xi_{II} + I_I)$$

$$x_{\xi II} = \left(x_{\xi \mu(m+1)}, \cdots, x_{\xi \mu(n)}\right)^T = \xi_{II}$$

and let

$$r_\xi \in \Re, \; r_\xi = \min\left((T_{II,I}x_{\xi I} + T_{II,II}\xi_{II} + I_{II}) * \xi_{II}\right). \quad (4.6.5)$$

III. For $\xi \in \Lambda_0 = B^n$, $C(\xi) = \{\xi\}$, let

$$x_\xi = \xi \quad (4.6.6)$$

and

$$r_\xi \in \Re, \; r_\xi = \min((T\xi + I) * \xi). \quad (4.6.7)$$

4.6. DISCRETE-TIME SYSTEMS

Assumption 4.6.2 Given Assumption 4.6.1, we assume that for $\xi \in \Lambda_m$, $0 \leq m < n$, $x_\xi \notin \partial C(\xi)$, i.e., $x_{\xi\mu(i)} \neq \pm 1$, for $i = 1, \cdots, m$. ∎

Remark 4.6.2 For fixed T, Assumption 4.6.2 is true for almost all vectors I in $\Re^n$. ∎

Lemma 4.6.1 Suppose that system (M_d) satisfies Assumptions 4.6.1 and 4.6.2. Then, for any $\xi \in \Lambda_m$, $0 \leq m < n$, $r_\xi \neq 1$.

Proof: Suppose that for some $\xi \in \Lambda_m$, $0 < m < n$, $r_\xi = 1$. Then from the notation given in (4.6.3)–(4.6.7), there is j, $1 \leq j \leq n - m$, such that the jth component of the vector $(T_{\text{II},\text{I}} x_{\xi\text{I}} + T_{\text{II},\text{II}} \xi_{\text{II}} + I_{\text{II}})$ is equal to ± 1. Without loss of generality, assume that $j = 1$. Take $\zeta \in \Lambda_{m+1}$ where $\zeta_{\mu(i)} = 0$ for $1 \leq i \leq m+1$ and $\zeta_{\mu(i)} = \xi_{\mu(i)}$ for $m+1 < i \leq n$. Then $x_\xi = x_\zeta \in \partial C(\xi)$ and this contradicts Assumption 4.6.2. Suppose that for some $\xi \in \Lambda_0$, $r_\xi = 1$. Then we can arrive at a contradiction in the same manner. ∎

Theorem 4.6.1 Suppose that (M_d) satisfies Assumptions 4.6.1 and 4.6.2. Then for any m, $0 \leq m \leq n$, and for any $\xi \in \Lambda_m$, with the notation given above, we have the following results:

Case I: $m = n$, $\xi = 0 \in \Lambda_n$.

1) If $x_\xi \notin C(\xi) = (D^n)^\circ$, there is no equilibrium point of system (M_d) in $(D^n)^\circ$.

2) If $x_\xi \in C(\xi) = (D^n)^\circ$, x_ξ is the unique equilibrium point of system (M_d) in $(D^n)^\circ$. In particular,
   i) if the eigenvalues of $T = T_{\text{I},\text{I}}$ satisfy $|\lambda_i| < 1$, $i = 1, \cdots, n$, then x_ξ is asymptotically stable and there are no other equilibrium points of system (M_d) in $\overline{C(\xi)} = D^n$; and
   ii) if there is at least one i such that $|\lambda_i| \geq 1$, then x_ξ is unstable.

Case II: $0 < m < n$, $\xi \in \Lambda_m$.

A) If $r_\xi < 1$, there is no equilibrium point of system (M_d) in $C(\xi)$.

B) If $r_\xi > 1$, we have that
1) if $x_\xi \notin C(\xi)$, there is no equilibrium point of system (M$_d$) in $C(\xi)$.
2) if $x_\xi \in C(\xi)$, x_ξ is the unique equilibrium point of system (M$_d$) in $C(\xi)$. In particular,
   i) if the eigenvalues of $T_{I,I}$ satisfy $|\lambda_i| < 1$, $i = 1,\cdots,m$, then x_ξ is asymptotically stable, and there are no other equilibrium points in $\overline{C(\xi)}$; and
   ii) if there is at least one i such that $|\lambda_i| \geq 1$, then x_ξ is unstable.

Case III: $\xi \in \Lambda_0 = B^n$. (Note: $C(\xi) = \{\xi\}$.)

A) If $r_\xi < 1$, $x_\xi = \xi$ is not an equilibrium point of (M$_d$).

B) If $r_\xi > 1$, $x_\xi = \xi$ is an asymptotically stable equilibrium point of system (M$_d$).

Proof: Case I: In this case, $\xi = 0$ and $C(\xi) = (D^n)°$, and from Definition 4.6.2, solutions of (M$_d$) on $C(0)$ are identical to solutions of (M$_d$) on $C(0)$ in the usual sense. Then the conclusions of Case I of the theorem follow directly from the theory of linear difference equations.

Case II: Consider $\xi \in \Lambda_m$, $0 < m < n$, and a constant function $\varphi \colon Z^+ \to C(\xi)$, $\varphi(k) = \tilde{x}$. If $\tilde{x}$ is an equilibrium point of (M$_d$) in $C(\xi)$, then by Definition 4.6.1, we have that

$$\tilde{x}_I = T_{I,I}\tilde{x}_I + T_{I,II}\xi_{II} + I_I$$

or

$$\tilde{x}_I = (E_m - T_{I,I})^{-1}(T_{I,II}\xi_{II} + I_I) = x_{\xi I}$$

and

$$\min\Big((T_{II,I}\tilde{x}_I + T_{II,II}\xi_{II} + I_{II}) * \xi_{II}\Big) \geq 1.$$

Since $\tilde{x} \in C(\xi)$, then $\tilde{x}_{II} = \xi_{II}$ and $x_\xi = \tilde{x} \in C(\xi)$. Also, $r_\xi \geq 1$ and by Lemma 4.6.1, $r_\xi > 1$. Thus, if $\tilde{x}$ is an equilibrium point of (M$_d$) in $C(\xi)$, then $\tilde{x} = x_\xi$ and $r_\xi > 1$.

4.6. DISCRETE-TIME SYSTEMS

On the other hand, if $x_\xi \in C(\xi)$ and $r_\xi > 1$, let $\varphi: Z^+ \to C(\xi)$ and $\varphi(k) = x_\xi$. Then φ satisfies (4.6.1) and (4.6.2). By Definition 4.6.1, φ is a solution of (M_d) and by Definition 4.6.3, $\varphi \equiv x_\xi$ is an equilibrium point of (M_d) in $C(\xi)$. Then, if $x_\xi \in C(\xi)$ and $r_\xi > 1$, $\varphi(k) \equiv x_\xi$ is an equilibrium point of (M_d) in $C(\xi)$.

Therefore, if $r_\xi > 1$ and $x_\xi \in C(\xi)$, then x_ξ is the unique equilibrium point of system (M_d) in $C(\xi)$. If $r_\xi < 1$, then clearly there is no equilibrium point of system (M_d) in $C(\xi)$. Also, if $r_\xi > 1$ and $x_\xi \notin C(\xi)$, then it is clear that there is no equilibrium of system (M_d) in $C(\xi)$.

Now suppose that x_ξ is an equilibrium point of (M_d). There is an open neighborhood U of x_ξ in $\Re^n$ such that

$$\min\Big((T_{\mathbb{II},\mathbb{I}}x_\mathbb{I} + T_{\mathbb{II},\mathbb{II}}\xi_\mathbb{II} + I_\mathbb{II}) * \xi_\mathbb{II}\Big) > 1$$

for all $x \in U \cap D^n$. If the eigenvalues of $T_{\mathbb{I},\mathbb{I}}$ satisfy $|\lambda_i| < 1$, $i = 1, \cdots, m$, then it can be proved by induction and by the theory of linear difference equations that all solutions of (M_d) starting in $U \cap D^n$ will monotonically converge to x_ξ as $k \to \infty$. Thus, x_ξ is an asymptotically stable equilibrium point of (M_d). On the other hand, if there is at least one i such that $|\lambda_i| \geq 1$, there is a $\delta_0 > 0$ such that $B(x_\xi, \delta_0) \cap D^n \subset U \cap D^n$, and for any $\varepsilon, 0 < \varepsilon < \delta_0$, there is a function $\varphi: \{0, \cdots, k_u\} \to C(\xi) \cap U$, $k_u \leq k_0$, such that $\varphi(0) \in C(\xi) \cap B(x_\xi, \varepsilon)$, $|\varphi(k_u) - x_\xi| > \delta_0$, and $\varphi_\mathbb{I}$ is a solution of the linear system $(M_{d\xi})$. Since $\varphi(\{0, \cdots, k_u\}) \subset U$, $\varphi_\mathbb{II}$ satisfies (4.6.2) and φ is a solution of system (M_d). Thus, x_ξ is an unstable equilibrium point of (M_d) by Definition 4.6.3.

Finally, for the purpose of contradiction, assume that x_ξ is an asymptotically stable equilibrium point of (M_d) and assume that x_ζ is another equilibrium point of (M_d) in $\overline{C(\xi)}$. Since x_ξ is the unique equilibrium point of (M_d) in $C(\xi)$, we must have $x_\zeta \in \overline{C(\xi)} - C(\xi)$. Then there is a k, $1 \leq k \leq m$, such that $\zeta_{\mu(k)} = 1$ or -1. By the theory of linear difference equations, the $\mu(k)$-th component of $Tx_\zeta + I$ starting at x_ζ points to x_ξ. Thus, $(Tx_\zeta + I)_{\mu(k)} * \zeta_{\mu(k)} < 1$ and $r_\zeta < 1$. This contradiction shows that x_ξ is the only equilibrium point of (M_d) in $\overline{C(\xi)}$.

138   CHAPTER 4.   LINEAR SYSTEMS ON A HYPERCUBE

Case III: If $r_\xi < 1$, $\varphi \equiv x_\xi$ does not satisfy (4.6.2) and x_ξ is not a solution of (M_d). If $r_\xi > 1$, then there is an open neighborhood U of x_ξ in $\Re^n$ such that

$$\min\bigl((T_{\mathbb{I},\mathbb{I}} x_\mathbb{I} + T_{\mathbb{I},\mathbb{II}} \xi_\mathbb{II} + I_\mathbb{I}) * \xi_\mathbb{II}\bigr) > 1$$

for all $x \in U \cap D^n$. It can be proved by induction and by the theory of linear difference equations that all solutions of (M_d) starting in $U \cap D^n$ will monotonically converge to x_ξ as $k \to \infty$. Thus, x_ξ is an asymptotically stable equilibrium point of (M_d) by Definition 4.6.3.

This concludes the proof of Theorem 4.6.1. ∎

Remark 4.6.3 1) Theorem 4.6.1 establishes an algorithm to locate all equilibrium points of (M_d) and to determine the stability properties of all equilibrium points.

2) In practice, due to noise, unstable equilibrium points cannot be used as memory locations. However, by investigating the locations of the unstable equilibrium points of (M_d), the domain of attraction of each asymptotically stable equilibrium point of (M_d) can be approximately determined.

3) If for some $\xi \in \Lambda$, the corresponding $T_{I,I}$ is singular, Theorem 4.6.1 can still be applied to other vectors in Λ. If Lemma 4.6.1 is not true, we need to consider the case $r_\xi = 1$. In fact, we can study this case using the same method as was employed in Theorem 4.6.1. In this case, the conclusions might be less straightforward. ∎

Theorem 4.6.2 If system (M_d) satisfies Assumptions 4.6.1 and 4.6.2, we have the following results.

1) There is at most one equilibrium point of (M_d) in each region $C(\xi)$, $\xi \in \Lambda$.

2) There are at most 3^n equilibrium points for system (M_d).

3) If for $\xi \in \Lambda$ the corresponding x_ξ is an asymptotically stable equilibrium point for system (M_d), then

   i) x_ξ is the unique equilibrium point of system (M_d) in $\overline{C(\xi)}$, and

4.6. DISCRETE-TIME SYSTEMS

ii) x_ξ is the unique asymptotically stable equilibrium point of system (M_d) in $\overline{C(\xi)} \cup C(\zeta)$, where $\zeta \in \Lambda$ such that $x_\xi \in \overline{C(\zeta)}$. In particular, if $\xi \in \Lambda_0 = B^n$ and $x_\xi = \xi$ is an asymptotically stable equilibrium point of system (M_d), then $x_\xi = \xi$ is the unique asymptotically stable equilibrium of system (M_d) in the region $\{x \in D^n: -1 < x_i\xi_i \leq 1,\ 1 \leq i \leq n\}$.

4) There are at most 2^n asymptotically stable equilibrium points for system (M_d).

Proof: Part 1 follows from Theorem 4.6.1. Part 2 follows from the fact that D^n is separated into 3^n regions by $C(\xi)$, $\xi \in \Lambda$. Part 3 has been proved in Theorem 4.6.1. Part 4 follows from Part 3. ∎

Remark 4.6.4 Theorem 4.6.2 is not only very useful to simplify the algorithm given in Theorem 4.6.1 for checking the locations of equilibrium points of system (M_d), but it is also useful to determine whether a given set of vectors can be synthesized as a set of asymptotically stable equilibria of system (M_d) or not (cf. [14]). ∎

Definition 4.6.4 If T is symmetric, then

1) the *energy function* $E\colon D^n \to \Re$ of system (M_d) is defined by

$$E(x) = -x^T(T - E_n)x - 2x^T I, \qquad (4.6.8)$$

where E_n is the $n \times n$ identity matrix, and

2) $x \in D^n$ is said to be a *(local) minimum* of the energy function E if there is an open neighborhood U of x in $\Re^n$ such that $E(x) \leq E(y)$, for any $y \in D^n \cap U$. ∎

Theorem 4.6.3 Suppose that system (M_d) satisfies Assumptions 4.6.1 and 4.6.2, and all the eigenvalues of system (M_d) satisfy $\lambda_i > -1$, $i = 1, \cdots, n$. Then it is true that

1) along nonequilibrium solutions of system (M_d), the energy function E given in (4.6.8) decreases monotonically; and

2) each nonequilibrium solution of (M_d) converges to an equilibrium point of (M_d).

Proof: 1) It is sufficient to consider the proof for local solutions of (M_d) as defined in Definition 4.6.1. Consider a nonconstant local solution of (M_d) given by $\varphi: \{l_i, \cdots, l_i + k_i\} \to C(\xi)$, $\xi \in \Lambda_m$. With the notation given above, we have, for $k = l_i, \cdots, l_i + k_i$,

$$E(k) = -\varphi(k)^T(T - E_n)\varphi(k) - 2\varphi(k)^T I$$
$$= -\varphi(k)^T T\varphi(k) + \varphi(k)^T \varphi(k) - 2\varphi(k)^T I.$$

Since T is symmetric, we can find an orthonormal matrix P such that $T = P^T Q P$, where $P^T = P^{-1}$, Q is a diagonal matrix, i.e., $Q = \text{diag}\{\lambda_1, \cdots, \lambda_n\}$. Hence, we have

$$\varphi(k+1) = T\varphi(k) + I = P^{-1}QP\varphi(k) + I.$$

Let

$$P\varphi(k) = \psi(k), \ PI = J.$$

Then

$$\psi(k+1) = Q\psi(k) + J,$$

or equivalently,

$$\psi_i(k+1) = \lambda_i \psi_i(k) + J_i, \quad i = 1, \cdots, n.$$

Then,

$$E(k) = -\varphi(k)^T P^T Q P \varphi(k) + \varphi(k)^T P^T P \varphi(k) - 2\varphi(k)^T P^T P I$$
$$= -\psi(k)^T Q \psi(k) + \psi(k)^T \psi(k) - 2\psi(k)^T J$$
$$= -\sum_{i=1}^{m} \lambda_{\mu(i)} \psi_{\mu(i)}(k)^2 + \sum_{i=1}^{m} \psi_{\mu(i)}(k)^2 - 2\sum_{i=1}^{m} J_{\mu(i)} \psi_{\mu(i)}(k)$$
$$- \sum_{i=m+1}^{n} \lambda_{\mu(i)} \psi_{\mu(i)}(k)^2 + \sum_{i=m+1}^{n} \psi_{\mu(i)}(k)^2$$
$$- 2\sum_{i=m+1}^{n} J_{\mu(i)} \psi_{\mu(i)}(k)$$

4.6. DISCRETE-TIME SYSTEMS

where $\psi_{\mathrm{II}}(k) = (\psi_{\mu(m+1)}(k), \cdots, \psi_{\mu(n)}(k))^T = \xi_{\mathrm{II}}$,

$$\begin{aligned}
E(k+1) - E(k) &= -\sum_{i=1}^{m} \lambda_{\mu(i)}[\psi_{\mu(i)}(k+1)^2 - \psi_{\mu(i)}(k)^2] \\
&\quad + \sum_{i=1}^{m}[\psi_{\mu(i)}(k+1)^2 - \psi_{\mu(i)}(k)^2] \\
&\quad - 2\sum_{i=1}^{m} J_{\mu(i)}[\psi_{\mu(i)}(k+1) - \psi_{\mu(i)}(k)] \\
&= -\sum_{i=1}^{m} \Big\{[\lambda_{\mu(i)}\psi_{\mu(i)}(k+1) + \lambda_{\mu(i)}\psi_{\mu(i)}(k)] \\
&\quad -[\psi_{\mu(i)}(k+1) + \psi_{\mu(i)}(k)] + 2J_{\mu(i)}\Big\} \\
&\quad \cdot [\psi_{\mu(i)}(k+1) - \psi_{\mu(i)}(k)] \\
&= -\sum_{i=1}^{m} \Big\{\psi_{\mu(i)}(k+2) + \psi_{\mu(i)}(k+1) - \psi_{\mu(i)}(k+1) \\
&\quad - \psi_{\mu(i)}(k)\Big\}[\psi_{\mu(i)}(k+1) - \psi_{\mu(i)}(k)] \\
&= -\sum_{i=1}^{m} \Big\{\lambda_{\mu(i)}[\psi_{\mu(i)}(k+1) - \psi_{\mu(i)}(k)] \\
&\quad + [\psi_{\mu(i)}(k+1) - \psi_{\mu(i)}(k)]\Big\} \\
&\quad \cdot [\psi_{\mu(i)}(k+1) - \psi_{\mu(i)}(k)] \\
&= -\sum_{i=1}^{m}(\lambda_i + 1)[\psi_{\mu(i)}(k+1) - \psi_{\mu(i)}(k)]^2 \\
&\leq 0
\end{aligned}$$

since $\lambda_i > -1$ by assumption. Moreover, $E(k+1) - E(k) = 0$ only at equilibrium points of $(\mathrm{M_d})$.

2) The proof of Part 2 of the theorem follows from the theory of ordinary difference equations (see, e.g., [15]). ∎

Remark 4.6.5 1) Theorem 4.6.3 shows that system $(\mathrm{M_d})$ has no oscillatory solutions.

2) In practice, due to noise, all solutions of system $(\mathrm{M_d})$ will only converge to asymptotically stable equilibrium points of $(\mathrm{M_d})$. ∎

Theorem 4.6.4 Suppose that system $(\mathrm{M_d})$ satisfies all assumptions of Theorems 4.6.1 and 4.6.3. Then there is a one-to-one correspondence between the set of local minima of the energy function E and the set of asymptotically stable equilibrium points of system $(\mathrm{M_d})$.

142　CHAPTER 4.　LINEAR SYSTEMS ON A HYPERCUBE

Proof: Suppose that $\tilde{x}$ is an asymptotically stable equilibrium point of system (M_d). Then there is an open neighborhood U of $\tilde{x}$ in $\Re^n$ such that all solutions of (M_d) starting in $U \cap D^n$ will converge to $\tilde{x}$ as $k \to \infty$. Since along any solution φ, the value of the energy function E decreases monotonically in k and the energy function E is continuous in x, we have that $E(\tilde{x}) < E(x)$ for $x \in U \cap D^n$. Thus $\tilde{x}$ is a local minimum of E.

On the other hand, suppose that $\tilde{x}$ is a local minimum of the energy function E. Then there is an open neighborhood U of $\tilde{x}$ in $\Re^n$ such that $E(\tilde{x}) \leq E(x)$, $x \in U \cap D^n$. By Theorem 4.6.3, $\tilde{x}$ is an equilibrium point of system (M_d). If $\tilde{x}$ is not asymptotically stable, then by assumption, it is unstable. Thus, there is a $\delta_0 > 0$ such that $B(\tilde{x}, \delta_0) \subset U$ and for any ε, $0 < \varepsilon < \delta_0$, there is a solution φ of (M_d) starting in $B(\tilde{x}, \varepsilon) \cap D^n$ which tends towards the exterior of $B(\tilde{x}, \delta_0) \cap D^n$. Since along solution φ, the energy function E decreases monotonically, we have that $E(\tilde{x}) > E(x_0)$ for some point $x_0 \in (\partial B(\tilde{x}, \delta_0)) \cap D^n \subset U \cap D^n$. This contradiction shows that $\tilde{x}$ is an asymptotically stable equilibrium point of system (M_d).　∎

Remark 4.6.6 Without $\lambda_i > -1$, $i = 1, \cdots, n$, we can not guarantee the global stability of system (M_d). As an example, let us consider the following system

$$\begin{cases} x_1(k+1) = -2x_1(k) + x_2(k) + 0.1 \\ x_2(k+1) = x_1(k) - 2x_2(k) + 0.1 \end{cases}$$

i.e.,

$$T = \begin{bmatrix} -2 & 1 \\ 1 & -2 \end{bmatrix}, \quad I = \begin{bmatrix} 0.1 \\ 0.1 \end{bmatrix}.$$

The eigenvalues of T are -1 and -3.

Using equations (4.6.3)–(4.6.7), we can find x_ξ's as

I. $m = 0$, $x_\xi = \begin{bmatrix} 0.05 \\ 0.05 \end{bmatrix}$.

II. $m = 1$,

$$x_{\xi 1} = \begin{bmatrix} 0.367 \\ 1 \end{bmatrix}, \quad x_{\xi 2} = \begin{bmatrix} -0.3 \\ -1 \end{bmatrix}, \quad x_{\xi 3} = \begin{bmatrix} 1 \\ 0.367 \end{bmatrix}, \quad x_{\xi 4} = \begin{bmatrix} -1 \\ -0.3 \end{bmatrix}.$$

4.6. DISCRETE-TIME SYSTEMS

III. $m = 2$,

$$x_{\xi 1} = \begin{bmatrix} 1 \\ 1 \end{bmatrix}, \ x_{\xi 2} = \begin{bmatrix} -1 \\ -1 \end{bmatrix}, \ x_{\xi 3} = \begin{bmatrix} 1 \\ -1 \end{bmatrix}, \ x_{\xi 4} = \begin{bmatrix} -1 \\ 1 \end{bmatrix}.$$

By Theorem 4.6.1,

Case I, when $m = 0$,

$$x_\xi = \begin{bmatrix} 0.05 \\ 0.05 \end{bmatrix}$$

is not an asymptotically stable equilibrium point.

Case II, when $m = 1$,

$$x_{\xi 1} = \begin{bmatrix} 0.367 \\ 1 \end{bmatrix},$$

we have $r_{\xi 1} = -1.533 < 1$, and $x_{\xi 1}$ is not asymptotically stable. For

$$x_{\xi 2} = \begin{bmatrix} -0.3 \\ -1 \end{bmatrix}, \ r_{\xi 2} = -1.533 < 1;$$

$$x_{\xi 3} = \begin{bmatrix} 1 \\ 0.367 \end{bmatrix}, \ r_{\xi 3} = -1.533 < 1;$$

$$x_{\xi 4} = \begin{bmatrix} -1 \\ -0.3 \end{bmatrix}; \ r_{\xi 4} = -1.8 < 1.$$

Thus $x_{\xi 2}$, $x_{\xi 3}$, and $x_{\xi 4}$ are not asymptotically stable either.

Case III, when $m = 2$,

$$x_{\xi 1} = \begin{bmatrix} 1 \\ 1 \end{bmatrix}, \ x_{\xi 2} = \begin{bmatrix} -1 \\ -1 \end{bmatrix}, \ x_{\xi 3} = \begin{bmatrix} 1 \\ -1 \end{bmatrix}, \ x_{\xi 4} = \begin{bmatrix} -1 \\ 1 \end{bmatrix}.$$

Correspondingly, we have, $r_{\xi 1} = -0.9 < 1$, $r_{\xi 2} = -1.1 < 1$, $r_{\xi 3} = -4.1 < 1$, $r_{\xi 4} = -3.1 < 1$. Thus $x_{\xi 1}$, $x_{\xi 2}$, $x_{\xi 3}$, and $x_{\xi 4}$ are not asymptotically stable equilibrium points.

In simulations of this system, none of the initial conditions within the unit square converged. ∎

4.7 Global Asymptotic Stability of Linear Continuous-Time Systems Operating on a Closed Hypercube

In addition to associative memories, recurrent neural networks have also been applied, e.g., in optimization problems (cf. [5], [17]). In such cases, it is usually required that the network possess only one equilibrium which is globally asymptotically stable.

In the present section we will address the global asymptotic stability of linear continuous-time systems operating on a closed hypercube. To this end, we will assume without loss of generality that $I = 0$ and, to be consistent with the notation used in the literature, we let $T = A$. Then (M) assumes the form

$$\frac{dx}{dt} = Ax \tag{4.7.1}$$

with the constraints

$$-1 \leq x_i \leq 1, \ i = 1, \cdots, n.$$

This system can equivalently be expressed as

$$\dot{x}(t) = h(Ax(t)) \tag{4.7.2}$$

where $x \in D^n$, $A = [a_{ij}] \in \Re^{n \times n}$, $\dot{x} = dx/dt$, $t \geq 0$,

$$h(Ax) = \left[h_1\left(\sum_{j=1}^{n} a_{1j}x_j\right), \cdots, h_n\left(\sum_{j=1}^{n} a_{nj}x_j\right) \right]^T \tag{4.7.3}$$

and

$$h_i\left(\sum_{j=1}^{n} a_{ij}x_j\right) = \begin{cases} 0, & |x_i| = 1 \text{ and } \left(\sum_{j=1}^{n} a_{ij}x_j\right)x_i \geq 0 \\ \sum_{j=1}^{n} a_{ij}x_j, & \text{otherwise.} \end{cases} \tag{4.7.4}$$

Since for system (4.7.2), $x \in D^n$ such that $h(Ax) = 0$ is an equilibrium, we note that in particular, $x = 0$, the trivial solution, is

4.7. CONTINUOUS-TIME RESULTS

an equilibrium of this system. Consistent with the definitions given in Section 3.2C, the following applies in the present case.

(i) The equilibrium $x = 0$ of (4.7.2) is *stable* if for every $\varepsilon > 0$ there is a $\delta = \delta(\varepsilon) > 0$ such that $|\varphi(t,x)| < \varepsilon$ for all $t \in [0, \infty)$ whenever $|x| < \delta$.

(ii) The equilibrium $x = 0$ of (4.7.2) is *asymptotically stable* if it is stable and there is an $\eta > 0$ such that $\lim_{t \to \infty} |\varphi(t,x)| = 0$ whenever $|x| < \eta$.

(iii) The equilibrium $x = 0$ of (4.7.2) is *globally asymptotically stable* if it is stable and if $\lim_{t \to \infty} |\varphi(t,x)| = 0$ whenever $x \in D^n$.

Also, we note that, in particular, Lemma 3.2.4 (see Section 3.2C) applies to system (4.7.4).

Returning now to the subject on hand, we first note that in order for the equilibrium $x = 0$ of system (4.7.2) to be globally asymptotically stable, it is *necessary* that A be Hurwitz stable (i.e., that all eigenvalues of A be in the left half of the complex plane). Accordingly, we will assume throughout this section that A is Hurwitz stable.

In the following, we will employ continuously differentiable Lyapunov functions $v : D^n \to \Re$ which satisfy the following hypotheses:

(A–1) v is positive definite on D^n,

$$\nabla v(x) = \left[\frac{\partial v(x)}{\partial x_1}, \ldots, \frac{\partial v(x)}{\partial x_n}\right]^T$$

exists for all $x \in D^n$, and $\nabla v(x)^T A x$ is negative definite on D^n. ∎

(A–2) For all $x \in D^n$ it is true that

$$\nabla v(x)^T h(Ax) \leq \nabla v(x)^T Ax. \qquad \blacksquare$$

To simplify our subsequent notation, we will let $\varphi(t, x_0, t_0) \triangleq x(t)$ denote a solution of (4.7.2), with $t_0 \geq 0$ and $x(t_0) = x_0 \in D^n$

146   CHAPTER 4. LINEAR SYSTEMS ON A HYPERCUBE

given. Since we are dealing with autonomous systems, we let without loss of generality $t_0 = 0$.

Theorem 4.7.1 The equilibrium $x = 0$ of system (4.7.2) is globally asymptotically stable if there exists a function v which satisfies Assumptions (A–1) and (A–2).

Proof: In view of Theorem 4.3.1 and Remark 4.3.3, $h(Ax(t))$ is continuous from the right with respect to t in the sense that $\lim_{t \to t_1, t > t_1} h(Ax(t)) = h(Ax(t_1))$ for any t_1. Therefore, along the solutions of system (4.7.2), the right-hand derivative of $v(x(t))$, given by

$$\dot{v}(t) \stackrel{\triangle}{=} D_{(4.7.2)}v(x(t)) = \nabla v(x(t))^T h\big(A(x(t))\big)$$

exists for all $t \geq t_0$. Now by Assumption (A–2), we have

$$D_{(4.7.2)}v(x(t)) \leq \nabla v(x(t))^T Ax(t) < 0$$

for all $x(t) \in D^n - \{0\}$. This shows that $x = 0$ is the only equilibrium of system (4.7.2).

We next show that $x = 0$ is asymptotically stable. It follows from (A–1) that v is positive definite and from (A–1) and (A–2) that $D_{(4.7.2)}v(x)$ is negative definite on D^n. Thus, there exist two functions $\psi_i: [0,1] \to \Re$ in class $\mathcal{K}$ such that $v(0) = 0$ and $v(x) \geq \psi_1(|x|)$ for all $x \in D^n$ and $D_{(4.7.2)}v(x) \leq \nabla v(x)^T Ax \leq -\psi_2(|x|)$ for all $x \in D^n$. It follows from Lemma 3.2.4 (see Section 3.2C) that the equilibrium $x = 0$ of system (4.7.2) is asymptotically stable.

To conclude the proof, we show that $x = 0$ is globally asymptotically stable. First, since $x = 0$ is asymptotically stable, we note that there exists $d > 0$ such that $|x(t)| < 1/2$ for all $t \geq t_0 \geq 0$ whenever $|x(0)| < d$ and $\lim_{t \to \infty} |x(t)| = 0$. Now let x_0 denote *any* initial point in D^n for the solution $x(t) = \varphi(t, x_0, 0)$. Then there must exist $t_1 > 0$ such that $|x(t_1)| < d$, and hence, $|x(t)| < 1/2$ for all $t \geq t_1$ and $\lim_{t \to \infty} |x(t)| = 0$; for otherwise, we must have $|x(t)| \geq d$ for all t, and then

$$v(x(t)) = v(x(0)) + \int_0^t D_{(4.7.2)}v(x(\tau))d\tau$$

4.7. CONTINUOUS-TIME RESULTS

$$\leq v(x(0)) - \int_0^t \psi_2(|x(\tau)|)d\tau$$

$$\leq v(x(0)) - t\psi_2(d)$$

and when t is sufficiently large, $v(x(t)) < 0$. But this is a contradiction, since by Assumption (A–1), $v(x(t)) \geq 0$.

We have shown that $x = 0$ of system (4.7.2) is asymptotically stable and the domain of attraction of $x = 0$ is all of D^n. ∎

In [6] and [10] it is shown by the use of specific examples that Assumption (A–1) (i.e., that A is stable) is *not sufficient* for the equilibrium $x = 0$ to be globally asymptotically stable, although it is obviously sufficient for the equilibrium to be (locally) asymptotically stable.

When system (4.7.2) operates in an *unsaturated mode*, it is described by the system of equations $\dot{x} = Ax$. It is well known that the equilibrium $x_e = 0$ of this system is asymptotically stable if and only if for every symmetric positive definite matrix $Q = [q_{ij}] \in \Re^{n \times n}$ there exists a symmetric positive definite matrix $P = [p_{ij}] \in \Re^{n \times n}$ such that

$$PA + A^T P = -Q. \tag{4.7.5}$$

This result is usually proved by utilizing a quadratic Lyapunov function of the form

$$v(x) = x^T P x \tag{4.7.6}$$

(refer, e.g., to [16]).

The above result suggests that an excellent choice of a Lyapunov function for the stability analysis of system (4.7.2) is a function of the form (4.7.6) which satisfies Assumption (A–1) and (A–2) of Theorem 4.7.1.

Theorem 4.7.2 Assume that there exist two symmetric positive definite matrices $P \in \Re^{n \times n}$ and $Q \in \Re^{n \times n}$ such that (4.7.5) is true and such that the condition

$$p_{ii} \geq \sum_{j=1, j\neq i}^{n} |p_{ji}|, \ i=1,\cdots,n \tag{4.7.7}$$

is satisfied. Then the Lyapunov function (4.7.6) satisfies Assumptions (A–1) and (A–2); therefore, the equilibrium $x = 0$ of system (4.7.2) is globally asymptotically stable.

Proof: Since v satisfies Assumption (A–1), we only need to show that it also satisfies Assumption (A–2). This is accomplished by considering two types of points in D^n.

Type 1: For any $x \in D^n$ such that $h(Ax) = Ax$, we have

$$D_{(4.7.2)}v(x) = \nabla v(x)^T Ax = x^T(PA + A^TP)x = -x^TQx$$

and therefore Hypothesis (A–2) is satisfied.

Type 2: Assume that $h(Ax) \neq Ax$ so that $x \in \partial D^n$. Let $\sigma\colon \{1,\cdots,n\} \to \{1,\cdots,n\}$ be a permutation such that for some $1 \leq m < n$, it is true that

$$\dot{x}_{\sigma(i)} = \sum_{j=1}^{n} a_{\sigma(i)j} x_j, \ i=1,\cdots,m \tag{4.7.8}$$

and

$$\dot{x}_{\sigma(i)} = 0, \ |x_{\sigma(i)}| = 1 \text{ and } \left(\sum_{j=1}^{n} a_{\sigma(i)j} x_j\right) x_{\sigma(i)} \geq 0. \tag{4.7.9}$$

Let $x_{\mathrm{I}} = \left(x_{\sigma(1)}, \cdots, x_{\sigma(m)}\right)^T$, $x_{\mathrm{II}} = \left(x_{\sigma(m+1)}, \cdots, x_{\sigma(n)}\right)^T$

$$\begin{aligned} A_{\mathrm{I},\mathrm{I}} &= [a_{\sigma(i)\sigma(j)}]_{1\leq i\leq m, 1\leq j\leq m} \\ A_{\mathrm{I},\mathrm{II}} &= [a_{\sigma(i)\sigma(j)}]_{1\leq i\leq m, m<j\leq n} \\ A_{\mathrm{II},\mathrm{I}} &= [a_{\sigma(i)\sigma(j)}]_{m<i\leq n, 1\leq j\leq m} \\ A_{\mathrm{II},\mathrm{II}} &= [a_{\sigma(i)\sigma(j)}]_{m<i\leq n, m<j\leq n}. \end{aligned} \tag{4.7.10}$$

Utilizing (4.7.8)–(4.7.10), we can represent system (4.7.2) equivalently as

$$\dot{x}_{\mathrm{I}} = A_{\mathrm{I},\mathrm{I}} x_{\mathrm{I}} + A_{\mathrm{I},\mathrm{II}} x_{\mathrm{II}}, \ \dot{x}_{\mathrm{II}} = 0. \tag{4.7.11}$$

4.7. CONTINUOUS-TIME RESULTS

If we define the matrix $S = [s_{ij}]$ as $s_{ij} = 1$ if $j = \sigma(i)$ and $s_{ij} = 0$ otherwise, then it is easily verified that

$$SS^T = E, \quad x = S \begin{bmatrix} x_{\mathrm{I}} \\ x_{\mathrm{II}} \end{bmatrix}$$

and

$$S^T A S = \begin{bmatrix} A_{\mathrm{I},\mathrm{I}} & A_{\mathrm{I},\mathrm{II}} \\ A_{\mathrm{II},\mathrm{I}} & A_{\mathrm{II},\mathrm{II}} \end{bmatrix} \quad (4.7.12)$$

where E is the identity matrix.

We now evaluate the derivative of v given in (4.7.6) with respect to t along the solutions of (4.7.2) as

$$\begin{aligned} D_{(4.7.2)} v(x(t)) &= 2x(t)^T P \dot{x}(t) \\ &= 2x(t)^T P h(Ax(t)) \\ &= 2x(t)^T PAx(t) - 2x(t)^T P[Ax(t) - h(Ax(t))] \\ &= -x(t)^T Q x(t) - 2[x_{\mathrm{I}}(t)^T, x_{\mathrm{II}}(t)^T] S^T P S \\ &\quad \cdot \begin{bmatrix} 0 \\ A_{\mathrm{II},\mathrm{I}} x_{\mathrm{I}}(t) + A_{\mathrm{II},\mathrm{II}} x_{\mathrm{II}}(t) \end{bmatrix} \\ &= -x(t)^T Q x(t) \\ &\quad - 2 \sum_{i=m+1}^n \left[\left(p_{\sigma(i)\sigma(i)} x_{\sigma(i)}(t) + \sum_{j=1, j \neq i}^n p_{\sigma(j)\sigma(i)} x_j(t) \right) \right. \\ &\quad \left. \cdot \left(\sum_{j=1}^n a_{\sigma(i)j} x_j(t) \right) \right]. \end{aligned}$$

$$(4.7.13)$$

Noticing that $|x_{\sigma(i)}| = 1$ for all $m < i \leq n$, we obtain

$$\begin{aligned} &\left(p_{\sigma(i)\sigma(i)} x_{\sigma(i)}(t) + \sum_{j=1, j \neq i}^n p_{\sigma(j)\sigma(i)} x_j(t) \right) \left(\sum_{j=1}^n a_{\sigma(i)j} x_j(t) \right) \\ &= \left(p_{\sigma(i)\sigma(i)} + \sum_{j=1, j \neq i}^n p_{\sigma(j)\sigma(i)} x_j(t) x_{\sigma(i)}(t) \right) \\ &\quad \cdot \left(\sum_{j=1}^n a_{\sigma(i)j} x_j(t) \right) x_{\sigma(i)}(t) \\ &\geq \left(p_{\sigma(i)\sigma(i)} - \sum_{j=1, j \neq i}^n |p_{\sigma(j)\sigma(i)}| \right) \left(\sum_{j=1}^n a_{\sigma(i)j} x_j(t) \right) x_{\sigma(i)}(t) \\ &\geq 0, \end{aligned}$$

$$(4.7.14)$$

for all $m < i \leq n$. In the last two steps we have made use of (4.7.7) and (4.7.9) and the fact that $p_{\sigma(j)\sigma(i)}$, $j = 1, \cdots, n$ is a rearrangement of $p_{j\sigma(i)}$, $j = 1, \cdots, n$. It now follows that

$$x(t)^T P[Ax(t) - h(Ax(t))]$$
$$= \sum_{i=m+1}^{n} \left[\left(p_{\sigma(i)\sigma(i)} x_{\sigma(i)} + \sum_{j=1, j \neq i}^{n} p_{\sigma(j)\sigma(i)} x_j(t) \right) \cdot \left(\sum_{j=1}^{n} a_{\sigma(i)j} x_j(t) \right) \right]$$
$$\geq 0$$
(4.7.15)

and therefore, in view of (4.7.13) and (4.7.15) we have that

$$D_{(4.7.2)} v(x(t)) \leq -x(t)^T Q x(t) = \nabla v(x(t))^T A x(t).$$

Therefore, Hypothesis (A–2) is satisfied. This concludes the proof of the theorem. ∎

Remark 4.7.1 We recall that a matrix $A \in \Re^{n \times n}$ is said to be *diagonally stable* if there exists a positive diagonal matrix P such that $(PA + A^T P) < 0$ (i.e., the matrix $PA + A^T P$ is negative definite). It follows from Theorem 4.7.2 that if A in (4.7.2) is diagonally stable, then the equilibrium $x_e = 0$ of system (4.7.2) is globally asymptotically stable. It has been shown (see, e.g., [1] and [3]) that in particular, the following classes of matrices are diagonally stable:

a) stable symmetric matrices (i.e., symmetric matrices with negative eigenvalues);

b) stable triangular matrices;

c) second-order stable matrices with negative diagonal entries;

d) any nonsingular matrix $A = [a_{ij}]$ which has nonpositive diagonal elements (i.e., $a_{ii} \leq 0$ for all $i = 1, \cdots, n$) and which has the property that $\mu(A)$ is an M-matrix, where $\mu(A) = [\Delta_{ij} |a_{ij}|]_{1 \leq i,j \leq n}$ and $\Delta_{ij} = 1$ if $i = j$ and $\Delta_{ij} = -1$ if $i \neq j$ (Recall that a matrix $H = [h_{ij}] \in \Re^{n \times n}$ is an M-matrix if $h_{ij} \leq 0$, $i \neq j$, and all successive principal minors of H are positive. For the general properties of M-matrices, refer, e.g., to [13].);

4.7. CONTINUOUS-TIME RESULTS

e) stable matrices with nonnegative off-diagonal entries; and

f) any matrix $A \in \Re^{n \times n}$ with the property that $\mu_\infty(A) < 0$, where $\mu_\infty(A)$ is the infinity matrix measure of A (refer, e.g., to [10]). ∎

We note that in [7], a computational method is provided for determining whether a matrix is diagonally stable or not.

In [10], the condition f) given in the remarks above is derived as a stability criterion for the global asymptotic stability of the equilibrium $x_e = 0$ of system (4.7.2). Since condition f) constitutes a *special case* of Theorem 4.7.2, the present results are in general less conservative than the corresponding results reported in [10].

We note that the conditions of Theorems 4.7.1 and 4.7.2 provide automatically sufficient conditions for the uniqueness of the equilibrium of system (4.7.2). However, it is frequently desirable to have uniqueness of equilibrium conditions which are independent of any other conditions, such as asymptotic stability. We conclude the present section with a result which provides sufficient conditions for the uniqueness of an equilibrium of system (4.7.2). In doing so, we require the following concept.

Definition 4.7.1 A matrix $B \in \Re^{n \times n}$ is said to be a $\mathcal{P}$-*matrix* if all of its principal minors are positive, or equivalently, if for each $x \in \Re^n$, $x \neq 0$, there is a component, say i, such that $x_i \neq 0$ and $x_i(Bx)_i > 0$. ∎

For properties of $\mathcal{P}$-matrices, refer to [2].

Theorem 4.7.3 System (4.7.2) has one and only one equilibrium (located at the origin) if the matrix $(-A)$ in (4.7.2) is a $\mathcal{P}$-matrix.

Proof: The proof is by contradiction. Suppose there exists $x \in D^n$, $x \neq 0$, such that x is an equilibrium of system (4.7.2), i.e., such that $h(Ax) = 0$. Then,

$(Ax)_i x_i \geq 0$ for those i such that $|x_i| = 1$, and

$(Ax)_i = 0$ for those i such that $|x_i| < 1$,

where $(Ax)_i$ denotes the ith component of Ax and thus, $(Ax)_i x_i \geq 0$ for all i. On the other hand, if $-A$ is a $\mathcal{P}$-matrix, then there exists an index i such that $(Ax)_i x_i < 0$. We have arrived at a contradiction. This proves the theorem. ∎

4.8 Global Asymptotic Stability of Linear Discrete-Time Systems Operating on a Closed Hypercube

In the present section we consider neural networks described by equations of the form

$$x(k+1) = \text{sat}[Ax(k)], \ k = 0, 1, 2, \cdots \qquad (4.8.1)$$

where $x(k) \in D^n$, $A \in \Re^{n \times n}$, $\text{sat}(x) = [\text{sat}(x_1), \cdots, \text{sat}(x_n)]^T$ and

$$\text{sat}(x_i) = \begin{cases} 1, & x_i > 1 \\ x_i, & -1 \leq x_i \leq 1 \\ -1, & x_i < -1. \end{cases}$$

We obtain system (4.8.1) as a special case of system (M_d) (see Section 4.6) by choosing without loss of generality, $I = 0$, and letting $T = A$.

When considering system (4.8.1) as a neural network with applications to optimization problems (cf. [5]), we wish to construct a network with a unique equilibrium which is globally asymptotically stable, in order to prevent convergence to local minima of an objective function (see, e.g., [17]). When the desired equilibrium x_d is located in the interior of D^n, the conditions for this equilibrium to be globally asymptotically stable will be identical to the conditions for the equilibrium $x = 0$ of (4.8.1) to be globally asymptotically stable since we can always consider $x_d = 0$ without loss of generality (cf. [15]).

4.8. DISCRETE-TIME RESULTS

Before establishing the desired results for system (4.8.1), we need to digress to recall certain aspects of the stability theory of systems described by difference equations. To this end we consider autonomous difference equations,

$$x(k+1) = f(x(k)), \ k = 0, 1, 2, \cdots \qquad (4.8.2)$$

where $x(k) \in \Re^n$ and $f: \Re^n \to \Re^n$ is assumed to be continuous. Note that (4.8.1) is a special case of (4.8.2).

A point $x_e \in \Re^n$ is said to be an equilibrium of (4.8.2) if

$$x_e = f(x_e).$$

We assume without loss of generality that $x_e = 0$. Consistent with Definition 4.6.3, we define various stability concepts for (4.8.2) as follows, letting $\varphi(k, x)$ denote a solution of (4.8.2):

(i) The equilibrium $x_e = 0$ of (4.8.2) is *stable* if for every $\varepsilon > 0$ there is a $\delta = \delta(\varepsilon) > 0$ such that $|\varphi(k, x)| < \varepsilon$ for all $k \in Z^+$ whenever $|x| < \delta$;

(ii) the equilibrium $x_e = 0$ of (4.8.2) is *asymptotically stable* if it is stable and if there is an $\eta > 0$ such that $\lim\limits_{k \to \infty} |\varphi(k, x)| = 0$ whenever $|x| < \eta$; and

(iii) the equilibrium $x_e = 0$ of (4.8.2) is *globally asymptotically stable* if it is stable and $\lim\limits_{k \to \infty} |\varphi(k, x)| = 0$ for all $x \in D^n$.

Next, we recall (see Section 3.2C) that a continuous function $\psi: \Re^+ \to \Re^+$ is said to belong to *class* $\mathcal{K}$ (i.e., $\psi \in \mathcal{K}$) if $\psi(0) = 0$ and $\psi(s)$ is monotonically increasing in s. Furthermore, we say that a function ψ belongs to *class* $\mathcal{KR}$ (i.e., $\psi \in \mathcal{KR}$) if $\psi \in \mathcal{K}$ and $\lim\limits_{r \to \infty} \psi(r) = \infty$.

To simplify our notation, we denote in the following a solution of (4.8.2) [resp., (4.8.1)] by $\varphi(k, x) = x(k)$. Also, for a continuous function $v: \Re^n \to \Re$, we define the first forward difference of v along the solutions of (4.8.2) by

$$\begin{aligned} D_{(4.8.2)} v(x(k)) &= v(x(k+1)) - v(x(k)) \\ &\triangleq v(f(x(k))) - v(x(k)). \end{aligned}$$

154 CHAPTER 4. LINEAR SYSTEMS ON A HYPERCUBE

We will rely on the following stability results.

Lemma 4.8.1 (cf. [15]) The equilibrium $x = 0$ of (4.8.2) is globally asymptotically stable if there exists a continuous function $v \colon \Re^n \to \Re$, two functions $\psi_1, \psi_2 \in \mathcal{KR}$ and a function $\psi_3 \in \mathcal{K}$ which satisfy the conditions

$$\psi_1(|x(k)|) \leq v(x(k)) \leq \psi_2(|x(k)|)$$

and

$$D_{(4.8.2)} v(x(k)) \leq -\psi_3(|x(k)|)$$

for all $x \in \Re^n$. ∎

The above result states that the equilibrium $x = 0$ of (4.8.2) is *globally asymptotically stable* if there exists a positive definite, radially unbounded function $v \colon \Re^n \to \Re$ whose first forward difference along the solutions of (4.8.2), $D_{(4.8.2)} v(x(k))$, is negative definite for all $x \in \Re^n$.

We now return to the subject on hand.

In establishing our results for system (4.8.1), we will make use of Lyapunov functions for the linear systems [corresponding to (4.8.1)], given by

$$w(k+1) = Aw(k), \quad k = 0, 1, 2, \cdots \qquad (4.8.3)$$

where $A \in \Re^{n \times n}$ is defined in (4.8.1). For such systems, we will make the following assumptions.

(A–1) Assume that for system (4.8.3) there exists a continuous function $v \colon \Re^n \to \Re$ with the following properties:

(i) v is positive definite and radially unbounded, and

$$D_{(4.8.3)} v(w(k))$$

is negative definite for all $w(k) \in \Re^n$ (and thus the eigenvalues of A are within the unit circle of the complex plane); and

(ii) for all $w \in \Re^n$ such that $w \notin D^n$, it is true that

$$v(\operatorname{sat}(w)) < v(w). \qquad ∎ \qquad (4.8.4)$$

4.8. DISCRETE-TIME RESULTS

An example of a function $v_1: \Re^2 \to \Re$ which satisfies (4.8.4) is given by $v_1(w) = d_1 w_1^2 + d_2 w_2^2$, $d_1 > 0$, $d_2 > 0$. On the other hand, the function $v_2: \Re^2 \to \Re$ given by $v_2(w) = w_1^2 + (2w_1 + w_2)^2$ does not satisfy (4.8.4). To see this, consider the point $w = (-0.99, 1.05)^T \notin D^2$ and note that $v_2(\text{sat}(w)) = 1.9405$ and $v_2(w) = 1.845$.

We are now in a position to prove the following result.

Theorem 4.8.1 If assumption (A–1) holds, then the equilibrium $x = 0$ of the system (4.8.1) is globally asymptotically stable.

Proof: Since assumption (A–1) is true, there exists a positive definite, radially unbounded function v for the system (4.8.3) such that (4.8.4) is true, which in turn implies that

$$v(\text{sat}(Aw)) \leq v(Aw), \text{ for all } w \in \Re^n.$$

Also, by (A–1),

$$v(Aw(k)) - v(w(k)) < 0, \text{ for all } w(k) \neq 0.$$

Therefore, along the solutions of the system (4.8.1), we have

$$\begin{aligned} D_{(4.8.1)} v(x(k)) &= v(x(k+1)) - v(x(k)) \\ &= v(\text{sat}[Ax(k)]) - v(x(k)) \\ &\leq v(Ax(k)) - v(x(k)) \\ &< 0 \end{aligned}$$

for all $x(k) \neq 0$ and $D_{(4.8.1)} v(x(k)) = 0$ if and only if $x(k) = 0$. Therefore, $v(x)$ is positive definite and radially unbounded, and $D_{(4.8.1)} v(x)$ is negative definite for all x. Hence, the equilibrium $x = 0$ of the system (4.8.1) is globally asymptotically stable. ∎

Remark 4.8.1 In particular, for fixed p, $1 \leq p \leq \infty$, let us choose

$$v(w) = |w|_p = \left(\sum_{i=1}^n |w_i|^p \right)^{1/p}$$

for system (4.8.3) and assume that $\|A\|_p < 1$, where $\|A\|_p$ denotes the norm induced by $|w|_p$. Under these conditions, (A–1) is true. To see this, note that v is positive definite and radially unbounded, that $v(Aw) = |Aw|_p \leq \|A\|_p |w|_p < |w|_p = v(w)$, and that $|\text{sat}(w)|_p < |w|_p$, for all $w \in \Re^n$ such that $w \notin D^n$.

Therefore, the equilibrium $x = 0$ of the system (4.8.1) is globally asymptotically stable if $\|A\|_p < 1$ for some p, $1 \leq p \leq \infty$. ∎

In order to generate quadratic form Lyapunov functions which satisfy Assumption(A–1) for systems described by (4.8.1), we will find it convenient to utilize the next assumption. (When using the term *positive definite matrix*, we will have in mind a *symmetric* matrix with positive eigenvalues.)

(A–2) Let $x_s = \text{sat}(x) = [\text{sat}(x_1), \cdots, \text{sat}(x_n)]^T$ for $x \in \Re^n$ and let $H \in \Re^{n \times n}$ denote a positive definite matrix. Assume that

$$x_s^T H x_s < x^T H x \tag{4.8.5}$$

whenever $x \notin D^n$, $x \in \Re^n$. ∎

An example of a matrix which satisfies (A–2) is any diagonal matrix with positive diagonal elements. On the other hand, the positive definite matrix H given by

$$H = \begin{pmatrix} 5 & 2 \\ 2 & 1 \end{pmatrix}$$

does not satisfy Assumption (A–2). (To see this, refer to the example following Assumption (A–1) by noting that $v_2(x) = x^T H x$.)

The next result gives a *necessary and sufficient* condition for matrices to satisfy Assumption (A–2). This result is very useful in applications.

Lemma 4.8.2 An $n \times n$ positive definite matrix $H = [h_{ij}]$ satisfies Assumption (A–2) *if and only if*

$$h_{ii} \geq \sum_{j=1, j \neq i}^{n} |h_{ij}|, \ i = 1, \cdots, n. \qquad \blacksquare$$

4.8. DISCRETE-TIME RESULTS

The proof of Lemma 4.8.2 follows along similar lines as the proof of Theorem 4.7.2 and will not be given here. For the details of the proof, refer to [11].

The following result is now a direct consequence of Theorem 4.8.1.

Corollary 4.8.1 The equilibrium $x = 0$ of the system (4.8.1) is globally asymptotically stable, if there exists a matrix H which satisfies (A–2), such that $Q \triangleq H - A^T H A$ is positive definite. ∎

By choosing $v(x) = x(k)^T H x(k)$, the proof follows from Theorem 4.8.1.

Remark 4.8.2 For *linear* system (4.8.3), the equilibrium $w = 0$ is globally asymptotically stable if and only if all eigenvalues of A are within the unit circle. Equivalently, the equilibrium $w = 0$ of system (4.8.3) is globally asymptotically stable if and only if for every positive definite matrix Q, there exists a positive definite matrix P, such that (cf. [15]),

$$Q = P - A^T P A. \qquad (4.8.6)$$

Corollary 4.8.1 tells us that the equilibrium $x = 0$ of the *nonlinear* system (4.8.1) is globally asymptotically stable if in addition to the conditions given above [for linear system (4.8.3)], Assumption (A–2) is satisfied, i.e., there exists a matrix H which satisfies (A–2) such that $H - A^T H A$ is positive definite. ∎

In the next result, Theorem 4.8.2, we show that Corollary 4.8.1 is actually true when Q is only positive semidefinite, still assuming that A is stable.

Theorem 4.8.2 The equilibrium $x = 0$ of the system (4.8.1) is globally asymptotically stable, if A is stable and if there exists a matrix H which satisfies (A–2), such that $Q \triangleq H - A^T H A$ is positive semidefinite.

158   CHAPTER 4. LINEAR SYSTEMS ON A HYPERCUBE

Proof: Let us choose $v(x(k)) = x(k)^T H x(k)$ for the system (4.8.1). The function v is clearly positive definite and radially unbounded. Also, since

$$\begin{aligned}
D_{(4.8.1)} v(x(k)) &= v(x(k+1)) - v(x(k)) \\
&= [\text{sat}(Ax(k))]^T H [\text{sat}(Ax(k))] - x(k)^T H x(k) \\
&\leq x(k)^T (A^T H A - H) x(k)
\end{aligned}$$

and since $H - A^T H A$ is positive semidefinite, $D_{(4.8.1)} v(x(k))$ is negative semidefinite for all $x(k)$. Therefore, the equilibrium $x = 0$ is stable. To show that it is asymptotically stable, we must show that $x(k) \to 0$ as $k \to \infty$.

Let us consider an n consecutive-step iteration for the system (4.8.1), from $n_0 \geq 0$ to $n + n_0$. Without loss of generality, assume that the system (4.8.1) saturates at $k = l$, $l \in [n_0, n + n_0)$. In view of (A–2), it follows that

$$\begin{aligned}
v(x(l+1)) &= x(l+1)^T H x(l+1) \\
&= [\text{sat}(Ax(l))]^T H [\text{sat}(Ax(l))] \\
&< [Ax(l)]^T H A x(l) \\
&\leq x(l)^T H x(l) \\
&= v(x(l)).
\end{aligned}$$

On the other hand, if no saturation occurs during this period, then, using the fact that if $H - A^T H A$ is positive semidefinite, it follows that $H - (A^T)^n H A^n$ is positive definite when A is stable (cf. [18]). We have

$$\begin{aligned}
v(x(n+n_0)) &= x(n+n_0)^T H x(n+n_0) \\
&= [A^n x(n_0)]^T H A^n x(n_0) \\
&= x(n_0)^T (A^T)^n H A^n x(n_0) \\
&< x(n_0)^T H x(n_0) \\
&= v(x(n_0)).
\end{aligned}$$

Therefore, we can conclude that for the sequence $\{k : k = 1, 2, \cdots\}$, there always exists an infinite subsequence $\{k_j : j = 1, 2, \cdots\}$, such that $D_{(4.8.1)} v(x(k_j))$ is negative for $x(k_j) \neq 0$, and that $v(x(k)) \leq v(x(k_j))$ for all $k \geq k_j$. Since v is a positive definite quadratic form, it follows that $v(x(k_j)) \to 0$ as $j \to \infty$, and therefore $v(x(k)) \to 0$

as $k \to \infty$. This in turn implies that $x(k) \to 0$ as $k \to \infty$. Thus the equilibrium $x = 0$ of (4.8.1) is globally asymptotically stable. ∎

4.9 Summary

In the present chapter we investigated local and global qualitative properties of continuous-time neural networks described by linear differential equations defined on a hypercube, given by

$$\frac{dx}{dt} = Tx + I \qquad \text{(M)}$$

with constraints

$$-1 \leq x_i \leq 1, \; i = 1, \cdots, n.$$

For such systems we first formulated a definition of solution which incorporates the notion of "solution in a saturated mode," and we studied some of the properties of such solutions. We showed in particular that (M) possesses for every $x \in \Re^n$ a unique solution $\varphi(t, x)$ which exists for all $t \geq t_0$.

Next, we introduced the concept of equilibrium for (M) and we established an algorithm which enables us to determine in a systematic manner the locations of all equilibria of (M) and their stability properties.

Next, we showed that system (M) has at most 3^n equilibrium points and that at most 2^n of these are asymptotically stable.

Next, we introduced an energy function for (M) of the form

$$E(x) = -\frac{1}{2}x^T T x - x^T I.$$

Assuming that T in (M) is symmetric, and using this function, we showed that there is a one-to-one correspondence between the set of local minima of E and the set of asymptotically stable equilibria of system (M).

Next, we showed that along each solution of (M), the energy function E decreases monotonically, and therefore, system (M) will not exhibit periodic solutions.

CHAPTER 4. LINEAR SYSTEMS ON A HYPERCUBE

In the present chapter we also investigated local and global qualitative properties of discrete-time neural networks described by linear difference equations defined on a hypercube, given by

$$x(k+1) = \text{sat}(Tx(k) + I), \quad k = 0, 1, 2, \cdots. \tag{M_d}$$

For such systems, we established results which are very similar to the ones described above for system (M). In doing so, we made use of an energy function for system (M_d) of the form

$$E(x) = -x^T(T - E_n)x - 2x^T I,$$

again under the assumption that T is symmetric.

In applications to optimization problems, neural networks with globally asymptotically stable equilibria have been employed. In the present chapter we also established sufficient conditions for the global asymptotic stability of the neural network (M_d), assuming without loss of generality that $I = 0$ and that $x = 0$ is the only equilibrium.

If we let $T = A$, system (M_d) assumes under the present assumptions the form

$$x(k+1) = \text{sat}(Ax(k)), \quad k = 0, 1, 2, \cdots. \tag{4.9.1}$$

We associated with (4.9.1) the linear system

$$w(k+1) = Aw(k), \quad k = 0, 1, 2, \cdots. \tag{4.9.2}$$

For system (4.9.1) we first established the following result: The equilibrium $x = 0$ of system (4.9.1) is globally asymptotically stable if there exists a function $v: \Re^n \to \Re$ with the following properties:

(i) v is continuous, positive definite, and radially unbounded, and $D_{(4.9.2)}v$ is negative definite for all $w(k) \in \Re^n$; and

(ii) for all $w \in \Re^n$ such that $w \notin D^n$, it is true that $v(\text{sat}(w)) < v(w)$.

As a next step, we obtained more explicit stability conditions by employing quadratic Lyapunov functions in the above result.

We also obtained sufficient conditions for the global asymptotic stability of system (M), assuming $I = 0$ and assuming that $x = 0$ is the equilibrium. These results are similar, and in the same spirit as the results described above for system (4.9.1). In addition, we obtained sufficient conditions for system (M) to have only one equilibrium, $x = 0$, (assuming $I = 0$), which are independent of any specific stability requirements.

4.10 Notes and References

The material presented in Sections 4.1 through and including 4.5 is based on results established in [9] while the results of Section 4.6 rely on the material presented in [14]. The global asymptotic stability results of Sections 4.7 and 4.8 are based on the results developed in [6] and [10], respectively. For related results involving systems with partial state saturation constraints (i.e., systems in which only some of the states are subjected to saturation constraints), refer to [12]. Systems with partial state saturation constraints arise in the modeling of control systems (e.g., process control systems), digital signal processing (digital filters), and other applications.

Bibliography

[1] GP Barker, A Berman, RJ Plemmons. Positive diagonal solutions to the Lyapunov equations. Linear and Multilinear Algebra 5:249–256, 1978.

[2] A Berman, RJ Plemmons. Nonnegative Matrices in the Mathematical Sciences. New York, NY: Academic Press, 1979.

[3] D Hershkowitz. Recent directions in matrix stability. Linear Algebra and its Applications 171:161–186, 1992.

[4] JJ Hopfield. Neurons with graded response have collective computational properties like those of two-state neurons. Proceedings of the National Academy of Sciences USA 81:3088–3092, 1984.

[5] JJ Hopfield, DW Tank. 'Neural' computation of decisions in optimization problems. Biological Cybernetics 52:141–152, 1985.

[6] L Hou, AN Michel. Asymptotic stability of systems with saturation constraints. IEEE Transactions on Automatic Control 43:1148–1154, 1998.

[7] HK Khalil. On the existence of positive diagonal P such that $PA + A^T P < 0$. IEEE Transactions on Automatic Control 27:181–184, 1982.

[8] JH Li, AN Michel, W Porod. Qualitative analysis and synthesis of a class of neural networks. IEEE Transactions on Circuits and Systems 35:976–987, 1988.

[9] JH Li, AN Michel, W Porod. Analysis and synthesis of a class of neural networks: Linear systems operating on a closed hypercube. IEEE Transactions on Circuits and Systems 36:1405–1422, 1989.

[10] D Liu, AN Michel. Asymptotic stability of systems operating on a closed hypercube. Systems & Control Letters 19:281–285, 1992.

[11] D Liu, AN Michel. Asymptotic stability of discrete-time systems with saturation nonlinearities with applications to digital filters. IEEE Transactions on Circuits and Systems-I: Fundamental Theory and Applications 39:798–807, 1992.

[12] D Liu, AN Michel. Stability analysis of systems with partial state saturation nonlinearities. IEEE Transactions on Circuits and Systems-I: Fundamental Theory and Applications 43:230–232, 1996.

[13] AN Michel, RK Miller. Qualitative Analysis of Large Scale Dynamical Systems. New York, NY: Academic Press, 1977.

[14] AN Michel, J Si, G Yen. Analysis and synthesis of a class of discrete-time neural networks described on hypercubes. IEEE Transactions on Neural Networks 2:32–46, 1991.

[15] AN Michel, K Wang, B Hu. Qualitative Theory of Dynamical Systems–The Role of Stability Preserving Mappings. Second Edition. New York, NY: Marcel Dekker, 2001.

[16] RK Miller, AN Michel. Ordinary Differential Equations. New York, NY: Academic Press, 1982.

[17] DW Tank, JJ Hopfield. Simple 'neural' optimization networks: An A/D converter, signal decision circuit, and a linear programming circuit. IEEE Transactions on Circuits and Systems 33:533–541, 1986.

[18] PP Vaidyanathan, V Liu. An improved sufficient condition for absence of limit cycles in digital filters. IEEE Transactions on Circuits and Systems 34:319–322, 1987.

Chapter 5

Qualitative Analysis of Hopfield-Type Neural Networks: Local Results

The analog Hopfield neural network model was introduced in Chapter 2 and its global qualitative properties were investigated in Chapter 3. In the present chapter we first study local qualitative properties under the assumption that the interconnecting structure of such networks is not necessarily symmetric. In our approach we view an analog Hopfield network as an interconnection of n free subsystems (consisting of the individual neurons with their associated dynamics) and our results are phrased in terms of the qualitative properties of the subsystems and the constraints imposed by the network interconnections. We use two general approaches in our analysis, employing scalar Lyapunov functions (consisting of a weighted sum of Lyapunov functions for the free subsystems) and vector Lyapunov functions (whose components are scalar Lyapunov functions for the free subsystems), respectively. In the latter approach, we invoke the comparison principle encountered in the stability theory of differential equations, making use of the properties of M-matrices. Issues that we address include asymptotic stability, exponential stability, and instability of an equilibrium; estimates of the domain of attraction of an asymptotically stable equilibrium; estimates of trajectory bounds (which provide estimates of the rate of convergence of trajectories to asymptotically stable equilibria); stability under structural perturbations in the network; and qualitative properties of analog Hopfield neural networks under the high gain limit assumption for the activation functions.

Next, we conduct a study of the local qualitative properties of synchronous discrete-time Hopfield neural networks. In doing so, we utilize the same approach as in the case of the analog Hopfield neural networks and we address in our analysis most of the issues enumerated above.

The chapter is concluded with an analysis of analog Hopfield-type neural networks which are endowed with saturation nonlinearities for activation functions. For such networks, we establish results which enable one to locate all equilibria and to determine their stability properties in a systematic manner. The approach used in arriving at these results is in the spirit of some of the local stability results developed in Chapter 4 for neural networks described by linear systems operating on a closed hypercube.

5.1 Notation

In the present section we establish some of the notation used throughout the present chapter.

Let V and W be arbitrary sets. Then $V \cup W$, $V \cap W$, and $V - W$ denote the union, intersection, and difference of V and W, respectively. If V is a subset of W, we write $V \subset W$ and if x is an element of V, we write $x \in V$. If f is a function from V into W, we write $f: V \to W$. Let $\emptyset$ denote the empty set. Let $\Re$ denote the set of real numbers, let $\Re^+ = [0, \infty)$, let Z denote the integers, let $Z^+ = \{0, 1, 2, \cdots\}$ and let $\Re^n$ be real n-space. If $x \in \Re^n$, then $x^T = (x_1, \cdots, x_n)$ denotes the transpose of x. If $V \subset \Re^n$, then $\overline{V}$, V° and ∂V represent the closure, interior and boundary of V in $\Re^n$, respectively. For $x \in \Re^n$, $|x|$ denotes any one of the equivalent vector

5.2. SOME BACKGROUND MATERIAL

norms on $\Re^n$. Let $B(x_0, r) = \{x \in \Re^n : |x - x_0| < r \text{ for some } r > 0\}$, let $B(r) = \{x \in \Re^n : |x| < r\}$, and let $\overline{B(r)} = \{x \in \Re^n : |x| \le r\}$. Let $B^n = \{x \in \Re^n : x_i = 1 \text{ or } -1, i = 1, \cdots, n\}$ and $D^n = \{x \in \Re^n : -1 \le x_i \le 1, i = 1, \cdots, n\}$. If $A = [a_{ij}]$ is an arbitrary matrix, then A^T denotes the transpose of A. If A is a square matrix, we use $\lambda(A)$ to denote eigenvalues of A, and $\|A\|$ to denote the matrix norm induced by a vector norm $|\cdot|$. Also, let $P(n)$ denote the set of all permutations on $\{1, \cdots, n\}$.

5.2 Some Background Material

In Chapter 3 (Section 3.2), we included some facts and results from the Lyapunov stability theory for systems described by ordinary differential equations which we required as background material. Presently, we add to these results. The present section is divided into two parts.

A. Systems Described by Ordinary Differential Equations

Continuing our discussion of Chapter 3, Section 3.2B, we consider once more systems of first order autonomous ordinary differential equations of the form

$$\dot{x} = f(x) \tag{E}$$

where $x \in \Re^n$, $f : \Re^n \to \Re^n$, and f is a C^1-function (i.e., the components of f are continuously differentiable on $\Re^n$ with respect to all variables). We assume without loss of generality that $x = 0$ is an isolated equilibrium of system (E), so that $f(0) = 0$.

In Chapter 3 (Section 3.2C) we defined the notions of *stability*, *asymptotic stability*, and *instability* of an equilibrium for (E). We now introduce the following additional characterization of an equilibrium (see, e.g., [19]):

The equilibrium $x = 0$ of system (E) is said to be *exponentially stable* if there is $k > 0$ and for every $\varepsilon > 0$ there exists $\eta = \eta(\varepsilon) > 0$

such that $|\varphi(t, t_0, x(t_0))| \leq \varepsilon e^{-k(t-t_0)}$ for all $t \geq t_0$ whenever $|x(t_0)| < \eta$. [As before, $\varphi(\cdot, t_0, x(t_0))$ denotes a solution of (E).]

The next result provides a set of sufficient conditions for exponential stability (see, e.g., [19]):

Lemma 5.2.1 The equilibrium $x = 0$ of (E) is *exponentially stable* if there exists a C^1-function $v: B(r) \to \Re$ for some $r > 0$ and three positive constants c_1, c_2, c_3 such that

$$c_1|x|^2 \leq v(x) \leq c_2|x|^2$$

and

$$D_{(E)}v(x) \leq -c_3|x|^2$$

for all $x \in B(r)$. [As before, $D_{(E)}v$ denotes the derivative of v with respect to t along the solutions of (E).] ∎

There are several different instability results among the principal Lyapunov results (see, e.g., [19]). In the following, we provide one of these which we will require later.

Lemma 5.2.2 The equilibrium $x = 0$ of (E) is *unstable* if there exists a C^1-function $v: B(r) \to \Re$ with the property that $D_{(E)}v(x)$ is negative definite and if every neighborhood of the origin contains at least one point x' where $v(x') < 0$. Moreover, in the case when $v(x)$ is negative definite, the equilibrium $x = 0$ of (E) is *completely unstable*. ∎

When the equilibrium $x = 0$ of (E) is completely unstable, all solutions of (E) with initial conditions sufficiently close to the origin, will tend away from the origin (see, e.g., [19]).

B. Systems Described by Ordinary Difference Equations

Next, we consider systems of first order, autonomous ordinary difference equations of the form

$$x(k+1) = h(x(k)), \quad k = 0, 1, 2, \cdots, \tag{D}$$

5.2. SOME BACKGROUND MATERIAL

where $x \in \Re^n$ and $h: \Re^n \to \Re^n$. We assume that h is continuous on $\Re^n$. Under these circumstances, (D) possesses for every $k_0 \in Z^+$ and for every $x(k_0) = x_0 \in \Re^n$ a unique solution $\varphi(k, k_0, x_0)$ which exists for all $k \geq k_0$ ($k \in Z^+$). Since (D) is autonomous, we can assume without loss of generality that $k_0 = 0$, and we denote a solution of (D) by $\varphi(k, x_0)$ or by $\varphi(k)$ when x_0 is clear from context.

A constant solution $\varphi(k, \tilde{x}) \equiv \tilde{x}$ is said to be an *equilibrium* of (D). Equivalently, any point $\tilde{x} \in \Re^n$ such that $\tilde{x} = h(\tilde{x})$ is an equilibrium of (D). An equilibrium $\varphi(k) \equiv \tilde{x}$ of (D) is said to be *isolated* if there is an $r > 0$ such that for any $x \in B(\tilde{x}, r) - \{\tilde{x}\}$, there is no other equilibrium of (D).

Similarly as in Section 3.2C, we have the following stability definitions for system (D) (see, e.g., [18]):

a) $\tilde{x}$ is said to be *stable* if for every $\varepsilon > 0$, there is a $\delta = \delta(\varepsilon) > 0$ such that $|\varphi(k, 0, x) - \tilde{x}| < \varepsilon$ for all $k \in \{0, 1, 2, \cdots\} = Z^+$ whenever $|x - \tilde{x}| < \delta$;

b) $\tilde{x}$ is said to be *asymptotically stable* if it is stable and if there is an $\eta > 0$ such that $\lim_{k \to \infty} |\varphi(k, 0, x) - \tilde{x}| = 0$ whenever $|x - \tilde{x}| < \eta$; and

c) $\tilde{x}$ is said to be *unstable* if it is not stable.

Given a continuous function $v: \Re^n \to \Re$, we define the function $D_{(D)}v: \Re^n \to \Re$ by $D_{(D)}v(x) = v(h(x)) - v(x)$ and we call $D_{(D)}v$ the *first forward difference of v* (with respect to k) *along the solutions of* (D).

In the following we assume without loss of generality that the origin is an isolated equilibrium of (D). Also, in what follows, we make use of functions of *class $\mathcal{K}$*, which we introduced and defined in Section 3.2C.

Lemma 5.2.3 The equilibrium $\tilde{x} = 0$ of (D) is *asymptotically stable* if there exists a continuous function $v: B(r) \to \Re$ for some $r > 0$ and functions $\psi_1, \psi_2 \in \mathcal{K}$ such that $v(0) = 0$,

$$v(x) \geq \psi_1(|x|)$$

and
$$D_{(D)}v(x) \leq -\psi_2(|x|)$$
for all $x \in B(r)$. ∎

The above result states that the equilibrium $x = 0$ of (D) is asymptotically stable if there exists a positive definite function v whose first forward difference evaluated along the solutions of (D) is negative definite. For additional stability results for system (D), refer to [18].

5.3 Analog Hopfield Model Viewed as an Interconnected System

In the present chapter we consider analog Hopfield neural networks described by equations of the form

$$\begin{cases} C_i du_i/dt = -u_i/R_i + \sum_{j=1}^{n} t_{ij} v_j + w_i(t) \\ v_i = g_i(u_i), \ i = 1, \cdots, n \end{cases} \quad (\text{H}_i)$$

where all symbols for (H$_i$) are defined in Section 2.2 [refer to (2.2.3)]. In particular, g_i is a sigmoidal function, i.e., $g_i \colon \Re \to (-1, 1)$, g_i is continuously differentiable and strictly monotonically increasing [i.e., $g_i(u'_i) > g_i(u''_i)$ if and only if $u'_i > u''_i$], $u_i g_i(u_i) > 0$ for all $u_i \neq 0$, $g_i(0) = 0$, $\lim_{u_i \to \infty} g_i(u_i) = 1$, and $\lim_{u_i \to -\infty} g_i(u_i) = -1$. We can rewrite (H$_i$) as

$$\dot{u}_i = -a_i u_i + \sum_{j=1}^{n} T_{ij} g_j(u_j) + I_i(t), \ i = 1, \cdots, n \quad (\text{H}'_i)$$

where $a_i > 0$, $T_{ij} \in \Re$ and $I_i \colon \Re^+ \to \Re$ are defined in the obvious way and $\dot{u}_i = du_i/dt$. We will view $I_i(\cdot)$ as an external input and we will assume that it is continuous, and is usually a constant.

In the literature it is frequently assumed that in particular,

$$g_i(u_i) = d_i \tan^{-1}(\lambda_i u_i) \quad (5.3.1)$$

5.3. ANALOG HOPFIELD MODEL

for some $d_i > 0$ and $\lambda_i > 0$. However, in our subsequent discussions, any sigmoidal function will do. [In Chapter 2, Eq. (2.2.1), we used, in particular, $v_i = g_i(\lambda u_i) = (2/\pi)\tan^{-1}((\pi/2)\lambda u_i)$.]

In the present chapter, we are interested in the qualitative behavior of solutions of (H$_i'$) near equilibrium points (rest positions where $\dot{u}_i \equiv 0$, $i = 1, \cdots, n$). By setting the *external inputs* $I_i(t)$, $i = 1, \cdots, n$, equal to zero, we define $u^* = (u_1^*, \cdots, u_n^*)^T \in \Re^n$ to be an *equilibrium* for (H$_i'$) provided that

$$-a_i u_i^* + \sum_{j=1}^{n} T_{ij} g_j(u_j^*) = 0, \; i = 1, \cdots, n. \tag{5.3.2}$$

Note that the above notion of equilibrium is consistent with the concept of equilibrium used in the preceding chapters, since in those cases, the systems in question were not subjected to external inputs. Note also that the locations of the equilibria of (H$_i'$) in $\Re^n$ are determined by the interconnection pattern of the neural network (i.e., by the parameters $T_{ij}, i, j = 1, \cdots, n$) as well as by the parameters a_i and the nature of the nonlinearities $g_i(\cdot)$, $i = 1, \cdots, n$.

Remark 5.3.1 In many neural network applications, the inputs $I_i(t)$ are held constant over some time interval of interest. For example, in analog-to-digital converters realized by neural networks, the input voltage sample is applied until a binary output is obtained. In such applications, it is customary to define an equilibrium point $u^* \in \Re^n$ as having the property that

$$-a_i u_i^* + \sum_{j=1}^{n} T_{ij} g_j(u_j^*) + c_i = 0, \; i = 1, \cdots, n \tag{5.3.3}$$

where the assumption $I_i(t) \equiv c_i$, $i = 1, \cdots, n$ has been made, with the constant c_i not necessarily equal to zero. Note that in this case the locations of the equilibria (H$_i'$) in $\Re^n$ are determined by the interconnection pattern of the neural network (i.e., by the parameters $T_{ij}, i, j = 1, \cdots, n$), by the parameters a_i, by the properties of the nonlinearities $g_i(\cdot)$, and the constant inputs c_i, $i = 1, \cdots, n$.

With all the assumptions given above still in tact, we show in the next paragraph that it is always possible to transform the equations in (5.3.3) to a set of equations of the *form* given in (5.3.2). In view of this, we will use (5.3.2) [rather than (5.3.3)] in defining the notion of equilibrium, and we will view $I_i(t) \equiv c_i$ as an external input. This is consistent with the convention used in the literature on Lyapunov stability of dynamical systems (see, e.g., [18], [19]).

To show that (5.3.3) can be transformed to a set of equations having the form (5.3.2), we let

$$u_i = y_i + \frac{c_i}{a_i}$$

and

$$\tilde{g}_i(y_i) = g_i\left(y_i + \frac{c_i}{a_i}\right).$$

Substituting these relations into (H'_i), we obtain the set of equations

$$\dot{y}_i = -a_i y_i + \sum_{j=1}^{n} T_{ij}\tilde{g}_j(y_j), \ i = 1, \cdots, n.$$

The right-hand side of this equation vanishes identically at the points y^* where

$$-a_i y_i^* + \sum_{j=1}^{n} T_{ij} g_j\left(y_j^* + \frac{c_i}{a_i}\right) = 0, \ i = 1, \cdots, n$$

which is of the form given in (5.3.2). ∎

Throughout the present chapter we will assume that a given equilibrium u^* being analyzed is an isolated equilibrium for (H'_i), i.e., there exists an $r > 0$ such that in the neighborhood $B(u^*, r)$ no equilibrium for (H'_i), other than $u = u^*$, exists. We have shown in Chapter 3 (resp., in [8]) that this is a reasonable assumption for the case of the systems considered herein.

When analyzing the stability properties of a given equilibrium point, we will be able to assume without loss of generality, that this

5.3. ANALOG HOPFIELD MODEL

equilibrium is located at the origin of $\Re^n$. To show this, assume that $u^* \neq 0$ is an equilibrium for (H'_i) [i.e., assume that for u^*, (5.3.2) is satisfied], and define

$$x_i = u_i - u_i^*, \quad h_i(u_i) = g_i(u_i) - g_i(u_i^*), \quad i = 1, \cdots, n. \quad (5.3.4)$$

Substituting (5.3.4) into (H'_i), we obtain

$$\dot{x}_i = -a_i x_i - a_i u_i^* + \sum_{j=1}^n T_{ij}[h_j(x_j + u_j^*) + g_j(u_j^*)] + I_i(t)$$

$$= -a_i x_i + \sum_{j=1}^n T_{ij} h_j(x_j + u_j^*) + \left[\sum_{j=1}^n T_{ij} g_j(u_j^*) - a_i u_i^*\right] + I_i(t)$$

$$= -a_i x_i + \sum_{j=1}^n T_{ij} h_j(x_j + u_j^*) + I_i(t).$$

Now define

$$G_j(x_j) \stackrel{\triangle}{=} h_j(x_j + u_j^*) = g_j(x_j + u_j^*) - g_j(u_j^*). \quad (5.3.5)$$

Then (H'_i) is equivalent, under the transformation (5.3.4) and (5.3.5), to the system

$$\dot{x}_i = -a_i x_i + \sum_{j=1}^n T_{ij} G_j(x_j) + I_i(t), \quad i = 1, \cdots, n \quad (\Sigma_i)$$

where $G_j(0) = 0$. In view of the preceding assumptions, the origin $x = (x_1, \cdots, x_n)^T = (0, \cdots, 0)^T$ is clearly an isolated equilibrium for system (Σ_i) [with $I_i(t) \equiv 0$, $i = 1, \cdots n$]. Furthermore, from the earlier assumptions, it follows that $a_i > 0$, $T_{ij} \in \Re$, $G_j: \Re \to (\gamma_1, \gamma_2) \subset (-2, 2)$ (where $\gamma_1 < 0 < \gamma_2$), G_j is continuously differentiable, G_j is strictly monotonically increasing in x_j, and $x_j G(x_j) > 0$ for all $x_j \neq 0$. Also, $I_i: \Re^+ \to \Re$ is a continuous function.

We recall from Chapter 3, that under the assumptions made above, for any $x_0 = (x_{10}, \cdots, x_{n0})^T \in \Re^n$ and for any specific allowable external input $I(t) = (I_1(t), \cdots, I_n(t))^T$, the system (Σ_i) will possess a unique solution

$$\varphi(t, t_0, x_0) = (\varphi_1(t, t_0, x_0), \cdots, \varphi_n(t, t_0, x_0))^T$$

with $\varphi(t_0, t_0, x_0) = x_0$, which exists for all $t \geq t_0 \geq 0$. On those occasions where the context is clear, we will frequently write $\varphi(t) = (\varphi_1(t), \cdots, \varphi_n(t))^T$ in place of $\varphi(t, t_0, x_0)$.

We will find it convenient to view system (Σ_i) as an interconnection of n *free subsystems* (or *isolated subsystems*) described by equations of the form

$$\dot{p}_i = -a_i p_i + T_{ii} G_i(p_i) + I_i(t). \qquad (\mathcal{S}_i)$$

Under this view point, the terms

$$h_i(x_1, \cdots, x_n) \triangleq \sum_{j=1, j \neq i}^{n} T_{ij} G_j(x_j), \ i = 1, \cdots, n \qquad (5.3.6)$$

make up the *interconnecting structure* of the system (Σ_i).

If we define $x \in \Re^n$ and $I: \Re^+ \to \Re^n$ as before, and if we let $T = [T_{ij}]$, $G(x) = (G_1(x_1), \cdots, G_n(x_n))^T$, and $A = \text{diag}[a_1, \cdots, a_n]$, then we can rewrite system (Σ_i) equivalently as

$$\dot{x} = -Ax + TG(x) + I(t). \qquad (\mathcal{S})$$

We refer to ($\mathcal{S}$) as an *interconnected system* or a *composite system with decomposition* (Σ_i) (see [16]).

Following the method of analysis advocated in [16], we will establish stability results for system ($\mathcal{S}$) which are phrased in terms of the qualitative properties of the free subsystems ($\mathcal{S}_i$) and in terms of the properties of the interconnecting structure given in (5.3.6). This method of analysis makes it often possible to circumvent difficulties that arise in the analysis of complex high-dimensional systems. Furthermore, results obtained in this manner frequently yield insights into the dynamic behavior of systems in terms of system components and interconnections.

5.4 Stability Analysis of the Single Neuron Subsystems

The stability results for the entire neural network $(\mathcal{S})$ (given in the next section) make use of the stability results for the individual free neuron subsystems $(\mathcal{S}_i)$. For this reason, we undertake a stability analysis of these subsystems first. In doing so, we will make use of the following hypotheses.

(H–1) For $(\mathcal{S}_i)$, $I_i(t) \equiv 0$ for all $t \geq t_0 \geq 0$. ∎

(H–2) For $(\mathcal{S}_i)$, the following conditions are true for $p_i \in B(r_i)$ for some $r_i > 0$:

$$T_{ii}G_i(p_i) - a_i p_i < 0, \ p_i > 0$$

$$T_{ii}G_i(p_i) - a_i p_i = 0, \ p_i = 0$$

$$T_{ii}G_i(p_i) - a_i p_i > 0, \ p_i < 0.$$ ∎

(H–3) For $(\mathcal{S}_i)$, the following conditions are true for $p_i \in B(r_i)$ for some $r_i > 0$:

$$T_{ii}G_i(p_i) - a_i p_i > 0, \ p_i > 0$$

$$T_{ii}G_i(p_i) - a_i p_i = 0, \ p_i = 0$$

$$T_{ii}G_i(p_i) - a_i p_i < 0, \ p_i < 0.$$ ∎

(H–4) For $(\mathcal{S}_i)$, the following conditions are true for $p_i \in B(r_i)$ for some $r_i > 0$:

$$T_{ii}G_i(p_i) - a_i p_i > 0, \ p_i > 0$$

$$T_{ii}G_i(p_i) - a_i p_i = 0, \ p_i = 0$$

$$T_{ii}G_i(p_i) - a_i p_i > 0, \ p_i < 0.$$ ∎

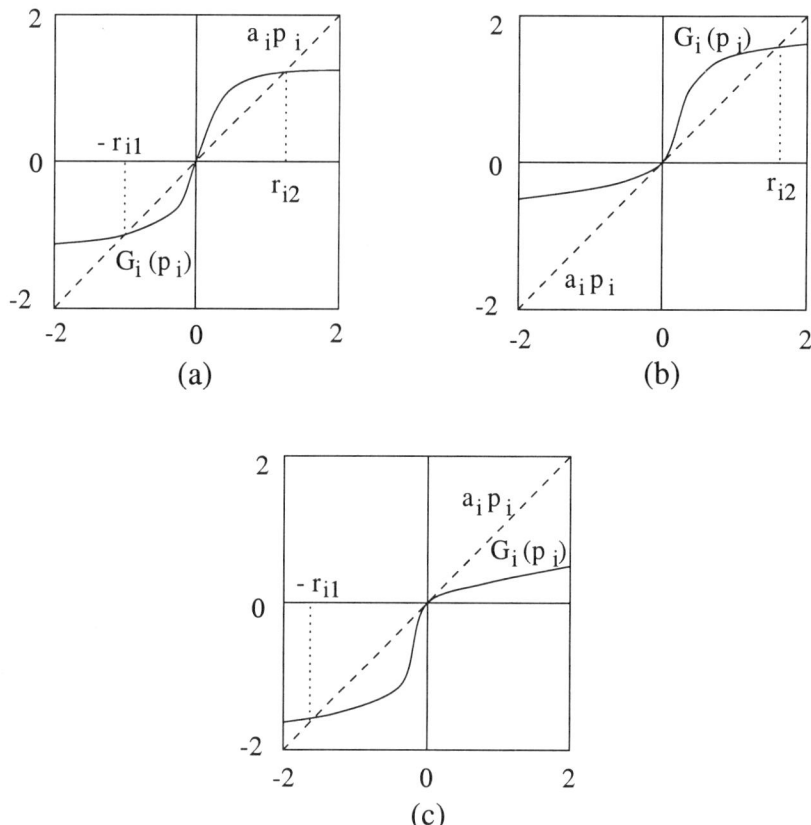

Figure 5.4.1: (a)–(c) Graphs of nonlinearities $G_i(p_i)$ corresponding to an unstable equilibrium $p_i = 0$.

(H–5) For $(\mathcal{S}_i)$, the following conditions are true for $p_i \in B(r_i)$ for some $r_i > 0$:

$$T_{ii}G_i(p_i) - a_i p_i < 0, \; p_i > 0$$

$$T_{ii}G_i(p_i) - a_i p_i = 0, \; p_i = 0$$

$$T_{ii}G_i(p_i) - a_i p_i < 0, \; p_i < 0.$$ ∎

5.4. SINGLE NEURON SUBSYSTEMS

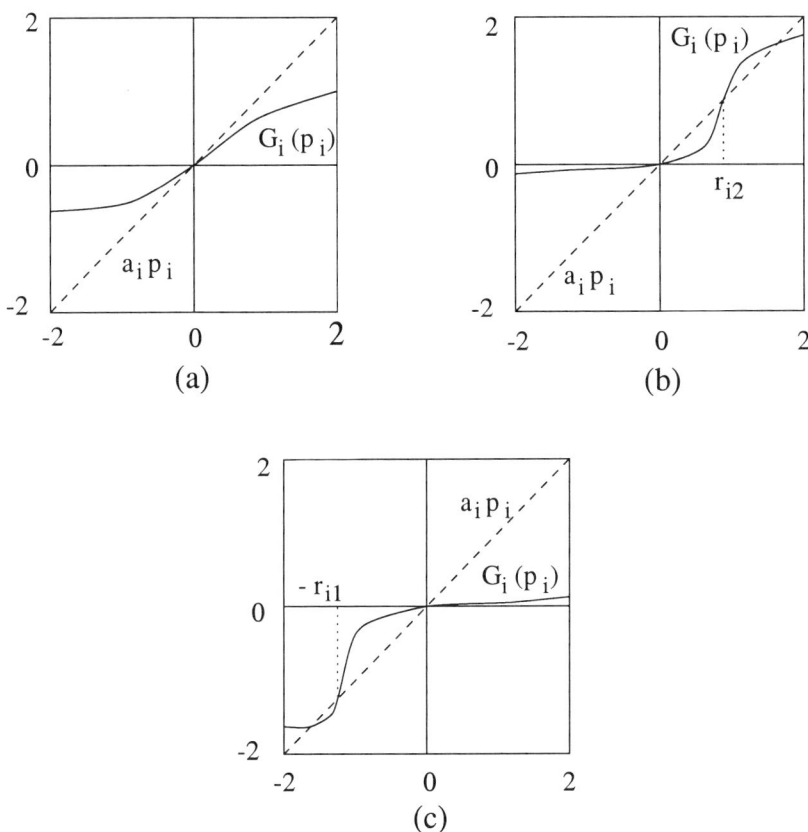

Figure 5.4.2: (a)–(c) Graphs of nonlinearities $G_i(p_i)$ corresponding to an asymptotically stable equilibrium $p_i = 0$.

Remark 5.4.1 Conditions corresponding to (H–5) are depicted in Fig. 5.4.1(c) with r_i defined in that figure. Also, conditions corresponding to (H–4) are shown in Fig. 5.4.1(b) with r_i again defined in that figure. Conditions satisfying (H–3) are illustrated in Fig. 5.4.1(a), where $r_i = \min\{|r_{i1}|, |r_{i2}|\}$ with r_{i1} and r_{i2} specified in that figure. Finally, various conditions corresponding to (H–2) are demonstrated in Fig. 5.4.2(a)–(c). In Fig. 5.4.2(a) we have $r_i = \infty$, in Fig. 5.4.2(b) we have $r_i = r_{i2}$ and in Fig. 5.4.2(c) we have $r_i = r_{i1}$, with r_{i2} and r_{i1} defined in theses figures, respectively. ∎

Remark 5.4.2 In view of the assumptions imposed on the functions $G_i(p_i)$ in Section 5.3, for $r_i > 0$ there exist constants $\sigma_{i1} > 0$ and $\sigma_{i2} > 0$ such that

$$\sigma_{i1} p_i^2 < p_i G_i(p_i) < \sigma_{i2} p_i^2, \quad -r_i < p_i < r_i \tag{5.4.1}$$

or equivalently, when $p_i \neq 0$,

$$\sigma_{i1} < \frac{G_i(p_i)}{p_i} < \sigma_{i2}, \quad -r_i < p_i < r_i. \tag{5.4.2}$$

∎

We will also require the next hypothesis.

(H–6) For $(\mathcal{S}_i)$ we have
$$(-a_i + T_{ii}\delta_i) < 0$$
where
$$\delta_i = \begin{cases} \sigma_{i1}, & \text{if } T_{ii} < 0 \\ \sigma_{i2}, & \text{if } T_{ii} > 0. \end{cases}$$
∎

We can now state and prove the following result.

Proposition 5.4.1 Assume that for $(\mathcal{S}_i)$ hypothesis (H–1) is true.
1) If (H–2) is true, then the equilibrium $p_i = 0$ is *asymptotically stable*.

2) If (H–2) and (H–6) are true, then $p_i = 0$ is *exponentially stable*.

5.4. SINGLE NEURON SUBSYSTEMS

3) If (H–3) is true, then the equilibrium $p_i = 0$ is *unstable*, in fact, *completely unstable*.

4) If (H–4) or (H–5) is true, then $p_i = 0$ is unstable.

Proof: (i) Choose the function

$$v_i(p_i) = \frac{1}{2}p_i^2. \tag{5.4.3}$$

Since (H–1) is true, then

$$D_{(S_i)}v_i(p_i) = p_i\dot{p}_i = p_i[-a_ip_i + T_{ii}G_i(p_i)]. \tag{5.4.4}$$

If (H–2) is true, then $v_i(p_i)$ is positive definite and $D_{(S_i)}v_i(p_i)$ is negative definite. Hence, $p_i = 0$ for (S_i) [with $I_i(t) \equiv 0$] is asymptotically stable.

(ii) Choose (5.4.3) as a Lyapunov function and assume that (H–1), (H–2), and (H–6) are true. Then

$$D_{(S_i)}v_i(p_i) \leq (-a_i + T_{ii}\delta_i)p_i^2$$

when $|p_i| < r_i$. Since $(-a_i + T_{ii}\delta_i) < 0$, it follows that the equilibrium $p_i = 0$ is exponentially stable.

(iii) Choose (5.4.3) as a Lyapunov function and assume that (H–1) and (H–3) are true. From inspection of (5.4.3) and (5.4.4) it follows that both $v_i(p_i)$ and $D_{(S_i)}v_i(p_i)$ are positive definite. Hence, the equilibrium $p_i = 0$ is completely unstable.

(iv) Choose as a Lyapunov function

$$v_i(p_i) = -\frac{1}{2}p_i^2 \tag{5.4.5}$$

and assume that (H–1) and (H–4) are true. Then

$$D_{(S_i)}v_i(p_i) = -p_i\left[-a_ip_i + T_{ii}G_i(p_i)\right]. \tag{5.4.6}$$

Thus when $p_i \in B(r_i)$ and $p_i > 0$, then $D_{(S_i)}v_i(p_i) < 0$ and $v_i(p_i) < 0$, and hence, $p_i = 0$ will be unstable.

In a similar manner, let us assume that (H–1) and (H–5) are true and choose the Lyapunov function (5.4.5). When $p_i \in B(r_i)$ and $p_i < 0$, then $v_i(p_i) < 0$ and $D_{(S_i)}v_i(p_i) < 0$ and hence, $p_i = 0$ will again be unstable. ∎

We conclude the present section by specifying the domain of attraction of $p_i = 0$ for (S_i) with $I_i(t) \equiv 0$, corresponding to the three cases shown in Fig. 5.4.2.

Fig. 5.4.2(a): $D_i = \Re$.

Fig. 5.4.2(b): $D_i = \{p_i \in \Re : p_i < r_{i2}\}$.

Fig. 5.4.2(c): $D_i = \{p_i \in \Re : p_i > -r_{i1}\}$.

5.5 Qualitative Analysis of the Analog Hopfield Neural Network Model: Local Results

In Chapter 3 we conducted a qualitative analysis of the class of neural networks (L) which includes the analog Hopfield neural network model (H_i') as a special case. In these results, we addressed primarily *global* qualitative properties of (H_i'), making use of an energy function of the form

$$E = -\frac{1}{2}\sum_{i=1}^{n}\sum_{j=1}^{n} T_{ij}v_i v_j - \sum_{i=1}^{n} I_i v_i + \sum_{i=1}^{n} \frac{1}{R_i}\int_0^{v_i} g_i^{-1}(\eta)d\eta.$$

Under the assumption that $T = [T_{ij}]$ is symmetric, we showed that (H_i') is globally stable, i.e., that all the trajectories of (H_i') tend to some asymptotically stable equilibrium (where E has a local minimum). When T is not symmetric, this global stability property will in general not hold. The results of Chapter 3 do not address local qualitative properties of (H_i').

Whether (H_i') is globally stable or not, an understanding of local qualitative properties of this network is of great importance. In the present section, we will address several of these properties, using the

5.5. HOPFIELD LOCAL RESULTS

interconnected system representation (Σ_i) for the network (H'_i), and employing the method of analysis indicated at the end of Section 5.3.

The present section is divided into nine parts. In the first three parts, we present various results for the asymptotic and exponential stability of equilibria of neural network (H'_i). In the fourth part, we establish estimates of trajectory bounds for (H'_i) while in the fifth part we determine estimates of the domain of attraction of an asymptotically stable equilibrium of (H'_i). In the sixth part we establish conditions for instability of an equilibrium for neural network (H'_i). In the seventh part we consider the stability of neural networks under structural changes. In the eighth part we address the question of stability under the conditions of the high gain limit. Finally, in the ninth part we illustrate some of the above results by means of a simple specific example.

A. General Stability Conditions

We will utilize the following hypotheses in our first result.

(A-1) For system (Σ_i), the external inputs are all identically zero, i.e.,
$$I_i(t) \equiv 0, \ i = 1, \cdots, n.$$ ∎

(A-2) For system (Σ_i), the interconnections satisfy the estimates
$$x_i T_{ij} G_j(x_j) \leq |x_i| a_{ij} |x_j|$$
for all $|x_i| < r_i$, $|x_j| < r_j$, $i,j = 1, \cdots n$, where the a_{ij} are real constants. ∎

(A-3) There exists an n-vector $\alpha > 0$ [i.e., $\alpha^T = (\alpha_1, \cdots, \alpha_n)$ and $\alpha_i > 0$, $i = 1, \cdots, n$] such that the *test matrix* $S = [s_{ij}]$, given by
$$s_{ij} = \begin{cases} \alpha_i(-a_i + a_{ii}), & i = j \\ (\alpha_i a_{ij} + \alpha_j a_{ji})/2, & i \neq j \end{cases}$$
is negative definite, where the a_i are defined in (Σ_i) and the a_{ij} are given in (A-2). ∎

We are now in a position to prove the following result.

Theorem 5.5.1 The equilibrium $x = 0$ of the neural network (S) with decomposition (Σ_i) is *exponentially stable* if hypotheses (A–1)–(A–3) are satisfied.

Proof: For system (Σ_i) [resp., system (S)], we choose the Lyapunov function

$$v(x) = \sum_{i=1}^{n} \frac{1}{2}\alpha_i x_i^2 \tag{5.5.1}$$

where the α_i are given in (A–3). This function is clearly positive definite. The time derivative of v along the solutions of (Σ_i) is given by

$$D_{(\Sigma_i)}v(x) = \sum_{i=1}^{n} \frac{1}{2}\alpha_i(2x_i)\left[-a_i x_i + \sum_{j=1}^{n} T_{ij}G_j(x_j)\right]$$

where (A–1) has been invoked. In view of (A–2) we have

$$\begin{aligned} D_{(\Sigma_i)}v(x) &\leq \sum_{i=1}^{n} \alpha_i\left(-a_i x_i^2 + |x_i|\sum_{j=1}^{n} a_{ij}|x_j|\right) \\ &= w^T R w \\ &= w^T \frac{R + R^T}{2} w \\ &= w^T S w \\ &\leq \lambda_M(S)|x|^2 \end{aligned} \tag{5.5.2}$$

for all $|x| < r$, where $r = \min_i(r_i)$, $w^T = (|x_1|, \cdots, |x_n|)^T$,

$$|x| = \sqrt{\sum_{i=1}^{n} x_i^2},$$

r_i is given in (A–2), $R = [r_{ij}]$ is given by

$$r_{ij} = \begin{cases} \alpha_i(-a_i + a_{ii}), & i = j \\ \alpha_i a_{ij}, & i \neq j, \end{cases}$$

S is the matrix given in (A–3), and $\lambda_M(S)$ denotes the largest eigenvalue of the real symmetric matrix S. Since S is by assumption

5.5. HOPFIELD LOCAL RESULTS

negative definite, we have $\lambda_M(S) < 0$. It follows from (5.5.1) and (5.5.2) that in some neighborhood of the origin $x = 0$, we have

$$c_1|x|^2 \leq v(x) \leq c_2|x|^2, \; D_{(\Sigma_i)}v(x) \leq -c_3|x|^2$$

where $c_1 = (1/2)\min_i \alpha_i > 0$, $c_2 = (1/2)\max_i \alpha_i > 0$, and $c_3 = -\lambda_M(S) > 0$. Hence, the equilibrium $x = 0$ of the neural network (Σ_i) is exponentially stable (see Section 5.2 or [19], Chapter 5). ∎

Remark 5.5.1 Consistent with the philosophy of viewing the neural network (S) as an interconnection of n free subsystems (S_i), we think of the Lyapunov function (5.5.1) as consisting of a weighted sum of Lyapunov functions for each free subsystem (S_i) [with $I_i(t) \equiv 0$]. There are two reasons for using the weighting vector $\alpha > 0$. First, it provides flexibility to emphasize the relative importance of the qualitative properties of the various individual subsystems. Secondly, as will be seen in the next subsection, it provides a vehicle for establishing additional and simpler results. ∎

Remark 5.5.2 It is emphasized that Theorem 5.5.1 does not require that the parameters T_{ij} in (Σ_i) form a symmetric matrix. ∎

Remark 5.5.3 Hypothesis (A–2) provides a measure of interaction between the various subsystems (S_i). ∎

In order to satisfy hypothesis (A–3), it is necessary that

$$-a_i + a_{ii} < 0, \quad i = 1, \cdots, n. \tag{5.5.3}$$

Now if we let $i = j$ in (A–2), we have

$$T_{ii}x_i G_i(x_i) \leq a_{ii}x_i^2$$

and if we apply the sector conditions (5.4.1), we obtain

$$a_{ii} = T_{ii}\delta_i$$

where
$$\delta_i = \sigma_{i2} \text{ when } T_{ii} > 0$$
and
$$\delta_i = \sigma_{i1} \text{ when } T_{ii} < 0.$$

Thus in order to satisfy (5.5.3), and hence (A–3), it is necessary that (H–6) be satisfied. It follows from Part 2) of Proposition 5.4.1 that (A–3) can only be satisfied if the equilibrium $p_i = 0$ of each free subsystem $(\mathcal{S}_i)$ [with $I_i(t) \equiv 0$] is exponentially stable.

If, as in Part 2) of Proposition 5.4.1 we choose for the free subsystem $(\mathcal{S}_i)$ [with $I_i(t) \equiv 0$] the Lyapunov function $v_i(p_i) = (1/2)p_i^2$, then we obtain under the above assumptions the estimate

$$D_{(\mathcal{S}_i)} v_i(p_i) \leq \sigma_i p_i^2$$

where
$$\sigma_i = -a_i + T_{ii}\delta_i.$$

This shows that the term $\sigma_i < 0$ constitutes a measure of the degree of stability for the free subsystem $(\mathcal{S}_i)$. The same reasoning shows that collectively, the numbers σ_i, $i = 1, \cdots, n$, will have stabilizing effects on the overall neural network while the off-diagonal terms in the matrix S in (A–3) *may* have destabilizing effects.

The above discussion shows that the conditions of Theorem 5.5.1 provide a means of analyzing a complex neural network in terms of the qualitative properties of the free subsystems $(\mathcal{S}_i)$ and in terms of the interconnecting structure of the network (Σ_i).

If in (A–2), we take absolute values of both sides of the inequality for $j \neq i$ and if we apply (5.4.1), we obtain

$$|x_i T_{ij} G_j(x_j)| \leq |x_i| \cdot |T_{ij}|\sigma_{j2}|x_j|.$$

In this case we may rephrase hypotheses (A–2) and (A–3) in the following manner.

(A–4) For system (Σ_i), the interconnections satisfy the estimates

$$x_i T_{ii} G_i(x_i) \leq \delta_i T_{ii} x_i^2$$

5.5. HOPFIELD LOCAL RESULTS

and
$$|x_i T_{ij} G_j(x_j)| \le |x_i| \cdot |T_{ij}|\sigma_{j2}|x_j|, \ i \ne j$$
where $\delta_i = \sigma_{i1}$ when $T_{ii} < 0$ and $\delta_i = \sigma_{i2}$ when $T_{ii} > 0$ for all $|x_i| < r_i$, $|x_j| < r_j$, $i, j = 1, \cdots, n$. ∎

(A–5) There exists an n-vector $\alpha > 0$ such that the test matrix $S = [s_{ij}]$ specified by

$$s_{ij} = \begin{cases} \alpha_i(-a_i + \delta_i T_{ii}), & i = j \\ (\alpha_i |T_{ij}|\sigma_{j2} + \alpha_j |T_{ji}|\sigma_{i2})/2, & i \ne j \end{cases}$$

is negative definite. ∎

Similarly as in Theorem 5.5.1, we now obtain the following result.

Corollary 5.5.1 The equilibrium $x = 0$ of the neural network (S) with decomposition (Σ_i) is exponentially stable if hypotheses (A–1), (A–4), and (A–5) are satisfied. ∎

B. Weak-Coupling Conditions

The test matrix S given in hypothesis (A–5) has off-diagonal terms which are nonnegative. For such cases, equivalent stability results may be obtained which are much easier to apply than, e.g., Theorem 5.5.1 or Corollary 5.5.1. Such results are called *weak-coupling conditions* in the literature [16], [19] since they involve sign-insensitive hypotheses for the interconnections of system (Σ_i).

In the proofs of several subsequent results, we will make use of some of the properties of M-matrices (see, e.g., [16], Chapter 2). In the following, we summarize those results which we will require.

Definition 5.5.1 A real $n \times n$ matrix $D = [d_{ij}]$ is said to be an M-matrix if $d_{ij} \le 0$, $i \ne j$, and if all successive principal minors of D are positive. ∎

Theorem 5.5.2 Let $D = [d_{ij}]$ be an $n \times n$ matrix with nonpositive off-diagonal elements. Then the following statements are true:

1) D is an M-matrix if and only if the real parts of all eigenvalues of D are positive.

2) D is an M-matrix if and only if D is nonsingular and all elements of D^{-1} are nonnegative. (In this case we write $D^{-1} \geq 0$.)

3) D is an M-matrix if and only if there exist positive constants λ_j, $j = 1, \cdots, n$, such that

$$\sum_{j=1}^{n} \lambda_j d_{ij} \geq 0, \; i = 1, \cdots, n. \tag{5.5.4}$$

[Inequality (5.5.4) is called a *row dominance condition*.]

4) D is an M-matrix if and only if there exist positive constants η_i, $i = 1, \cdots, n$, such that

$$\sum_{i=1}^{n} \eta_i d_{ij} \geq 0, \; j = 1, \cdots, n. \tag{5.5.5}$$

[Inequality (5.5.5) is called a *column dominance condition*.]

5) D is an M-matrix if and only if there exists a diagonal matrix $\tilde{A} = \text{diag}[\alpha_1, \cdots, \alpha_n]$, $\alpha_i > 0$, $i = 1, \cdots, n$, such that the matrix

$$B = \tilde{A} D + D^T \tilde{A} \tag{5.5.6}$$

is positive definite. ∎

In the first result of the present subsection we will require the following hypothesis.

(A–6) The successive principal minors of the $n \times n$ test matrix $D = [d_{ij}]$ are all positive, where

$$d_{ij} = \begin{cases} a_i - \delta_i T_{ii}, & i = j \\ -|T_{ij}|\sigma_{j2}, & i \neq j \end{cases}$$

where a_i is defined in Eq. (Σ_i) and $\delta_i T_{ii}$ and $|T_{ij}|\sigma_{j2}$ are defined in (A–4). ∎

5.5. HOPFIELD LOCAL RESULTS

Theorem 5.5.3 The equilibrium $x = 0$ of the neural network $(\mathcal{S})$ with decomposition (Σ_i) is *exponentially stable* if hypotheses (A–1), (A–4), and (A–6) are satisfied.

Proof: Since by assumption $d_{ij} \leq 0$ when $i \neq j$, and since the successive principal minors of matrix D in (A–6) are all positive, D is an M-matrix. In view of Part 5) of Theorem 5.5.2, there exists a diagonal matrix $\tilde{A} = \text{diag}[\alpha_1, \cdots, \alpha_n] > 0$ such that the matrix

$$-2S \triangleq \tilde{A}D + D^T \tilde{A}$$

is positive definite. But the matrix S is precisely the test matrix specified in (A–5). Furthermore, if $-2S$ is positive definite, then S will be negative definite. Therefore, if the hypotheses of the present theorem are satisfied, then the hypotheses of Corollary 5.5.1 are also satisfied. Hence, the equilibrium $x = 0$ for $(\mathcal{S})$ will be exponentially stable. ∎

Remark 5.5.4 From Theorem 5.5.2 it follows that any of the following assumptions are equivalent to hypothesis (A–6):

(A–7) The real parts of the eigenvalues of the matrix D given in (A–6) are positive.

(A–8) For the matrix D in (A–6) there exist positive constants λ_j, $j = 1, \cdots, n$, such that

$$(a_i - T_{ii}\delta_i) - \sum_{j=1, j \neq i}^{n} \frac{\lambda_j}{\lambda_i} |T_{ij}| \sigma_{j2} > 0, \ i = 1, \cdots, n. \tag{5.5.7}$$

(A–9) For the matrix D in (A–6) there exist positive constants η_i, $i = 1, \cdots, n$, such that

$$(a_j - T_{jj}\delta_j) - \sum_{i=1, i \neq j}^{n} \frac{\eta_i}{\eta_j} |T_{ij}| \sigma_{i2} > 0, \ j = 1, \cdots, n. \tag{5.5.8}$$

∎

Remark 5.5.5 Under the assumptions of Theorem 5.5.3 [i.e., under the assumptions (A-1), (A-4), and (A-6)] it can be shown, independently of Theorem 5.5.1 or Corollary 5.5.1, that the equilibrium $x_e = 0$ of (Σ_i) is asymptotically stable. In doing so, we use as a Lyapunov function a generalized Hamming distance from the equilibrium $x_e = 0$ of the neural network to the state x. Specifically, we let

$$v(x) = \sum_{i=1}^{n} \alpha_i |x_i| \qquad (5.5.9)$$

where the $\alpha_i > 0$, $i = 1, \cdots, n$ are weighting factors.

Along the solutions of system $(\mathcal{S})$, with $I(t) \equiv 0$, we have, letting $-Ax + TG(x) = F(x)$,

$$\begin{aligned} D_{(\mathcal{S})} v(x) &= \lim_{h \to 0+} \sup \frac{v[x + h \cdot F(x)] - v(x)}{h} \\ &\leq \sum_{i=1}^{n} \alpha_i \left[-a_i |x_i| + \delta_i T_{ii} |x_i| + \sum_{j=1, j\neq i}^{n} |T_{ij}| \sigma_{j2} |x_j| \right] \\ &\leq -\alpha^T D w \end{aligned}$$

where $\alpha^T = (\alpha_1, \cdots, \alpha_n)$, $w^T = (|x_1|, \cdots, |x_n|)$, and $D = [d_{ij}]$ is the test matrix given in hypothesis (A-6). Since $d_{ij} \leq 0$ for all $j \neq i$, and since by assumption the successive principal minors of D are positive, it follows that D is an M-matrix. Hence, D^{-1} exists and $D^{-1} \geq 0$ (i.e., $[D^{-1}]_{ij} \geq 0$ for all $i, j = 1, \cdots, n$), by Part 2) of Theorem 5.5.2. If we let

$$y^T = \alpha^T D$$

then

$$\alpha = (D^{-1})^T y. \qquad (5.5.10)$$

Now choose a vector $y > 0$ (i.e., $y_i > 0$, $i = 1, \cdots, n$). Then $\alpha > 0$ and $v(x)$ is positive definite and

$$D_{(\mathcal{S})} v(x) \leq -y^T w$$

is negative definite in some neighborhood of the origin. Hence, the equilibrium $x = 0$ of system $(\mathcal{S})$ is asymptotically stable (see [16], Theorem 2.2.23).

5.5. HOPFIELD LOCAL RESULTS

In other words, the above argument shows that if the hypotheses of Theorem 5.5.3 are satisfied, then the Lyapunov function $v(x)$ given in (5.5.9), which may be viewed as a generalized Hamming distance of the state vector x from the origin, will decrease with time and approach the origin as $t \to \infty$. ∎

Remark 5.5.6 Clearly, Theorem 5.5.3 is easier to apply than Theorem 5.5.1. ∎

It is possible to improve Theorem 5.5.3 by utilizing an alternative hypothesis to (A–6):

(A–10) The successive principal minors of the $n \times n$ test matrix $D = [d_{ij}]$ are all positive, where

$$d_{ij} = \begin{cases} a_i/\sigma_{i2} - T_{ii}, & i = j \\ -|T_{ij}|, & i \neq j \end{cases}$$

where a_i and T_{ij} are defined in (Σ_i) and σ_{i2} is defined in (5.4.2). ∎

Note that when $T_{ii} > 0$, then (A–10) and (A–6) are equivalent. However, when $T_{ii} < 0$, then (A–10) is easier to satisfy than (A–6).

Corollary 5.5.2 The equilibrium $x = 0$ of the neural network ($\mathcal{S}$) with decomposition (Σ_i) is *asymptotically stable* if hypotheses (A–1), (A–4), and (A–10) are true.

Proof: Once more we choose the Lyapunov function (5.5.9). Along the solutions of ($\mathcal{S}$) we have

$$\begin{aligned}
D_{(\mathcal{S})}v(x) &\leq \sum_{i=1}^{n} \alpha_i \bigg[-a_i|x_i| + \frac{T_{ii}G_i(x_i)}{x_i}|x_i| \\
&\quad + \sum_{j=1, j\neq i}^{n} |T_{ij}|\frac{G_j(x_j)}{x_j}|x_j| \bigg] \\
&\leq \sum_{i=1}^{n} \alpha_i \bigg[\left(-\frac{a_i}{\sigma_{i2}} + T_{ii}\right)\frac{G_i(x_i)}{x_i}|x_i| \\
&\quad + \sum_{j=1, j\neq i}^{n} |T_{ij}|\frac{G_j(x_j)}{x_j}|x_j| \bigg] \\
&= -\alpha^T D w
\end{aligned}$$

where

$$w^T = \left[\frac{G_1(x_1)}{x_1}|x_1|, \cdots, \frac{G_n(x_n)}{x_n}|x_n|\right] = (w_1, \cdots, w_n),$$

$w = 0$ if and only if $x = 0$ and $w_i > 0$, $i = 1, \cdots, n$ when $x \neq 0$. The vector α is defined in (5.5.9) and the matrix $D = [d_{ij}]$ is defined in (A–10). Following the argument given in Remark 5.5.5, we conclude that $D_{(S)}v(x)$ is negative definite. ∎

C. Application of the Comparison Principle to Vector Lyapunov Functions

In the present subsection we show how the comparison principle, when applied to vector Lyapunov functions, can be used in the stability analysis of neural networks (S). To this end, we consider the system of ordinary differential equations

$$\dot{x} = g(x) \tag{A}$$

where $x \in \Re^n$, $g: B(r) \to \Re^n$ for some $r > 0$, g is continuous, and $x = 0$ is an isolated equilibrium for (A). We also consider the *comparison system*

$$\dot{y} = H(y) \tag{VC}$$

where $y \in \Re^l$, $l \leq n$, $H: B(r) \to \Re^l$ for some $r > 0$, H is continuous, and $y = 0$ is an isolated equilibrium for (VC).

Definition 5.5.2 A function $H(y) = [H_1(y), \cdots, H_l(y)]^T$ is said to be *quasimonotonically increasing* if for each component H_j, $j = 1, \cdots, l$, the inequality $H_j(y) \leq H_j(z)$ is true whenever $y_i \leq z_i$ for all $j \neq i$ and $y_j = z_j$. ∎

Now let $v_i: \Re^n \to \Re$, $i = 1, \cdots, l$, denote l locally Lipschitz continuous Lyapunov functions having the property that $v_i(0) = 0$. Let

$$V(x) = [v_1(x), \cdots, v_l(x)]^T. \tag{5.5.11}$$

We call V a *vector Lyapunov function*. Such functions have been found useful in stability analysis (see, e.g., [16]), using comparison theorems. An example of such a comparison result is as follows.

5.5. HOPFIELD LOCAL RESULTS

Theorem 5.5.4 Let g and H be continuous on their respective domains of definition and let H be quasimonotonically increasing. Let $V(x)$ be a continuous nonnegative vector Lyapunov function of dimension l [i.e., $v_i(x) \geq 0$, $i = 1, \cdots, l$ for all x] such that $|V(x)|$ is positive definite (where $|\cdot|$ is any one of the equivalent norms on $\Re^l$). Assume that along the solutions of (A), the differential vector inequality

$$D_{(A)}V(x) \leq H[V(x)] \qquad (5.5.12)$$

holds componentwise, i.e., if $\varphi(t)$ is a solution of (A), then

$$Dv_i(\varphi(t)) = \lim_{k \to 0+} \tfrac{1}{k}\{v_i[\varphi(t+k)] - v_i[\varphi(t)]\}$$
$$\leq H_i[V(\varphi(t))], \ i = 1, \cdots, l.$$

If there are constants $a > 0$ and $b > 0$ such that $a|x|^b \leq |V(x)|$ and if the equilibrium $y = 0$ of system (VC) is exponentially stable, then the trivial solution of system (A) is also *exponentially stable*. ∎

Returning now to the analysis of the neural network, we associate with system ($\mathcal{S}$) equation (A) above, we let $l = n$, and we pick as a vector Lyapunov function

$$V(x) = [v_1(x), \cdots, v_n(x)]^T = [|x_1|, \cdots, |x_n|]^T.$$

Now assume that for system ($\mathcal{S}$), hypotheses (A–1), (A–4), and (A–6) are satisfied. Then along the solutions of ($\mathcal{S}$) we have

$$D_{(\mathcal{S})}V(x) = \begin{bmatrix} Dv_1(x) \\ \vdots \\ Dv_n(x) \end{bmatrix}$$
$$\leq \begin{bmatrix} -a_1|x_1| + \delta_1 T_{11}|x_1| + \sum_{j=2}^{n} |T_{1j}|\sigma_{j2}|x_j| \\ \vdots \\ -a_n|x_n| + \delta_n T_{nn}|x_n| + \sum_{j=1}^{n-1} |T_{nj}|\sigma_{j2}|x_j| \end{bmatrix}$$
$$= PV(x)$$

where $P = [p_{ij}] = -D$ and D is as defined in hypothesis (A–6).

Next, we consider the n-dimensional comparison equation

$$\dot{y} = H(y) \stackrel{\triangle}{=} Py. \qquad (\text{VC}')$$

Since $p_{ij} \geq 0$ for all $i \neq j$, we see that $H(y)$ in (VC') is quasimonotonically increasing. Finally, if we now assume that hypothesis (A–6) is satisfied, then it follows from Part 1) of Theorem 5.5.2 that all eigenvalues of $D = -P$ have positive real parts. Hence the equilibrium $y = 0$ of (VC') is exponentially stable. Since all conditions of Theorem 5.5.4 are now satisfied, we can conclude that the equilibrium $x = 0$ of the neural network $(\mathcal{S})$ is also exponentially stable. In other words, if hypotheses (A–1), (A–4), and (A–6) are satisfied, then the equilibrium $x = 0$ of $(\mathcal{S})$ is exponentially stable. But this is precisely Theorem 5.5.3, i.e., *we have proved Theorem 5.5.3 yet by another method, namely, by applying a comparison principle to vector Lyapunov functions.*

Remark 5.5.7 Our presentation thus far indicates that several equivalent weak coupling conditions (Corollary 5.5.1, Theorem 5.5.3) can be arrived at in a variety of *different* ways, including (a) usage of scalar quadratic Lyapunov functions [Eq. (5.5.1)]; (b) usage of a generalized Hamming distance [Eq. (5.5.9)]; (c) certain properties of M-matrices (see the proof of Theorem 5.5.3); and (d) applications of the comparison principle (e.g., Theorem 5.5.4) to vector Lyapunov functions [Eq. (5.5.11)]. This suggests that under certain circumstances the present results may yield reasonably good stability conditions. ∎

Remark 5.5.8 In arriving at the present results, experiments were conducted with a variety of Lyapunov functions $v(x)$ for composite system (Σ_i), including a weighted sum of energy functions for the free subsystems (single neurons). Such functions yield results which are more complicated but not less conservative than the ones presented herein. The explanation for this lies in the fact that in the vicinity of an equilibrium point, the neural network (Σ_i) is nearly linear [i.e., the terms $G_i(x_i)$ near $x_i = 0$ are nearly linear]. But for linear systems, quadratic Lyapunov functions (resp., norm Lyapunov functions) yield the best possible stability results, namely, necessary and

5.5. HOPFIELD LOCAL RESULTS

sufficient conditions (c.f. [19], Section 5.10). This observation is consistent with Sandberg's original work [21] and the work reported in [16] (pp. 82–83) in the analysis of a class of nonlinear transistor-linear resistor networks. ∎

D. Estimates of Trajectory Bounds

In general, one is not only interested in questions concerning the stability of an equilibrium of the system (S), but also in performance. One way of assessing the qualitative properties of the neural system (S) is by investigating solution bounds near an equilibrium of interest. We present here such a result by assuming that the hypotheses of Corollary 5.5.2 are satisfied. (Similar results can be established by assuming that, e.g., Theorem 5.5.3 is satisfied.)

In the following, *we will not require that the external inputs $I_i(t)$, $i = 1, \cdots, n$ be zero.* However, we will need to make the additional assumptions enumerated below.

(A–11) Assume that there exist $\lambda_i > 0$, $i = 1, \cdots, n$, and $\varepsilon > 0$ such that

$$\left(\frac{a_i}{\sigma_{i2}} - T_{ii}\right) - \sum_{j=1, j\neq i}^{n} \left(\frac{\lambda_j}{\lambda_i}\right)|T_{ji}| \geq \varepsilon > 0, \quad i = 1, \cdots, n \quad (5.5.13)$$

where a_i and T_{ij} are defined in (Σ_i) and σ_{i2} is defined in (5.4.2). ∎

(A–12) Assume that for system (Σ_i),

$$\sum_{i=1}^{n} \lambda_i |I_i(t)| \leq k, \text{ for all } t \geq 0 \quad (5.5.14)$$

for some constant $k > 0$ where the λ_i, $i = 1, \cdots, n$ are defined in (A–11). ∎

In the proof of our next theorem, we will once again make use of a comparison result. This time we consider a scalar comparison equation of the form

$$\dot{y} = G(y) \quad (C)$$

where $y \in \Re$, $G: B(r) \to \Re$ for some $r > 0$, and G is continuous on $B(r)$.

Theorem 5.5.5 Let $p(t)$ denote the maximal solution of (C) with $p(t_0) = y_0 \in B(r)$, $t \geq t_0 > 0$. If $r(t)$, $t \geq t_0 \geq 0$ is a continuous function such that $r(t_0) \leq y_0$, if $r(t)$ satisfies the differential inequality

$$Dr(t) = \lim_{h \to 0+} \frac{1}{h} \sup[r(t+h) - r(t)] \leq G(r(t))$$

almost everywhere, then

$$r(t) \leq p(t), \text{ for } t \geq t_0 \geq 0$$

for as long as both $r(t)$ and $p(t)$ exist. ∎

For the proof of the above result, as well as other comparison theorem, see e.g., [16] and [19].

Notation In the following, we let

$$\delta = \min_i \sigma_{i1} \quad (5.5.15)$$

where σ_{i1} is defined in (5.4.2), we let

$$c = \varepsilon\delta \quad (5.5.16)$$

where ε is given in (A–11), and we let

$$\varphi(t, t_0, x_0) = [\varphi_1(t, t_0, x_0), \cdots, \varphi_n(t, t_0, x_0)]^T$$

denote the solution of ($\mathcal{S}$) with $\varphi(t_0, t_0, x_0) = x_0 = (x_{10}, \cdots, x_{n0})^T$ for some $t_0 \geq 0$. ∎

We are now in a position to prove the following result.

Theorem 5.5.6 Assume that hypotheses (A–11) and (A–12) are satisfied. Then

$$\|\varphi(t, t_0, x_0)\| \stackrel{\triangle}{=} \sum_{i=1}^n \lambda_i |\varphi_i(t, t_0, x_0)|$$
$$\leq \left(\alpha - \frac{k}{c}\right) e^{-c(t-t_0)} + \frac{k}{c}, \ t \geq t_0 \geq 0 \quad (5.5.17)$$

5.5. HOPFIELD LOCAL RESULTS

provided that $\alpha > k/c$ and

$$\|x_0\| = \sum_{i=1}^{n} \lambda_i |x_{i0}| \leq \alpha$$

where the λ_i, $i = 1, \cdots, n$ are given in (A–11) and k is given in (A–12).

Proof: For $(\mathcal{S})$ we choose the Lyapunov function

$$v(x) = \sum_{i=1}^{n} \lambda_i |x_i|. \qquad (5.5.18)$$

Along the solutions of $(\mathcal{S})$ we obtain

$$D_{(\mathcal{S})} v(x) \leq \lambda^T D w + \sum_{i=1}^{n} \lambda_i |I_i(t)| \qquad (5.5.19)$$

where

$$w^T = \left[\frac{G_1(x_1)}{x_1} |x_1|, \cdots, \frac{G_n(x_n)}{x_n} |x_n| \right],$$

$$\lambda = (\lambda_1, \cdots, \lambda_n)^T,$$

and $D = [d_{ij}]$ is the test matrix given in (A–10). Note that when (A–11) is satisfied, as in the present theorem, then (A–10) is automatically satisfied. Note also that $w \geq 0$ (i.e., $w_i \geq 0$, $i = 1, \cdots, n$) and $w = 0$ if and only if $x = 0$.

Using manipulations involving (5.5.13)–(5.5.16) and (5.5.19), it is easy to show that

$$D_{(\mathcal{S})} v(x) \leq -cv(x) + k.$$

The above inequality yields now the comparison equation

$$\dot{y} = -cy + k. \qquad (C')$$

The unique solution of eq. (C') is given by

$$p(t, t_0, p_0) = \left(p_0 - \frac{k}{c} \right) e^{-c(t-t_0)} + \frac{k}{c}, \quad t \geq t_0$$

where the notation of Theorem 5.5.5 has been used. If we let $r = v$, then we obtain from Theorem 5.5.5 that

$$\begin{aligned} p(t) &\geq r(t) \\ &= v(\varphi(t, t_0, x_0)) \\ &= \sum_{i=1}^{n} \lambda_i |\varphi_i(t, t_0, x_0)| \\ &= \|\varphi(t, t_0, x_0)\| \end{aligned}$$

i.e., the desired estimate given by (5.5.17) is true, provided that

$$|r(t_0)| = \sum_{i=1}^{n} \lambda_i |x_{i0}| = \|x_0\| \leq \alpha \text{ and } \alpha > k/c. \quad \blacksquare$$

We conclude the present subsection by noting that methods for determining the optimal choice of the λ_i in Theorem 5.5.6, to obtain the least conservative estimate in (5.5.17), do not seem to have been determined at this time.

E. Estimates of the Domain of Attraction of an Equilibrium

Neural networks of the type considered herein have many equilibrium points. If a given equilibrium is asymptotically stable, or exponentially stable, then the extent of this stability is of interest. As usual, we assume that $x = 0$ is the equilibrium of interest. If $\varphi(t, t_0, x_0)$ denotes a solution of the network (S) with $\varphi(t_0, t_0, x_0) = x_0$, then we would like to know for which points x_0 it is true that $\varphi(t, t_0, x_0)$ tends to the origin as $t \to \infty$. As noted earlier, the set of all such points x_0 makes up the *domain of attraction* (*the basin of attraction*) of equilibrium $x = 0$. In general, one cannot determine such a domain in its entirety. However, several techniques have been devised to estimate subsets of a domain of attraction. We apply one such method to neural networks, making use, e.g., of Theorem 5.5.1. This technique is applicable to our other results as well, by making obvious modifications.

We assume that the hypotheses (A–1)–(A–3) are satisfied and for the free subsystem (S_i) we choose the Lyapunov function

$$v_i(p_i) = \frac{1}{2} p_i^2.$$

5.5. HOPFIELD LOCAL RESULTS

Then
$$D_{(S_i)}v_i(p_i) \leq (-a_i + a_{ii})p_i^2, \quad |p_i| < r_i$$
for some $r_i > 0$. If (A-3) is satisfied, we must have $(-a_i + a_{ii}) < 0$ and $D_{(S_i)}v_i(p_i)$ is negative definite over $B(r_i)$. Let
$$C_{v_{0i}} = \left\{ p_i \in \Re : v_i(p_i) = \frac{1}{2}p_i^2 < \frac{1}{2}r_i^2 \triangleq v_{0i} \right\}.$$
Then $C_{v_{0i}}$ is contained in the domain of attraction of the equilibrium $p_i = 0$ for (S_i).

To obtain an estimate for the domain of attraction of $x = 0$ for the neural network (S), we use the Lyapunov function
$$v(x) = \sum_{i=1}^{n} \frac{1}{2}\alpha_i x_i^2 = \sum_{i=1}^{n} \alpha_i v_i(x_i).$$
It is now an easy matter to show that the set
$$C_\lambda = \left\{ x \in \Re^n : v(x) = \sum_{i=1}^{n} \alpha_i v_i(x_i) < \lambda \right\}$$
will be a subset of the domain of attraction of $x = 0$ for the neural network (S), where
$$\lambda = \min_{1 \leq i \leq n}(\alpha_i v_{0i}) = \sum_{1 \leq i \leq n} \left(\frac{1}{2}\alpha_i r_i^2 \right).$$

In order to obtain the best estimate of the domain of attraction of $x = 0$ by the present method, we must choose the α_i in an optimal fashion. The reader is referred to [12], [17], [20] where several methods to accomplish this are discussed.

F. Instability Results

Some of the equilibrium points in a neural network (S) may be unstable. We present here a sample instability result which may be viewed as a counterpart to Corollary 5.5.2. Instability results, formulated as counterparts to other stability results of the type considered herein may be obtained by making appropriate modifications.

(A–13) The successive principal minors of the $n \times n$ test matrix $D = [d_{ij}]$ given by
$$d_{ij} = \begin{cases} \sigma_i, & i = j \\ -|T_{ij}|, & i \neq j \end{cases}$$
are positive, where
$$\sigma_i = \frac{a_i}{\sigma_{i2}} - T_{ii} \text{ when } i \in F_s,$$
$$\sigma_i = \frac{-a_i}{\sigma_{i1}} + T_{ii} \text{ when } i \in F_u,$$
$F = F_s \cup F_u$ and $F = \{1, \cdots, n\}$. Here, a_i and T_{ij} are defined in (Σ_i) and σ_{i1} and σ_{i2} are specified in (5.4.2). ∎

Remark 5.5.9 To be able to satisfy (A–13), it is necessary that
$$\frac{a_i}{\sigma_{i2}} - T_{ii} > 0 \text{ when } i \in F_s, \tag{5.5.20}$$
and
$$-\frac{a_i}{\sigma_{i1}} + T_{ii} > 0 \text{ when } i \in F_u. \tag{5.5.21}$$
In particular, since $a_i/\sigma_{i1} > 0$, we must have $T_{ii} > 0$ when $i \in F_u$. ∎

Remark 5.5.10 We assume that for a free subsystem $(\mathcal{S}_i)$, either (5.5.20) or (5.5.21) is satisfied. If $i \in F_u$, choose a Lyapunov function of the form
$$v_i(p_i) = -|p_i|.$$
It is easily verified that
$$D_{(\mathcal{S}_i)} v_i(p_i) \leq -\sigma_i \frac{G_i(p_i)}{p_i} |p_i|, \quad |p_i| < r_i$$
where $G_i(p_i)$ is defined in (Σ_i) and σ_i is given in (A–13) and (5.5.21). Since in this case both $v_i(p_i)$ and $D_{(\mathcal{S}_i)} v_i(p_i)$ are negative definite, it follows that the equilibrium $p_i = 0$ for $(\mathcal{S}_i)$ will be completely unstable.

5.5. HOPFIELD LOCAL RESULTS

Similarly, when $i \in F_s$, we choose a Lyapunov function of the form
$$v_i(p_i) = |p_i|.$$
Then
$$D_{(\mathcal{S}_i)} v_i(p_i) \leq -\sigma_i \frac{G_i(p_i)}{p_i}|p_i|, \quad |p_i| < r_i$$
where σ_i is defined in (A–13) and (5.5.20). In this case, the equilibrium $p_i = 0$ for the free subsystem $(\mathcal{S}_i)$ will be asymptotically stable, since $v_i(p_i)$ is positive definite and $D_{(\mathcal{S}_i)} v_i(p_i)$ is negative definite.

Summarizing, in order for (A–13) to be satisfied, it is necessary that the equilibrium $p_i = 0$ of a free subsystem $(\mathcal{S}_i)$ be asymptotically stable when $i \in F_s$ and unstable when $i \in F_u$. ∎

We are now in a position to prove the following result.

Theorem 5.5.7 The equilibrium $x = 0$ of the neural network $(\mathcal{S})$ with decomposition (Σ_i) is *unstable* if hypotheses (A–1), (A–4), and (A–13) are satisfied. If in addition, $F_s = \emptyset$ ($\emptyset$ denotes the empty set), then the equilibrium $x = 0$ of $(\mathcal{S})$ is *completely unstable*.

Proof: For $(\mathcal{S})$ we choose the Lyapunov function
$$v(x) = \sum_{i \in F_u} \alpha_i(-|x_i|) + \sum_{i \in F_s} \alpha_i |x_i|$$
where $\alpha_i > 0$, $i = 1, \cdots, n$. Along the solutions of $(\mathcal{S})$ we have (following the proof of Corollary 5.5.2),
$$D_{(\mathcal{S})} v(x) \leq -\alpha^T D w \text{ for all } x \in B(r), \quad r = \min_i r_i$$
where $\alpha^T = (\alpha_1, \cdots, \alpha_n)$, D is defined in (A–13), and
$$w^T = \left[\frac{G_1(x_1)}{x_1}|x_1|, \cdots, \frac{G_n(x_n)}{x_n}|x_n| \right].$$

Again, using an argument similar to the one given in Corollary 5.5.2, we conclude that $D_{(\mathcal{S})} v(x)$ is negative definite over $B(r)$. Since every neighborhood of the origin $x = 0$ contains at least one point x' where

$v(x') < 0$, it follows that the equilibrium $x = 0$ for $(\mathcal{S})$ is unstable. Moreover, when $F_s = \emptyset$, then the function $v(x)$ is negative definite and the equilibrium $x = 0$ of $(\mathcal{S})$ is in fact completely unstable (refer to Lemma 5.2.2 and see, e.g., [19], Chapter 5). ∎

G. Stability Under Structural Perturbations

In specific applications involving adaptive schemes for learning algorithms in neural networks, the interconnection patterns (and external inputs) are changed to yield an evolution of different sets of desired asymptotically stable equilibrium points with appropriate domains of attraction. The present diagonal dominance conditions [see, e.g., (5.5.13) in (A–11)] can be used as constraints to guarantee that the desired equilibria always have the desired stability properties.

To be more specific, we assume that a given neural network has been designed with a set of interconnections whose strengths can be varied from zero to some specified values. We express this by writing in place of Eq. (Σ_i),

$$\dot{x}_i = -a_i x_i + \sum_{j=1}^{n} \theta_{ij} T_{ij} G_j(x_j) + I_i(t), \quad i = 1, \cdots, n \qquad (\Sigma'_i)$$

where $0 \leq \theta_{ij} \leq 1$. We also assume that in the given neural network things have been arranged in such a manner that for some given desired value $\Delta > 0$, it is true that

$$\Delta = \min_{i} \left(\frac{a_i}{\sigma_{i2}} - \theta_{ii} T_{ii} \right).$$

From what has been said in Part B of the present section, it should now be clear that if $I_i(t) \equiv 0$, $i = 1, \cdots, n$ and if the diagonal dominance conditions

$$\Delta - \sum_{j=1, j \neq i}^{n} \left(\frac{\lambda_j}{\lambda_i} \right) |\theta_j T_{ij}| > 0, \quad i = 1, \cdots, n \qquad (5.5.22)$$

are satisfied for some $\lambda_i > 0$, $i = 1, \cdots, n$, then the equilibrium $x = 0$ of system (Σ'_i) will be asymptotically stable. It is important

5.5. HOPFIELD LOCAL RESULTS

to recognize that condition (5.5.22) constitutes a single stability condition for the neural network under structural perturbations. Thus, the strengths of interconnections of the neural network may be rearranged in any manner to achieve some desired set of equilibrium points. If (5.5.22) is satisfied, then these equilibria will be asymptotically stable. (Stability under structural perturbations is addressed in great detail in [4], [24].)

H. The High Gain Limit

As mentioned at the beginning of the present section, the popular method of designing neural networks involves an energy function of the form

$$E = -\frac{1}{2}\sum_{i=1}^{n}\sum_{j=1}^{n}T_{ij}v_iv_j - \sum_{i=1}^{n}I_iv_i + \sum_{i=1}^{n}\frac{1}{R_i}\int_0^{v_i}g_i^{-1}(\eta)d\eta.$$

The first two terms of this equation are chosen in the design process to correspond to a quadratic cost function which when minimized over the range of v_i, $i = 1, \cdots, n$, will yield desired solutions to the problem of interest. The last term of the above equation is not used in this design process. The usual justification for ignoring this term is that the integral vanishes in the "high gain limit."

The term "high gain limit" (see Section 3.5) refers to the limit of the slope of $g_i(x_i)$ approaching infinity at $x_i = 0$, i.e.,

$$\left.\frac{dg_i(x_i)}{dx_i}\right|_{x_i=0} \to \infty.$$

For the specific nonlinearity given in (5.3.1), this corresponds to the case when $\lambda_i \to \infty$. The graph of $g_i(\cdot)$ is depicted in Fig. 5.5.1 for $\lambda_i = 1.4$. In general, as the slope increases, the function $g_i(\cdot)$ will approach the sign function given by

$$\text{sgn}(x_i) = \begin{cases} -1, & x_i < 0 \\ 0, & x_i = 0 \\ +1, & x_i > 0. \end{cases}$$

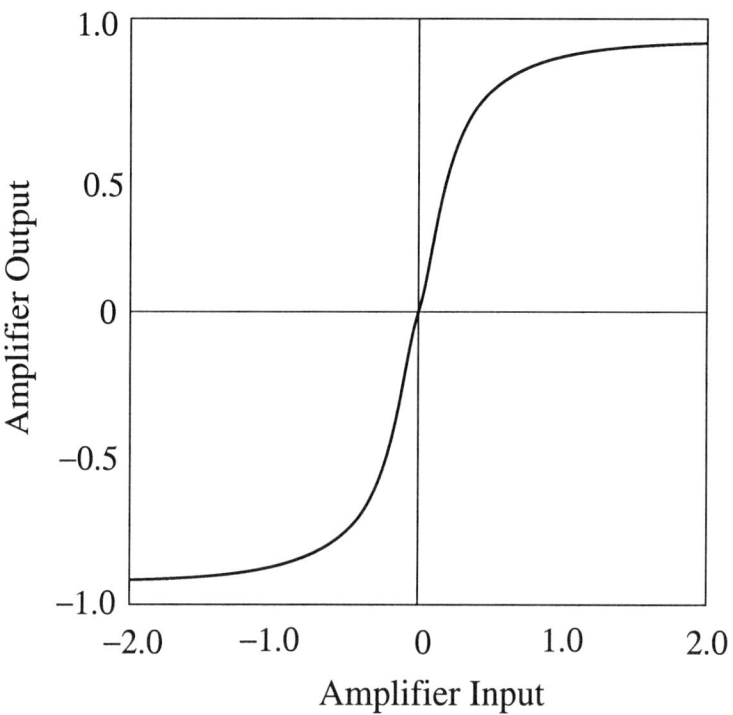

Figure 5.5.1: Sigmoidal nonlinearity $g_i(x_i)$.

5.5. HOPFIELD LOCAL RESULTS

In terms of the sector bounds σ_{i1} and σ_{i2} defined in (5.4.1), the high gain limit corresponds to

$$\sigma_{i2} \to \infty \quad \text{if } u_i^* = 0 \tag{5.5.23}$$

and

$$\left.\begin{array}{c}\sigma_{i1} \to 0 \\ \sigma_{i2} \to 0\end{array}\right\} \text{ if } u_i^* \neq 0 \tag{5.5.24}$$

where $u^* = (u_1^*, \cdots, u_n^*)^T$ is defined in (5.3.2).

When (5.5.23) applies, assumption (A–10) and Corollary 5.5.2 suggest that for asymptotic stability, the parameter a_i has relatively little effect but that T_{ii} is required to be negative for all $i = 1, \cdots, n$.

In the case when (5.5.24) applies, hypotheses (A–5) and (A–6) along with Corollary 5.5.1 and Theorem 5.5.3, respectively, show that the asymptotic stability of an equilibrium, with no component equal to zero, will depend only on the sign of a_i which is always assumed to be positive for each $i = 1, \cdots, n$. Thus in this case the matrix D in (A–6) approaches the diagonal matrix $D' = \text{diag}[a_1, \cdots, a_n]$, and D' has positive successive principal minors.

The above observations suggest the following. If for an equilibrium u^*, $u_i^* \neq 0$ for all $i = 1, \cdots, n$, then this equilibrium will be stable in the high gain limit. In this case, it is necessary to use only the first two terms of the energy function E in the design. On the other hand, if any component of the equilibrium is equal to zero, then the asymptotic stability of that equilibrium is not guaranteed. In this case, a design which neglects the third term of the energy function E may fail.

I. A Specific Example

To illustrate the applicability of some of the results established above, we consider the example in Hopfield [6]. For this case

$$T = \begin{bmatrix} 0 & 1 \\ 1 & 0 \end{bmatrix} \text{ and } g_i(x_i) = \frac{2}{\pi} \tan^{-1}\left(\frac{\lambda \pi}{2} x_i\right)$$

where $\lambda = 1.4$. Since specific values for a_1 and a_2 are not specified in [6], we chose $a_1 = a_2 = 1.1$. Thus (Σ_i) assumes the form

$$\begin{aligned}\dot{x}_1 &= -1.1x_1 + g_2(x_2) + I_1(t) \\ \dot{x}_2 &= g_1(x_2) - 1.1x_2 + I_2(t).\end{aligned} \qquad (\Sigma_i')$$

Letting $I_1(t) = I_2(t) \equiv 0$, we obtain three equilibrium points for (Σ_i'): $(0,0)$, $(0.454, 0.454)$, and $(-0.454, -0.454)$.

For the equilibrium at $(-0.454, -0.454)$, the translated free subsystems assume the form

$$\dot{p}_i = -1.1 p_i + I_i(t), \ i = 1, 2 \qquad (\mathcal{S}_i)$$

where $p_i = x_i + 0.454$. With $I_i(t) \equiv 0$, the equilibrium $p_i = 0$ for $(\mathcal{S}_i)$ will be globally asymptotically stable.

The nonlinearities $G_i(p_i)$, $i = 1, 2$, are given by

$$\begin{aligned}G_i(p_i) &= \tfrac{2}{\pi} \tan^{-1}\left(\tfrac{\lambda \pi}{2}(p_i - 0.454)\right) \\ &+ \tfrac{2}{\pi} \tan^{-1}\left(\tfrac{\lambda \pi}{2}(0.454)\right).\end{aligned}$$

For this case, relation (5.4.2) assumes the form

$$0 < \frac{G_i(p_i)}{p_i} < \sigma_{i2}, \ \ \sigma_{i2} < 1.1 \text{ when } |p_i| < 0.454. \qquad (5.5.25)$$

All hypotheses of Corollary 5.5.2 are satisfied. In particular, the test matrix D of that result assumes the form

$$D = \begin{bmatrix} \frac{1.1}{\sigma_{i2}} & -1 \\ -1 & \frac{1.1}{\sigma_{i2}} \end{bmatrix}.$$

Since all successive principal minors of D are positive, the equilibrium $(-0.454, -0.454)$ is asymptotically stable.

The equilibrium $(0.454, 0.454)$ can be analyzed by Corollary 5.5.2 in an identical manner. For illustration purposes, however, we analyze this equilibrium by Theorem 5.5.1. After translating this equilibrium point to the origin, relation (5.4.2) assumes once more the

5.5. HOPFIELD LOCAL RESULTS

form (5.5.25), where now $p_i = x_i - 0.454$. All hypotheses of Theorem 5.5.1 are satisfied. In particular, the matrix S for this case assumes the form

$$S = \begin{bmatrix} -1.1\alpha_1 & (\alpha_1\sigma_{22} + \alpha_2\sigma_{12})/2 \\ (\alpha_1\sigma_{22} + \alpha_2\sigma_{12})/2 & -1.1\alpha_2 \end{bmatrix}.$$

If we choose $\alpha_1 = \alpha_2 = 1$, then S will be negative definite. Thus either Theorem 5.5.1 or Corollary 5.5.1 may be applied to conclude that the equilibrium $(0.454, 0.454)$ is exponentially stable.

We can generate an estimate for the domain of attraction of the equilibrium $(0.454, 0.454)$ by determining the largest constant μ such that set

$$A = \{(x_1, x_2) \in \Re^2 \colon (x_1 - 0.454)^2 + (x_2 - 0.454)^2 < \mu\}$$

is a subset of the region where the time derivative of

$$v(x) = \frac{1}{2}\left[(x_1 - 0.454)^2 + (x_2 - 0.454)^2\right]$$

for the present system is negative definite. We obtain for this specific example $\mu = (0.64)^2$.

Not all equilibrium points of a neural system can be handled by our results. To illustrate this, consider the equilibrium of (Σ_i') at the origin $(0, 0)$. In this case $G_i(x_i) = g_i(x_i)$ and (5.4.2) assumes the form

$$0 < \frac{g_i(x_i)}{x_i} \leq \sigma_{i2} = 1.4, \quad i = 1, 2;\ x_i \in \Re.$$

The test matrix D in hypothesis (A–10) is given by

$$D = \begin{bmatrix} 1.1/1.4 & -1 \\ -1 & 1.1/1.4 \end{bmatrix}.$$

Since the successive principal minors of D are not positive, Corollary 5.5.2 is not applicable. In fact, none of the results for asymptotic or exponential stability will apply. Our instability results do not apply either, since the free subsystems $(\mathcal{S}_i)$, $i = 1, 2$ both have an exponentially stable equilibrium at the origin.

We can prove that the equilibrium at the origin is in fact unstable, using *Lyapunov's first method* (see [19], section 6.2). In doing so, we let $I_1(t) = I_2(t) \equiv 0$ in (Σ_i') and linearize, to obtain

$$\dot{q} = Aq$$

where $q = (q_1, q_2)^T$, $A = J(x)|_{x=0}$ = Jacobian matrix for (Σ_i) evaluated at the origin, and

$$A = \begin{bmatrix} -1.1 & 1.4 \\ 1.4 & -1.1 \end{bmatrix}.$$

Since A has one positive and one negative eigenvalue, it follows that the equilibrium $(0,0)$ is unstable.

We conclude by noting that we could have analyzed the equilibrium points $\pm(0.454, 0.454)$ by the first method of Lyapunov as well. However, such an analysis would not yield as much useful information as the present results (concerning, e.g., dominance conditions, forms of Lyapunov functions, estimates of domain of attraction, estimates of trajectory bounds, etc.).

5.6 Analysis of Synchronous Discrete-Time Hopfield-Type Neural Networks

In [11] (see also [3]) a detailed stochastic analysis of the memory capacity of discrete-time Hopfield-type neural networks is presented. The analysis in [11] is applicable to both synchronous and asynchronous systems with symmetric interconnection matrices. Among several issues, the analysis in [11] points to the need of methods to test the stability and attractivity of patterns that are to be stored as memories by such networks. Such tests are the topic of discussion in the present section. These tests will be applicable to synchronous discrete-time Hopfield-type neural networks, having interconnection matrices that need not necessarily be symmetric. Additionally, we will present a result for estimating the rate of convergence of a trajectory to an equilibrium.

5.6. SYNCHRONOUS HOPFIELD NETWORKS

The results which we will develop in the present section are in the same spirit as those established in the preceding sections. Thus, we will not pursue Hopfield's global energy function approach, but instead, we will develop a local qualitative theory for fully interconnected synchronous discrete-time Hopfield-type neural networks. Similarly as in Section 5.3, we will view such networks as an interconnection of n simple processes (subsystems) and we will analyze the networks in terms of the qualitative properties of the free subsystems and the properties of the interconnecting structure. The local results that we will establish will yield sufficient conditions for the asymptotic stability of an equilibrium, and estimates for the bounds of the trajectories for such networks.

By confining our attention to networks that switch synchronously, we are able to arrive at deterministic conditions in our analysis. Synchronous models of this type are suitable when straightforward neural network implementations by means of parallel digital processors are desired. This is frequently the case in engineering applications (e.g., pattern recognition applications) for which we desire fast responses. Synchronous models of this type are usually not suitable in cases where we wish to mimic biological systems.

A. The Synchronous Discrete-Time Hopfield Model as an Interconnected System

In the present section we consider synchronous discrete-time Hopfield-type neural networks described by equations of the form [refer to Chapter 2, Section 2.3, Eq. (2.3.4)]

$$\begin{cases} u_i(k+1) = \sum_{j=1}^{n} T_{ij} v_j(k) + (1 - \Delta T \cdot b_i) u_i(k) + I_i \\ \qquad\quad = \sum_{j=1}^{n} T_{ij} v_j(k) - a_i u_i(k) + I_i, \\ v_i(k) = g_i(u_i), \ i = 1, \cdots, n; \ k = 0, 1, 2, \cdots \end{cases} \quad (5.6.1)$$

where $a_i = 1 - \Delta T \cdot b_i$ [refer to equation (2.3.3) for the origin of the sampling period ΔT]. The function $g_i : \Re \to \Re$ is a monotone increasing, continuously differentiable function with $g_i(0) = 0$, which satisfies for $d_{i2} \geq d_{i1} > 0$ the sector condition

$$d_{i1} \leq g_i(\sigma)/\sigma \leq d_{i2} \tag{5.6.2}$$

for all $\sigma \in B(r_i) - \{0\}$ for some $r_i > 0$.

Defining $T = [T_{ij}] \in \Re^{n \times n}$, $A = \text{diag}[a_1, \cdots, a_n] \in \Re^{n \times n}$, $I = (I_1, \cdots, I_n)^T$, $g = (g_1, \cdots, g_n)^T \colon \Re^n \to \Re^n$, $u = (u_1, \cdots, u_n)^T$, and $v = (v_1, \cdots, v_n)^T$, equation (5.6.1) assumes the form

$$\begin{cases} u(k+1) = Tv(k) + Au(k) + I \\ v(k) = g(u(k)), \ k = 0, 1, 2, \cdots \end{cases} \tag{5.6.3}$$

In general, this network will have many equilibria, and at most one of these will be located at the origin $u = 0$. By definition, each equilibrium must satisfy the relation

$$u(k) = Tv(k) + Au(k) + I,$$

or equivalently,

$$0 = Tv(k) + Bu(k) + I \tag{5.6.4}$$

where $B = A - E$ and E denotes the $n \times n$ identity matrix. We are able to translate any equilibrium of (5.6.3) into the origin in the following manner. Let

$$\begin{cases} p(k) = u(k) - u^* \\ G(p(k)) = g(u(k)) - g(u^*) \end{cases} \tag{5.6.5}$$

where u^* satisfies (5.6.4), and $G = [G_1, \cdots, G_n]^T$. Then

$$\begin{aligned} p(k+1) + u^* &= Tg(p(k) + u^*) + A(p(k) + u^*) + I \\ &= T(G(p(k)) + g(u^*)) + Ap(k) + Au^* + I \\ &= TG(p(k)) + Ap(k) + Tg(u^*) + Au^* + I. \end{aligned}$$

Thus,

$$p(k+1) = TG(p(k)) + Ap(k) + Tg(u^*) + Bu^* + I$$

or, using (5.6.4),

$$p(k+1) = TG(p(k)) + Ap(k) \tag{W}$$

5.6. SYNCHRONOUS HOPFIELD NETWORKS

which has an equilibrium at $p(k) \equiv 0$.

Henceforth, we will use (W) to represent the neural network under study. We will assume that all equilibria of (W) are isolated. In the next subsection, we will conduct a stability analysis of arbitrary given equilibrium points. In our approach, *we will assume without loss of generality that a given equilibrium under investigation is located at the origin.*

We conclude by noting that due to the relationship between $G_i(x)$ and $g_i(x)$, it follows that $G_i(x)$ is also a monotonically increasing, continuously differentiable function with $G_i(0) = 0$. Furthermore, G_i will satisfy a sector condition

$$c_{i1} \leq G_i(\sigma)/\sigma \leq c_{i2} \tag{5.6.6}$$

for all $\sigma \in B(r_i) - \{0\}$ for some $r_i > 0$, $i = 1, \cdots, n$, where c_{i1} and c_{i2} are two positive real numbers that need not be the same as the d_{i1}, d_{i2} given in (5.6.2).

We rewrite (W) in the form

$$p_i(k+1) = \sum_{j=1}^{n} T_{ij} G_j(p_j(k)) + a_i p_i(k), \; i = 1, \cdots, n. \tag{Ω_i}$$

System (Ω_i) may be viewed as an interconnection of n *free* (*isolated*) *subsystems* represented by the equations

$$x_i(k+1) = T_{ii} G_i(x_i(k)) + a_i x_i(k), \; i = 1, \cdots, n, \tag{W$_i$}$$

with the *interconnecting structure* specified by

$$h_i(x_1, \cdots, x_n) \triangleq \sum_{j=1, j \neq i}^{n} T_{ij} G_j(x_j(k)), \; i = 1, \cdots, n. \tag{5.6.7}$$

Following the method of analysis advocated in [16], we will establish in the next subsection stability results for system (W) that are phrased in terms of the qualitative properties of the free subsystems (W$_i$) and in terms of the properties of the interconnecting structure given in (5.6.7).

B. Stability Analysis

The stability results of the entire neural network (W) are determined by the stability results of the individual single neuron subsystems (W_i) and the properties of the interconnecting structure (5.6.7) of the neural network. In the present subsection we first analyze the stability of the free subsystems. Next, we state and prove the desired stability results for the entire system (W).

To analyze the stability of a free subsystem (W_i), we need the following assumption:

(B–1) For (W_i),
$$0 < \sigma_i \triangleq (|a_i| + |T_{ii}|c_{i2}) < 1$$
where c_{i1} and c_{i2} are defined in (5.6.6). ∎

Proposition 5.6.1 If (B–1) is true, then the equilibrium $x_i = 0$ of (W_i) is asymptotically stable.

Proof: Choose $v_i(x_i(k)) = |x_i(k)|$ as a Lyapunov function for (W_i). Then the first forward difference of v_i along the solutions of (W_i) is given by

$$\begin{aligned}
D_{(W_i)}v(x_i(k)) &= v_i(x_i(k+1)) - v_i(x_i(k)) \\
&= |a_i x_i(k) + T_{ii}G_i(x_i(k))| - |x_i(k)| \\
&\leq (|a_i| - 1)|x_i(k)| + |T_{ii}G_i(x_i(k))| \\
&\leq [(|a_i| - 1) + |T_{ii}|c_{i2}]|x_i(k)|.
\end{aligned}$$

Clearly, v_i is positive definite and $D_{(W_i)}v_i$ is negative definite if (B–1) is true. Therefore, the equilibrium $x_i = 0$ is asymptotically stable (cf. [18] or Section 5.2B). ∎

In our next result, we will require the following hypothesis.

(B–2) Given σ_i of (B–1), the successive principal minors of the matrix $D = [d_{ij}]$ are all positive, with

$$d_{ij} = \begin{cases} -(\sigma_i - 1), & i = j \\ -\sigma_{ij}, & i \neq j \end{cases}$$

5.6. SYNCHRONOUS HOPFIELD NETWORKS

where $\sigma_{ij} = |T_{ij}|c_{j2}$ [c_{j2} is defined in (5.6.6)]. ∎

Theorem 5.6.1 If (B–1) and (B–2) are true, then the equilibrium $p = 0$ of (W) is asymptotically stable.

Proof: We choose a Lyapunov function for (W),

$$v(p(k)) = \sum_{i=1}^{n} \lambda_i |p_i(k)|$$

where $\lambda_i > 0$ for $i = 1, \cdots, n$. Then the first forward difference of v along the solutions of (W) [resp., (Ω)] is given by

$$\begin{aligned}
D_{(\Omega)}v(p(k)) &= v(k+1) - v(k) \\
&= \sum_{i=1}^{n} \lambda_i \left[|p_i(k+1)| - |p_i(k)| \right] \\
&= \sum_{i=1}^{n} \lambda_i \left[\left| a_i p_i(k) + \sum_{j=1}^{n} T_{ij} G_j(p_j(k)) \right| - |p_i(k)| \right] \\
&\leq \sum_{i=1}^{n} \lambda_i \left[|a_i| \cdot |p_i(k)| + \sum_{j=1}^{n} |T_{ij}| \cdot |G_j(p_j(k))| - |p_i(k)| \right] \\
&\leq \sum_{i=1}^{n} \lambda_i \left[(|a_i| - 1)|p_i(k)| + \sum_{j=1}^{n} |T_{ij}| \cdot |G_j(p_j(k))| \right] \\
&\leq \sum_{i=1}^{n} \lambda_i \left[(|a_i| - 1)|p_i(k)| + \sum_{j=1}^{n} |T_{ij}|c_{j2}|(p_j(k))| \right] \\
&= \sum_{i=1}^{n} \lambda_i \left(|a_i| - 1 + |T_{ii}|c_{i2} \right) |p_i(k)| \\
&\quad + \sum_{i=1}^{n} \lambda_i \sum_{j=1,\, j\neq i}^{n} |T_{ij}|c_{i2}|p_j(k)| \\
&= \sum_{i=1}^{n} \lambda_i(\sigma_i - 1)|p_i(k)| + \sum_{i=1}^{n} \lambda_i \sum_{j=1\, j\neq i}^{n} \sigma_{ij}|p_j(k)| \\
&= -\lambda^T D w
\end{aligned}$$

where $\lambda = (\lambda_1, \cdots, \lambda_n)^T$ and $w = (|p_1|, \cdots, |p_n|)^T$. Since by (B–2) $d_{ij} \leq 0$ when $i \neq j$, and the successive principal minors of matrix D are all positive, D is an M-matrix. By the properties of M-matrices, D^{-1} exists and each element of D^{-1} is nonnegative. Hence there exists a vector $y = (y_1, \cdots, y_n)^T$, with $y_i > 0$ for $i = 1, \cdots, n$, such that (refer to the argument in Remark 5.5.5; or see [16])

$$-y^T w < 0, \quad \text{where } y^T = \lambda^T D$$

$$\lambda = (D^{-1})^T y > 0.$$

Therefore, $D_{(\Omega)} v$ is negative definite, v is positive definite, and the equilibrium $p = 0$ of (W) is asymptotically stable (cf. [8] or Section 5.2B). ∎

The Lyapunov function in the proof of Theorem 5.6.1 is a generalized Hamming distance. Thus, if for an equilibrium x^* the translation (5.6.5) is applied and the assumptions of Theorem 5.6.1 are found to be true, then Theorem 5.6.1 shows that for initial conditions sufficiently near x^*, the generalized Hamming distance from x^* to solutions of (5.6.3) will asymptotically approach zero. The weighting vector λ is included to increase the applicability and to decrease the conservatism of Theorem 5.6.1. One method for choosing λ is shown in the proof of Theorem 5.6.1. Since the value of λ is not unique, [12] and [20] consider methods for choosing λ in an optimal fashion.

(B–3) Given c_{i1} and c_{i2} in (5.6.6), we define δ_i by

$$\delta_i = \begin{cases} 1/c_{i1}, & \text{if } |a_i| \geq 1 \\ 1/c_{i2}, & \text{if } |a_i| < 1. \end{cases}$$ ∎

(B–4) The successive principal minors of the $n \times n$ test matrix $D = [d_{ij}]$ are all positive where

$$d_{ij} = \begin{cases} -\delta_i(|a_i| - 1) - |T_{ii}|, & i = j \\ -|T_{ij}|, & i \neq j. \end{cases}$$ ∎

Similarly as in Theorem 5.6.1, we now obtain the following result.

Corollary 5.6.1 The equilibrium $p = 0$ of (W) is asymptotically stable if (B–1), (B–3), and (B–4) are satisfied.

Proof: We choose a Lyapunov function for (W) [resp., (Ω)] as

$$v(p(k)) = \sum_{i=1}^{n} \lambda_i |p_i(k)|, \text{ with } \lambda_i > 0.$$

5.6. SYNCHRONOUS HOPFIELD NETWORKS

Then

$$\begin{aligned}
D_{(\Omega)}v(p(k)) &= v(k+1) - v(k) \\
&= \sum_{i=1}^{n} \lambda_i \left[|p_i(k+1)| - |p_i(k)| \right] \\
&\leq \sum_{i=1}^{n} \lambda_i \left[(|a_i| - 1)|p_i(k)| + \sum_{j=1}^{n} |T_{ij}| \cdot |G_j(p_j(k))| \right] \\
&\leq \sum_{i=1}^{n} \lambda_i \left[(|a_i| - 1)\frac{p_i(k)}{G_i(p_i(k))} |G_i(p_i(k))| \right. \\
&\quad\left. + \sum_{j=1}^{n} |T_{ij}| \cdot |G_j(p_j(k))| \right] \\
&\leq \sum_{i=1}^{n} \lambda_i \left\{ [\delta_i(|a_i| - 1) + |T_{ii}|] |G_i(p_i(k))| \right. \\
&\quad\left. + \sum_{j=1, j\neq i}^{n} |T_{ij}| \cdot |G_j(p_j(k))| \right\} \\
&= -\lambda^T D w \\
&< 0, \quad \text{by proper choice of } \lambda,
\end{aligned}$$

where $\lambda = (\lambda_1, \cdots, \lambda_n)^T$ and $w = (|G_1(p_1)|, \cdots, |G_n(p_n)|)^T$. Therefore, the equilibrium is asymptotically stable. ∎

C. Estimates of Trajectory Bounds

In the previous subsection we presented methods for determining the stability properties of the various equilibria of (W). Usually we also desire information about network performance. One critical performance issue concerns the network's rate of convergence from an initial condition to the final state. The present section develops trajectory bound estimates that allow one to predict the rate of convergence near the asymptotically stable equilibria of the network.

In the case where (B-2) is satisfied, D is an M-matrix. Properties of M-matrices are discussed in [16] (see Section 5.5B). The particular property of M-matrices that will be used in the sequel is given in assumption (B-5).

(B-5) For the matrix $D = [d_{ij}]$ [as defined in (B-2)], there exist constants $\lambda_i > 0$, $i = 1, \cdots, n$, such that

$$d_{ii} + \sum_{j=1, j\neq i}^{n} \frac{\lambda_j}{\lambda_i} d_{ji} \geq \varepsilon > 0, \ i = 1, \cdots, n. \qquad \blacksquare$$

The condition for D to be an M-matrix [to satisfy (B–2)] only requires (B–5) to be satisfied with $\varepsilon = 0$. Thus (B–5) is slightly more stringent than (B–2). Using (B–5), we can prove the following.

Theorem 5.6.2 If (B–5) is satisfied, then

$$\|u(k) - u^*\| = \|p(k)\| \leq \mu^k \|p(0)\|$$

for all $\|p\| < r = \min(\lambda_i r_i)$, where $\|p\| = \sum_{i=1}^{n} \lambda_i |p_i|$, r_i is defined in connection with (5.6.6), and λ_i are given by (B–5).

Proof: Choose $v(p(k)) = \sum_{i=1}^{n} \lambda_i |p_i|$. Then

$$\begin{aligned}
D_{(\Omega)} v(p(k)) &= v(p(k+1)) - v(p(k)) \\
&= \sum_{i=1}^{n} \lambda_i (|p_i(k+1)| - |p_i(k)|) \\
&= \sum_{i=1}^{n} \lambda_i \left[\left| a_i p_i(k) + \sum_{j=1}^{n} T_{ij} G(p_i(k)) \right| - |p_i(k)| \right] \\
&\leq \sum_{i=1}^{n} \lambda_i \left[|a_i| \cdot |p_i(k)| - |p_i(k)| + \sum_{j=1}^{n} |T_{ij}| c_{j2} |p_j(k)| \right] \\
&= - \sum_{i=1}^{n} \lambda_i \left[d_{ii} |p_i(k)| + \sum_{j=1, j\neq i}^{n} d_{ij} |p_j(k)| \right] \\
&= - \sum_{i=1}^{n} \sum_{j=1}^{n} \lambda_i d_{ij} |p_j(k)| \\
&= - \sum_{j=1}^{n} \lambda_j \left(\sum_{i=1}^{n} \frac{\lambda_i}{\lambda_j} d_{ij} \right) |p_j(k)| \\
&\leq -\varepsilon \sum_{j=1}^{n} \lambda_j |p_j(k)| \\
&= -\varepsilon v(p(k))
\end{aligned}$$

i.e.,

$$D_{(\Omega)} v(p(k)) \leq -\varepsilon v(p(k)). \qquad (5.6.8)$$

5.6. SYNCHRONOUS HOPFIELD NETWORKS

At this point we invoke the comparison principle for ordinary difference equations (see [18]). Inequality (5.6.8) gives rise to the comparison equation

$$v_{k+1} - v_k' = -\varepsilon v_k. \tag{5.6.9}$$

The solution of (5.6.9) is

$$v_k = (1-\varepsilon)^k v_0.$$

It now follows from the comparison principle that

$$v(p(k)) \le \mu^k v(p(0))$$

where $\mu = (1-\varepsilon)$. From (B-5), $0 < \varepsilon < 1$, which implies that $1 > \mu > 0$. ∎

By the use of Theorem 5.6.2, we are able to compute an exponential bound for the rate of convergence from an initial state within the domain of attraction of u^*.

In the translation (5.6.5) and the subsequent analysis, we have assumed that the input I is constant. Our model can be generalized by the addition of a time-varying input $\hat{I}(k)$, resulting in the network description,

$$u(k+1) = Tg(u(k)) + Au(k) + I + \hat{I}(k). \tag{5.6.10}$$

With the following assumption, Theorem 5.6.2 can now be extended to apply to (5.6.10), as presented in the following.

(B–6) Assume that for (5.6.10)

$$\sum_{i=1}^{n} \lambda_i |\hat{I}_i(k)| \le M, \text{ for all } k \ge 0$$

for some $M > 0$. ∎

Corollary 5.6.2 If (B-5) and (B-6) are true, then

$$\|p(k)\| \le \left(\alpha - \frac{M}{\varepsilon}\right)\mu^{-k} + \frac{M}{\varepsilon},$$

provided that $\alpha > M/\varepsilon$ and $\|p(0)\| \le \alpha$. ∎

The proof of this corollary follows the same approach as the proof of Theorem 5.6.2.

We conclude the present section by noting that similarly as in Section 5.5, it is possible to establish estimates of the domain of attraction of an asymptotically stable equilibrium of system (W) and conditions for the instability of an equilibrium of system (W).

5.7 Analysis of Analog Hopfield Neural Networks with Saturation Nonlinearities as Activation Functions

In the present section we consider neural networks described by equations of the form
$$\begin{cases} \dot{x} = -Ax + Ty + I \\ y = \text{sat}(x). \end{cases} \quad (5.7.1)$$

This model, which was originally introduced in Section 2.2 [refer to equation (2.2.6)], is frequently employed in cellular neural network applications. We recall that in (5.7.1), $x \in \Re^n$ is the state vector, $\dot{x} = dx/dt$, $y \in D^n = \{x \in \Re^n : -1 \leq x_i \leq 1, \ i = 1, \cdots, n\}$ denotes the output vector, $A = \text{diag}[a_1, \cdots, a_n]$ with $a_i > 0$ for $i = 1, \cdots, n$, $T = [T_{ij}] \in \Re^{n \times n}$ is the coefficient (or connection) matrix, $I = (I_1, \cdots, I_n)^T \in \Re^n$ is a bias vector, and $\text{sat}(x) = (\text{sat}(x_1), \cdots, \text{sat}(x_n))^T$ represents the activation function vector with

$$\text{sat}(x_i) = \begin{cases} 1, & x_i > 1 \\ x_i, & -1 \leq x_i \leq 1 \\ -1, & x_i < -1. \end{cases}$$

We assume that the initial states of system (5.7.1) satisfy the condition $|x_i(t_0)| \leq 1$, $i = 1, \cdots, n$, where $t_0 \geq 0$ denotes initial time. It is not difficult to show that for every such initial condition, the system (5.7.1) possesses a unique solution $\varphi(t, t_0, x_0)$ which exists for all $t \geq t_0$ with $\varphi(t_0, t_0, x_0) = x_0$.

As noted in Chapter 2, system (5.7.1) is a variant to the analog Hopfield neural network model, using $\text{sat}(\cdot)$ as activation functions.

5.7. SATURATION HOPFIELD NETWORKS

In the analog Hopfield model [6] one usually requires that T be symmetric. We do not make this assumption for (5.7.1).

In the present section we conduct a (local) stability analysis of system (5.7.1). In doing so, we will employ an alternative representation of (5.7.1) which is in the same spirit as the representation given in Chapter 4, Definition 4.3.1, for linear systems operating on a closed hypercube. To accomplish this, we will utilize a notation which is identical or similar to some of the notation that was used in formulating the alternative representation given in Definition 4.3.1 for linear systems operating on a closed hypercube.

For each integer m, $0 \leq m \leq n$, let

$$\Lambda_m = \{\, \xi = (\xi_1, \cdots, \xi_n)^T \in \Lambda : \xi_{\sigma(i)} = 0,\ 1 \leq i \leq m,\ \text{and}\ \xi_{\sigma(i)} = \pm 1,\ m < i \leq n \text{ for some } \sigma \in P(n)\}$$

where $\Lambda = \{\xi = \{\xi_1, \cdots, \xi_n\}^T : \xi_i = \pm 1 \text{ or } 0,\ 1 \leq i \leq n\}$ and $P(n)$ denotes the set of all permutations on $\{1, \cdots, n\}$. [Recall that there are $n!$ elements in $P(n)$.] For each $\xi \in \Lambda$, let

$$C(\xi) = \{\, x = (x_1, \cdots, x_n)^T \in \Re^n : |x_i| < 1 \text{ if } \xi_i = 0,\\ x_i \geq 1 \text{ if } \xi_i = 1,\ \text{and } x_i \leq -1 \text{ if } \xi_i = -1\}.$$

From the notation given above, we have

Lemma 5.7.1

1) $\Lambda = \bigcup_{m=0}^{n} \Lambda_m$.

2) $\Lambda_0 = B^n$ and $C(\xi) = \{x \in \Re^n : |x_i| \geq 1,\ x_i \xi_i > 0,\ i = 1, \cdots, n\}$ for any $\xi \in \Lambda_0$.

3) $\Lambda_n = \{0\}$ and $C(0) = (D^n)^\circ = \{x \in \Re^n : -1 < x_i < 1,\ i = 1, \cdots, n\}$.

4) $\Re^n = \bigcup_{m=0}^{n} \{C(\xi),\ \xi \in \Lambda_m\}$.

5) For any $\xi, \eta \in \Lambda$, $\xi \neq \eta$, $C(\xi) \cap C(\eta) = \emptyset$. ∎

Suppose that $\xi \in \Lambda_m$ and $\sigma \in P(n)$ such that

$$\xi_{\sigma(i)} = 0,\ 1 \leq i \leq m \text{ and } \xi_{\sigma(i)} = \pm 1,\ m < i \leq n. \tag{5.7.2}$$

We denote

$$A_\mathrm{I} = \mathrm{diag}\left[a_{\sigma(1)}, \cdots, a_{\sigma(m)}\right]$$

$$A_\mathrm{II} = \mathrm{diag}\left[a_{\sigma(m+1)}, \cdots, a_{\sigma(n)}\right]$$

$$T_{\mathrm{I,I}} = \left[T_{\sigma(i)\sigma(j)}\right]_{1 \leq i,j \leq m}$$

$$T_{\mathrm{I,II}} = \left[T_{\sigma(i)\sigma(j)}\right]_{1 \leq i \leq m, m < j \leq n}$$

$$T_{\mathrm{II,I}} = \left[T_{\sigma(i)\sigma(j)}\right]_{m < i \leq n, 1 \leq j \leq m}$$

$$T_{\mathrm{II,II}} = \left[T_{\sigma(i)\sigma(j)}\right]_{m < i,j \leq n}$$

$$I_\mathrm{I} = \left(I_{\sigma(1)}, \cdots, I_{\sigma(m)}\right)^T$$

$$I_\mathrm{II} = \left(I_{\sigma(m+1)}, \cdots, I_{\sigma(n)}\right)^T$$

$$\xi_\mathrm{I} = \left(\xi_{\sigma(1)}, \cdots, \xi_{\sigma(m)}\right)^T$$

and

$$\xi_\mathrm{II} = \left(\xi_{\sigma(m+1)}, \cdots, \xi_{\sigma(n)}\right)^T.$$

Remark 5.7.1 For a given $\xi \in \Lambda_m$, there may exist different elements in $P(n)$ for which (5.7.2) is true. For these different permutations, the notation given above will be the same up to different orders in the components. Thus, the subsequent analysis and conclusions will be identical for any of the permutations used. ∎

Remark 5.7.2 If $m = n$, we have $A_\mathrm{I} = A$, $T_{\mathrm{I,I}} = T$, $I_\mathrm{I} = I$, $\xi_\mathrm{I} = \xi$ and the A_{II}, $T_{\mathrm{I,II}}, T_{\mathrm{II,I}}$, $T_{\mathrm{II,II}}$, I_II, ξ_II do not exist. If $m = 0$, we have $A_\mathrm{II} = A$, $T_{\mathrm{II,II}} = T$, $I_\mathrm{II} = I$, $\xi_\mathrm{II} = \xi$ and the A_I, $T_{\mathrm{I,I}}$, $T_{\mathrm{I,II}}$, $T_{\mathrm{II,I}}$, I_I, ξ_I do not exist. ∎

5.7. SATURATION HOPFIELD NETWORKS

Consider now $\xi \in \Lambda_m$, $0 < m < n$, with $\sigma \in P(n)$ such that $\xi_{\sigma(i)} = 0$, $1 \leq i \leq m$, and $\xi_{\sigma(i)} = \pm 1$, $m < i \leq n$. We can rewrite the first equation of system (5.7.1) as

$$\begin{cases} \dot{x}_{\text{I}} = -A_{\text{I}} x_{\text{I}} + T_{\text{I},\text{I}} x_{\text{I}} + T_{\text{I},\text{II}} \xi_{\text{II}} + I_{\text{I}} \\ \dot{x}_{\text{II}} = -A_{\text{II}} x_{\text{II}} + T_{\text{II},\text{I}} x_{\text{I}} + T_{\text{II},\text{II}} \xi_{\text{II}} + I_{\text{II}} \end{cases} \quad (5.7.3)$$

where $\xi_{\text{II}} = \left(\xi_{\sigma(m+1)}, \cdots, \xi_{\sigma(n)}\right)^T$, $x_{\text{I}} = \left(x_{\sigma(1)}, \cdots, x_{\sigma(m)}\right)^T$ with $-1 < x_{\sigma(i)} < 1$ for $1 \leq i \leq m$, and $x_{\text{II}} = (x_{\sigma(m+1)}, \cdots, x_{\sigma(n)})^T$ with $\xi_{\sigma(i)} x_{\sigma(i)} \geq 1$ for $m < i \leq n$. We will call (5.7.3) an *equivalent linear representation of (5.7.1) over the region* $C(\xi)$.

When $m = n$, $\Lambda_n = \{0\}$. In this case, for $x \in C(0) = (D^n)^\circ$, system (5.7.1) assumes the form

$$\dot{x} = (T - A)x + I. \quad (5.7.4)$$

When $m = 0$, $\Lambda_0 = B^n$. In this case, for $\xi \in \Lambda_0$, $x \in C(\xi)$, system (5.7.1) can be expressed as

$$\dot{x} = -Ax + T\xi + I. \quad (5.7.5)$$

We will have occasion to make use of the following hypotheses for system (5.7.1).

(C-1) For any m, $0 < m \leq n$, and for any $\xi \in \Lambda_m$, the $m \times m$ matrix $T_{\text{I},\text{I}} - A_{\text{I}} = [T_{\sigma(i)\sigma(j)}]_{1 \leq i,j \leq m} - \text{diag}[a_{\sigma(i)}, \cdots, a_{\sigma(m)}]$ is non-singular, where $\sigma \in P(n)$ so that $\xi_{\sigma(i)} = 0$, $1 \leq i \leq m$ and $\xi_{\sigma(i)} = \pm 1$, $m < i \leq n$. ∎

For system (5.7.1) satisfying Assumption (C-1) we will employ the following notation.

1) If $\xi = 0 \in \Lambda_n$ ($m = n$), let

$$x_\xi = (A - T)^{-1} I. \quad (5.7.6)$$

2) For $\xi \in \Lambda_m$, $0 < m < n$, with $A_{\text{I}}, A_{\text{II}}, T_{\text{I},\text{I}}, \cdots, T_{\text{II},\text{II}}, I_{\text{I}}, I_{\text{II}}$ defined above, let

$$x_\xi = (x_{\xi 1}, \cdots, x_{\xi n})^T \in \Re^n \quad (5.7.7)$$

where
$$x_{\xi\mathrm{I}} = \left(x_{\xi\sigma(1)}, \cdots, x_{\xi\sigma(m)}\right)^T$$
$$= (A_\mathrm{I} - T_{\mathrm{I},\mathrm{I}})^{-1}(T_{\mathrm{I},\mathrm{II}}\xi_\mathrm{II} + I_\mathrm{I}),$$
and
$$x_{\xi\mathrm{II}} = \left(x_{\xi\sigma(m+1)}, \cdots, x_{\xi\sigma(n)}\right)^T$$
$$= A_\mathrm{II}^{-1}(T_{\mathrm{II},\mathrm{I}}x_{\xi\mathrm{I}} + T_{\mathrm{II},\mathrm{II}}\xi_\mathrm{II} + I_\mathrm{II}).$$

3) For $\xi \in \Lambda_0 = B^n$ ($m = 0$), let
$$x_\xi = A^{-1}(T\xi + I). \tag{5.7.8}$$

4) For the x_ξ defined above, let $y_\xi = \mathrm{sat}(x_\xi)$.

(C–2) With the notation given above, assume that for any $\xi \in \Lambda_m$, $0 \leq m \leq n$, $x_\xi \notin \partial(C(\xi))$. ∎

The following result enables us to determine the location of all equilibria for system (5.7.1) in a systematic manner and to ascertain the stability properties for these equilibria. Furthermore, this result will serve as the theoretical basis of synthesis procedures which we will present in Chapters 8 and 9.

Theorem 5.7.1 Suppose that system (5.7.1) satisfies Assumptions (C–1) and (C–2). For any m, $0 \leq m \leq n$, and for any $\xi \in \Lambda_m$, we have:

Case I: $m = n$, $\xi = 0 \in \Lambda_n$. [Note that in this case $C(\xi) = (D^n)^\circ$.]

1) If $x_\xi \notin (D^n)^\circ$, there is no equilibrium point of system (5.7.1) in $(D^n)^\circ$.

2) If $x_\xi \in (D^n)^\circ$, x_ξ is the unique equilibrium point of system (5.7.1) in $(D^n)^\circ$. In particular,

   (i) if $T - A$ has one or more eigenvalues with non-negative real parts, x_ξ is unstable, and

   (ii) if all eigenvalues of $T - A$ have negative real parts, x_ξ is asymptotically stable.

5.7. SATURATION HOPFIELD NETWORKS

Case II: $0 < m < n$, $\xi \in \Lambda_m$.
1) If $x_\xi \notin C(\xi)$, there is no equilibrium point of system (5.7.1) in $C(\xi)$.
2) If $x_\xi \in C(\xi)$, x_ξ is the unique equilibrium point of system (5.7.1) in $C(\xi)$. In particular.

   (i) if $T_{I,I} - A_I$ has one or more eigenvalues with non-negative real parts, x_ξ is unstable, and

   (ii) if all eigenvalues of $T_{I,I} - A_I$ have negative real parts, x_ξ is asymptotically stable.

Case III: $m = 0$, $\xi \in \Lambda_0 = B^n$.
1) If $x_\xi \notin C(\xi)$, there is no equilibrium point of system (5.7.1) in $C(\xi)$.
2) If $x_\xi \in C(\xi)$, x_ξ is an asymptotically stable equilibrium point of system (5.7.1).

Proof: For each $\xi \in \Lambda_m$, $0 \leq m \leq n$, consider (5.7.3)–(5.7.5). Using similar arguments as in the proof of Theorem 4.4.1, the conclusions of this theorem follow directly from the theory of linear differential equations. ∎

If x_ξ is an asymptotically stable equilibrium point of system (5.7.1), $y_\xi \stackrel{\triangle}{=} \text{sat}(x_\xi)$ is said to be a *memory vector* of system (5.7.1). A memory vector y_ξ is said to be *reachable* if there exists a neighborhood V of y_ξ such that for any $x(0) \in V \cap D^n \neq \emptyset$, the output vector $y(t)$ to system (5.7.1) tends to y_ξ asymptotically as $t \to \infty$. Using the results given in Theorem 5.7.1, it can easily be shown that a memory vector $y_\xi \in (D^n)°$ or $y_\xi \in B^n = \{x \in \Re^n : x_i = 1 \text{ or } -1, i = 1, \cdots, n\}$ is always reachable. When a memory vector $y_\xi \in \partial(D^n) - B^n$, y_ξ is reachable if and only if for *every* neighborhood U of y_ξ, the set $U \cap D^n$ has a non-empty intersection with the domain of attraction of the corresponding asymptotically stable equilibrium point x_ξ. In synthesis procedures that we will present in Chapters 8 and 9, the objective is to store patterns in B^n. If we can guarantee that a desired set of bipolar patterns is stored as a set of memory vectors, then such vectors will always be reachable. Therefore, we will drop the modifier "reachable" when the context is clear.

Remark 5.7.3 With T symmetric, the function $E: D^n \to \Re$ defined by
$$E(y) = -\frac{1}{2}y^T T y + \frac{1}{2}y^T A y - y^T I \qquad (5.7.9)$$
can be shown to be monotonically decreasing in time t along the solutions of (5.7.1). To see this, we follow the same procedure as in Sections 4.3 and 4.5 by defining a *local solution* for system (5.7.1); or, we can follow the procedure in [1], by defining the derivatives dy_i/dx_i at the breaking points $|x_i| = 1$ to be zero. This shows that system (5.7.1) will neither oscillate nor become chaotic. When T is nonsymmetric, the function E defined in (5.7.9) is not necessarily monotonically decreasing, and oscillatory solutions for (5.7.1) may exist. ∎

Remark 5.7.4 It is possible to generalize Theorem 5.7.1 to a result which does not require Assumption (C–2). However, for such a case, the conclusions of the theorem will be less straightforward. ∎

Several important conclusions can be drawn from Theorem 5.7.1 which are given in the following.

Corollary 5.7.1 Suppose that in system (5.7.1)
$$T_{ii} \geq a_i \text{ for } i = 1, \cdots, n. \qquad (5.7.10)$$
Then, every asymptotically stable equilibrium point
$$x_e = (x_{e1}, \cdots, x_{en})^T$$
of system (5.7.1) satisfies the conditions
$$|x_{ei}| > 1, \ i = 1, \cdots, n. \qquad (5.7.11)$$

Proof: In Eq. (5.7.3), the trace $\text{tr}(-A_I + T_{I,I})$ of the coefficient matrix $-A_I + T_{I,I}$ is nonnegative since $T_{I,I} \geq a_i$. On the other hand,

5.7. SATURATION HOPFIELD NETWORKS

since the trace of a real-valued matrix equals the sum of the real parts of its eigenvalues, we have

$$\sum_{i=1}^{m} Re(\lambda_i) \geq 0 \qquad (5.7.12)$$

where λ_i, $i = 1, \cdots, m$, are the eigenvalues of $(-A_\mathrm{I} + T_{\mathrm{I,I}})$. Inequality (5.7.12) indicates that at least one eigenvalue of $(-A_\mathrm{I} + T_{\mathrm{I,I}})$ has a nonnegative real part. Therefore, the equilibrium of (5.7.3) is not stable, or at least not attractive. Similar arguments as above can be applied to (5.7.4). Therefore, stable memories (i.e., output vectors corresponding to asymptotically stable equilibrium points) of system (5.7.1) exist only in the case of the equivalent (or reduced) linear system given by (5.7.5), where the corresponding output vector $y = \mathrm{sat}(x)$ has the property given by $y \in B^n$ since $x \in F(\xi) = \{x \in \Re^n : x_i \xi_i > 1,\ i = 1, \cdots, n\}$ and $\xi \in B^n$.

To determine the exact location of the asymptotically stable equilibrium points and stable memory vectors, Case III of Theorem 5.7.1 should be applied. This proves the theorem. ∎

We point out that similar results as Corollary 5.7.1 have been obtained for cellular neural networks (with *symmetric* interconnections) in [1] and [9], using different approaches. The present result is less conservative than those given in [1] and [9].

Corollary 5.7.2 Suppose that β is an asymptotically stable equilibrium point and $\alpha = \mathrm{sat}(\beta)$ is a memory vector of system (5.7.1) with parameters $\{A, T, I\}$. Then, α and β will also be a pair of memory vector and asymptotically stable equilibrium point of system (5.7.1) with parameters $\{kA, kT, kI\}$ for every real number $k > 0$.

Proof: The proof can easily be established by considering (5.7.6)–(5.7.8) and Theorem 5.7.1. ∎

Remark 5.7.5 The significance of Corollary 5.7.2 is that we can increase the speed of evolution of a given neural network (5.7.1) by multiplying A, T, and I by a constant $k > 1$, without changing any of its asymptotically stable equilibrium points and any of its memory vectors. Since the speed of evolution of (5.7.1) depends on the eigenvalues of $T - A$ and $T_{I,I} - A_I$, it is also clear that the larger the k is, the faster the evolution will be. ∎

5.8 Summary

In the present chapter we first investigated local qualitative properties of analog Hopfield neural networks described by equations of the form

$$\begin{cases} \dot{u}_i = -a_i u_i + \sum_{j=1}^{n} T_{ij} g_j(u_j) + I_i(t) \\ v_i = g_i(u_i), \ i = 1, \cdots, n. \end{cases} \quad (5.8.1)$$

Given an equilibrium $u^* = (u_1^*, \cdots, u_n^*)^T \neq 0$ of (5.8.1) to be studied, we first showed that it is always possible to perform a translation $x_i = u_i - u_i^*$, $i = 1, \cdots, n$, which transforms (5.8.1) into the equivalent system described by the equations

$$\dot{x}_i = -a_i x_i + \sum_{j=1}^{n} T_{ij} G_j(x_j) + I_i(t), \ i = 1, \cdots, n \quad (\Sigma_i)$$

having the property that the equilibrium to be studied becomes now $x = (x_1, \cdots, x_n)^T = 0$. In (Σ_i), we have $G_i(x_i) = g_i(x_i + u_i^*) - g_i(u^*)$, and therefore $G_i(0) = 0$, $\sigma G_i(\sigma) > 0$ for $\sigma \neq 0$, and it is assumed that for some $r_i > 0$, there exist constants $\sigma_{i2} \geq \sigma_{i1} > 0$ such that

$$\sigma_{i1} p_i^2 < p_i G_i(p_i) < \sigma_{i2} p_i^2, \ -r_i < p_i < r_i. \quad (5.8.2)$$

In our analysis we view (Σ_i) as an *interconnected* or *composite system* consisting of an interconnection of n *free subsystems* described by equations of the form

$$\dot{p}_i = -a_i p_i + T_{ii} G_i(p_i) + I_i(t), \ i = 1, \cdots, n, \quad (\mathcal{S}_i)$$

with the system *interconnecting structure* given by

$$h_i(x_1, \cdots, x_n) = \sum_{j=1, j \neq i}^{n} T_{ij} G_j(x_j), \ i = 1, \cdots, n. \quad (5.8.3)$$

5.8. SUMMARY

Rewriting (Σ_i) in vector form as

$$\dot{x} = -Ax + TG(x) + I(t), \qquad (\mathcal{S})$$

we speak under the present viewpoint of *composite system* ($\mathcal{S}$) *with decomposition* (Σ_i).

The aim in the present chapter was to analyze system ($\mathcal{S}$) in terms of the qualitative properties of the subsystems ($\mathcal{S}_i$) (representing the individual neurons with their associated dynamics) and the system interconnecting structure (representing the interactions of the neurons). To accomplish this, we first conducted a stability analysis of the free subsystems ($\mathcal{S}_i$) under the assumption that $I_i(t) \equiv 0$. For such systems we established sufficient conditions for the asymptotic stability, exponential stability, and instability (resp., complete instability) of the equilibrium $p_i = 0$.

Next, we used *scalar Lyapunov functions*, consisting of a weighted sum of quadratic Lyapunov functions for the free subsystems, given by

$$v(x) = \sum_{i=1}^{n} \frac{1}{2}\alpha_i x_i^2, \qquad (5.8.4)$$

to establish sufficient conditions for asymptotic stability (resp., exponential stability) of the equilibrium $x = 0$ of system ($\mathcal{S}$). These results, as well as all the subsequent stability results, involve three basic ingredients. The first characterizes the qualitative properties of the free subsystems; the second specifies constraints on the interconnecting structure of ($\mathcal{S}$); and the third combines information from the first two to form a *test matrix* with certain desired definiteness properties. A specific sample result follows.

Assume that the following hypotheses hold for system ($\mathcal{S}$):

1) $I_i(t) \equiv 0$, $i = 1, \cdots, n$;
2) there are $a_{ij} \in \Re$, $i, j = 1, \cdots, n$, such that

$$x_i T_{ij} G_j(x_j) \leq |x_i| a_{ij} |x_j|$$

for all $|x_i| < r_i$, $|x_j| < r_j$, $i, j = 1, \cdots, n$; and

3) there exists an n-vector $\alpha^T = (\alpha_1, \cdots, \alpha_n)$, $\alpha_i > 0$, $i = 1, \cdots, n$, such that the $n \times n$ test matrix $S = [s_{ij}]$ given by

$$s_{ij} = \begin{cases} \alpha_i(-a_i + a_{ii}), & i = j \\ (\alpha_i a_{ij} + \alpha_j a_{ji})/2, & i \neq j \end{cases}$$

is negative definite.

Then the equilibrium $x = 0$ of the composite system $(\mathcal{S})$ with decomposition (Σ_i) is *asymptotically stable*.

Next, when the off-diagonal elements of a test matrix are nonnegative, we were able to simplify results of the type described above by invoking the properties of M-matrices. For example, a typical result of this type requires that hypothesis 3) above be replaced by the following assumption:

3') the successive principal minors of the $n \times n$ test matrix $D = [d_{ij}]$ are all positive, where

$$d_{ij} = \begin{cases} a_i - \delta_i T_{ii}, & i = j \\ -|T_{ij}|\sigma_{j2}, & i \neq j \end{cases}$$

where $\delta_i = \sigma_{i2}$ when $T_{ii} > 0$, $\delta_i = \sigma_{i1}$ when $T_{ii} < 0$, and σ_{i1}, σ_{i2} are defined in (5.8.2).

Next, by invoking the *comparison principle* (for the stability theory of ordinary differential equations), and by making use of *vector Lyapunov functions*, $V(x) = (v_1(x), \cdots, v_n(x))^T$ (whose components are scalar Lyapunov functions for the subsystems), we established several additional results for asymptotic and exponential stability of the equilibrium $x = 0$ of system $(\mathcal{S})$. These results, as well as the results discussed above, are in many instances equivalent.

Using the stability results described above, we established next estimates for trajectory bounds. Results of this type provide a measure of the speed of convergence of trajectories sufficiently close to the (asymptotically stable) equilibrium $x = 0$ of $(\mathcal{S})$. The estimates for trajectory bounds that we obtained are of the form

$$\|\varphi(t, t_0, x_0)\| \triangleq \sum_{i=1}^{n} \lambda_i |\varphi_i(t, t_0, x_0)|$$
$$\leq (\alpha - k/c)e^{-c(t-t_0)} + k/c, \quad t \geq t_0 \geq 0,$$

5.8. SUMMARY

provided that $\alpha > k/c$ and $\|x_0\| = \sum_{i=1}^{n} \lambda_i |x_{i0}| \leq \alpha$. In the above estimate, k is determined by $\sum_{i=1}^{n} \lambda_i |I_i(t)| \leq k$ for all $t \geq 0$; c is determined by $c = \varepsilon \delta$, where $\varepsilon > 0$ is given in hypothesis 4) below and δ is defined by $\delta = \min_i \sigma_{i1}$; and where the λ_i, $i = 1, \cdots, n$, are also given in hypothesis 4) below:

4) assume there exist $\lambda_i > 0$, $i = 1, \cdots, n$ and $\varepsilon > 0$ such that

$$\left(\frac{a_i}{\sigma_{i2}} - T_{ii}\right) - \sum_{j=1, j\neq i}^{n} \left(\frac{\lambda_j}{\lambda_i}\right) |T_{ij}| \geq \varepsilon > 0, \; i = 1, \cdots, n.$$

Next, we demonstrated how to determine an estimate of the domain of attraction of the equilibrium $x = 0$ of system $(\mathcal{S})$, when this equilibrium is asymptotically stable. Specifically, we showed that if the assumptions 1), 2), and 3) given earlier are true, then the set C_λ is a subset of the domain of attraction of the equilibrium $x = 0$ of the neural network $(\mathcal{S})$, where

$$C_\lambda = \left\{x \in \Re^n : v(x) = \sum_{i=1}^{n} \alpha_i v_i(x_i) < \lambda\right\},$$

where

$$\lambda = \min_{1 \leq i \leq n} \{\alpha_i v_{0i}\} = \sum_{i=1}^{n} \left(\alpha_i r_i^2\right),$$

where α_i is given in hypothesis 3) and r_i is given in hypothesis 2).

We also established instability (resp., complete instability) results for system $(\mathcal{S})$. These results are similar in form and spirit to the stability results discussed above.

We concluded our qualitative analysis of system $(\mathcal{S})$ with brief discussions concerning issues of stability under structural perturbations of the analog Hopfield neural network, and concerning interpretations of network behavior when the neuron gains become arbitrarily large.

Next, we turned our attention to the analysis of synchronous discrete-time Hopfield-type neural networks described by equations of the form

$$\begin{cases} u_i(k+1) = \sum_{j=1}^{n} T_{ij} v_j(k) - a_i u_i(k) + I_i \\ v_i(k) = g_i(u_i(k)), \; i = 1, \cdots, n; \; k = 0, 1, 2, \cdots. \end{cases} \quad (5.8.5)$$

For system (5.8.5) we established results that are analogous to many of the results that we discussed thus far, using the same methodology as was used in analyzing the analog Hopfield model.

The present chapter was concluded with an analysis of the analog Hopfield-type neural network model with saturation nonlinearities as activation functions, described by equations of the form

$$\begin{cases} \dot{x} = -Ax + Ty + I \\ y = \text{sat}(x). \end{cases} \quad (5.8.6)$$

For system (5.8.6) we established results that enable one to locate in a systematic manner the locations and the stability properties of all the equilibria. The method of analysis that was used in the present case is similar to that used in Chapter 4 (to prove Theorem 4.4.1).

For all networks considered in this chapter, we generally imposed no restrictions (such as symmetry) on the interconnection matrix T, and in cases when this was required, we explicitly stated so.

5.9 Notes and References

The results presented in Sections 5.3 through and including 5.5 are based on material established in [13]. For additional local stability results for analog Hopfield-type networks which are in the spirit of the results reported in Section 5.5, refer to [15] and [5]. The networks considered in [15] are endowed with interconnecting structure that is in lower block triangular form while the results in [5] provide additional insight into the qualitative properties of networks subjected to structural variations.

The results presented in Section 5.6 rely on material developed in [14]. For additional local stability results for discrete-time Hopfield-type networks that are in the spirit of the results reported in Section 5.6, refer to [22] and [23]. The networks considered in [22] are endowed with a nonlinear interconnecting structure while the results in [23] address networks having multi-threshold activation functions.

Additional sources dealing with the qualitative analysis of interconnected systems include the monographs [4] and [24]. For further references on M-matrices, see [2]. Also, extensive treatments of the comparison principle are provided in [7] and [18].

Finally, the results presented in Section 5.7 are based on results given in [9].

Bibliography

[1] LO Chua, L Yang. Cellular neural networks: Theory. IEEE Transactions on Circuits and Systems 35:1257–1272, 1988.

[2] M Fiedler, V Ptak. On matrices with non-positive off-diagonal elements and positive principal minors. Czechoslovak Mathematical Journal 12:382–400, 1962.

[3] EG Goles, G Vichniac. Lyapunov functions for parallel neural networks. IEEE Transactions on Circuits and Systems 36:165–181, 1989.

[4] LT Grujić, AA Martynyuk, M Ribbens-Pavella. Stability of Large-Scale Systems Under Structural and Singular Perturbations. Kiev, USSR: Nauka Dumka, 1984.

[5] LT Grujić, AN Michel. Exponential stability and trajectory bounds of neural networks under structure variations. IEEE Transactions on Circuits and Systems 38:1182–1192, 1991.

[6] JJ Hopfield. Neurons with graded response have collective computational properties like those of two-state neurons. Proceedings of the National Academy of Sciences USA 81:3088–3092, 1984.

[7] V Lakshmikantham, S Leela. Differential and Integral Inequalities, vol 1 and vol 2. New York, NY: Academic Press, 1969.

[8] JH Li, AN Michel, W Porod. Qualitative analysis and synthesis of a class of neural networks. IEEE Transactions on Circuits and Systems 35:976–987, 1988

[9] D Liu, AN Michel. Sparsely interconnected neural networks for associative memories with applications to cellular neural networks. IEEE Transactions on Circuits and Systems-II: Analog and Digital Signal Processing 41:295–307, 1994.

[10] M Marcus, H Minc. A Survey of Matrix Theory and Matrix Inequalities, Boston, MA: Allyn and Bacon, 1964.

[11] RJ McEliece, EC Posner, ER Rodemich, SS Venkatesh. The capacity of the Hopfield associative memory. IEEE Transactions on Information Theory 33:461–482, 1987.

[12] AN Michel. On the status of stability of interconnected systems. IEEE Transactions on Automatic Control 28:639–653, 1983.

[13] AN Michel, JA Farrell, W Porod. Qualitative analysis of neural networks. IEEE Transactions on Circuits and Systems 36:229–243, 1989.

[14] AN Michel, JA Farrell, HF Sun. Analysis and synthesis techniques for Hopfield type synchronous discrete time neural networks with applications to content addressable memory. IEEE Transactions on Circuits and Systems 37:1356–1366, 1990.

[15] AN Michel, DL Gray. Analysis and synthesis of neural networks with lower block triangular interconnecting structure. IEEE Transactions on Circuits and Systems 37:1267–1283, 1990.

[16] AN Michel, RK Miller. Qualitative Analysis of Large Scale Dynamical Systems, New York, NY: Academic Press, 1977.

[17] AN Michel, NR Sarabudla, RK Miller. Stability analysis of complex dynamical systems: Some computational methods. Circuits, Systems and Signal Processing 1:171–202, 1982.

[18] AN Michel, K Wang, B Hu. Qualitative Theory of Dynamical Systems–The Role of Stability Preserving Mappings. Second Edition. New York, NY: Marcel Dekker, 2001.

[19] RK Miller, AN Michel, Ordinary Differential Equations. New York, NY: Academic Press, 1982.

[20] MA Pai. Power System Stability. Amsterdam, The Netherlands: North Holland, 1981.

[21] IW Sandberg. Some theorems on the dynamic response of nonlinear transistor networks. The Bell System Technical Journal 48:35–54, 1969.

[22] J Si, AN Michel. Analysis and synthesis of a class of discrete-time neural networks with nonlinear interconnections. IEEE Transactions on Circuits and Systems-I: Fundamental Theory and Applications 41:52–58, 1994.

[23] J Si, AN Michel. Analysis and synthesis of a class of discrete-time neural networks with multilayer threshold neurons. IEEE Transactions on Neural Networks 6:105–116, 1995.

[24] DD Siljak. Large-Scale Dynamical Systems: Stability and Structure. New York, NY: North Holland, 1978.

Chapter 6

Qualitative Effects of Parameter Perturbations

6.1 Introduction

In the present chapter we will concern ourselves with artificial recurrent neural networks which can be described by systems of first order ordinary differential equations given by

$$\dot{x} = -Bx + TS(x) + I \qquad (S)$$

where x is a real n-vector (denoting the neuron variables), $\dot{x}$ denotes the time derivative of x, B is a real $n \times n$ diagonal matrix with positive elements (representing self-feedback), T is a real $n \times n$ matrix (representing the interconnections among the neurons), I is a real n-vector (representing bias terms), and the real n-vector valued function $S(x)$ (representing the neurons) will assume one of the following forms:

A) each component $s_i(x_i)$ of $S(x) = (s_1(x_1), \cdots, s_n(x_n))^T$ is a *sigmoidal function* [i.e., s_i maps the real numbers $\Re$ into the real interval $(-1, 1)$, it is smooth, it is monotonically increasing, and $s_i(0) = 0$]; or

B) each component of $S(x)$ is a *hard limiter* represented by the *saturation function*

$$\operatorname{sat}(x_i) = \begin{cases} 1, & x_i > 1 \\ x_i, & -1 \leq x_i \leq 1 \\ -1, & x_i < -1. \end{cases} \quad (6.1.1)$$

When the activation functions $s_i(x_i)$ are sigmoidal functions and the matrix T is symmetric, system (S) constitutes the *Hopfield model*. When the components of $S(x)$ are saturation functions, system (S) has been used, among other applications, to store bipolar memories and as cellular neural networks.

In the *implementation process* of artificial neural networks, parameter errors are unavoidably encountered. For system (S), such errors may include perturbations of interconnection weights, $T + \Delta T$; perturbations of the activation functions, $S + \Delta S$; perturbations of the self-feedback terms, $B + \Delta B$; and perturbations of the external inputs, $I + \Delta I$. We will assume that these parameter errors give rise to a *perturbation model* of system (S), given by

$$\dot{x} = -(B + \Delta B)x + (T + \Delta T)(S(x) + \Delta S(x)) + (I + \Delta I) \quad (\tilde{S})$$

where $\tilde{B} = B + \Delta B$ is a real $n \times n$ diagonal matrix with positive elements, $\tilde{T} = T + \Delta T$ is a real $n \times n$ matrix, and $\tilde{I} = I + \Delta I$ is a real n-vector. When the s_i are saturation functions, we will usually assume that $\Delta S(x) = 0$ and when the s_i are sigmoidal functions, we will assume that all components of $\tilde{S}(x) = S(x) + \Delta S(x) \triangleq (S + \Delta S)(x)$ are also sigmoidal functions.

The parameter inaccuracies introduced into system (S), resulting in system ($\tilde{S}$), will in general result in errors of the desired stable memories (or corresponding asymptotically stable equilibria), or can even result in the disappearance of stable memories, or the introduction of spurious states. Accordingly, an understanding of the qualitative robustness properties of system (S) with respect to parameter variations is of great importance.

In the present chapter we first study the robustness properties of a *general class of nonlinear systems* by addressing the following question: Given a nonlinear system with specified asymptotically stable equilibria, under what conditions will a perturbed model of the system possess asymptotically stable equilibria that are close (in distance) to the asymptotically stable equilibria of the unperturbed system? In arriving at our results, we establish robustness stability results for the perturbed system considered (Sections 6.3 and 6.4) and we determine conditions that ensure the existence of asymptotically stable equilibria of the perturbed system that are near the asymptotically stable equilibria of the original unperturbed system. These results involve quantitative estimates of the distance between the corresponding equilibrium points of the unperturbed and perturbed systems (Section 6.4). Next, we apply the above results in the qualitative analysis of neural networks (S) [and ($\tilde{S}$)] for the case when the activation functions s_i are sigmoidal functions and the matrix T is symmetric, i.e., for the case of Hopfield neural networks (Section 6.5).

Next, when the activation functions are saturation functions, for a network (S) with nominal parameters which stores a set of desired bipolar memories, we establish sufficient conditions under which the same set of bipolar memories is also stored in ($\tilde{S}$), the network with perturbed parameters (Section 6.6). In later chapters (Chapters 8 and 9), this result will be used to establish a synthesis procedure for neural networks whose stored memories are invariant under perturbations. This synthesis procedure is capable of generating artificial neural networks with prespecified sparsity constraints on the interconnecting structure and with nonsymmetric and symmetric interconnecting matrices (see Chapter 9).

6.2 Notation

As before, let $\Re$ denote the set of real numbers, let $\Re^{n \times n}$ denote the set of real $n \times n$ matrices, let $\Re^+ = [0, \infty)$, and let $\Re^n$ denote real n-space. If $x \in \Re^n$, then $x^T = (x_1, \cdots, x_n)$ denotes the transpose of x.

If X and Y are subsets of $\Re^n$ and $\Re^m$, respectively, we let $C(X,Y)$ denote the set of all continuous functions from X to Y. When X is an open subset of $\Re^n$, we let $C^N(X,Y)$ denote the set of all functions from X to Y, whose partial derivatives up to order N are continuous, $N \geq 1$.

In $\Re^n$, we let $|\cdot|$ denote any norm. The norms $|\cdot|_p$, $p \geq 1$ are defined by

$$|x|_p = \left(\sum_{i=1}^n |x_i|^p \right)^{1/p}$$

and in particular when $p = \infty$, it turns out that

$$|x|_\infty = \max_{1 \leq i \leq n} |x_i|.$$

Let $A = [a_{ij}]_{n \times n}$ denote an $n \times n$ matrix and let A^T denote the transpose of A. The matrix norms $\|\cdot\|_p$, $1 \leq p \leq \infty$, induced by the norms $|\cdot|_p$ on $\Re^n$, are defined as

$$\|A\|_p = \sup_{0 \neq x \in \Re^n} \frac{|Ax|_p}{|x|_p}.$$

In particular, we have

$$\|A\|_1 = \max_{1 \leq j \leq n} \sum_{i=1}^n |a_{ij}|$$

and

$$\|A\|_\infty = \max_{1 \leq i \leq n} \sum_{j=1}^n |a_{ij}|.$$

6.3 Robust Stability: Perturbed Systems with Fixed Equilibria

In the present section we address the robust stability of a class of nonlinear systems whose equilibrium locations are *invariant* under the influence of perturbations (Propositions 6.3.1 and 6.3.2). We utilize

6.3. SYSTEMS WITH FIXED EQUILIBRIA

these results (in Section 6.4) to study robust stability properties of systems whose equilibrium locations are *not invariant* under perturbations. We apply the above results in the perturbation analysis of a class of artificial feedback neural networks in Section 6.5.

The class of systems with uncertainty and perturbations which we consider is described by equations of the form

$$\dot{x} = f(x) + h(x) \qquad (6.3.1)$$

where $f, h \in C^1(U, \Re^n)$, $f(0) = 0$ and $U \subset \Re^n$ is a neighborhood of the origin $x = 0$. In Proposition 6.3.1, we will assume that $h(0) = 0$. Later, in Section 6.4, we will remove this restriction.

We will view system (6.3.1) as a perturbation model of systems described by equations of the form

$$\dot{x} = f(x). \qquad (6.3.2)$$

Thus, $h(x)$ in (6.3.1) represents uncertainties or perturbation terms.

Proposition 6.3.1 For system (6.3.1), assume that

1) The Jacobian matrix

$$\left. \frac{\partial f}{\partial x}(x) \right|_{x=0} \stackrel{\triangle}{=} Df(0) \stackrel{\triangle}{=} A$$

is Hurwitz stable (i.e., all eigenvalues of A have negative real parts); and

2) The Jacobian matrix $(\partial h/\partial x)|_{x=0} \stackrel{\triangle}{=} Dh(0) \stackrel{\triangle}{=} \Delta A$ satisfies the condition ■

$$\|\Delta A\|_\infty + \|\Delta A\|_1 < \frac{1}{\|P\|_\infty} \qquad (6.3.3)$$

where $P = P^T$ is a positive definite matrix determined by the matrix equation

$$PA + A^T P = -E \qquad (6.3.4)$$

where $E \in \Re^{n \times n}$ denotes the identity matrix.

Then the trivial solution $x = 0$ of (6.3.1) is *exponentially stable*.

Proof: We apply Lyapunov's Second Method with the choice of Lyapunov function given by $v(x) = x^T P x$.

Since $f, h \in C^1(U, \Re^n)$, we have that

$$f(x) + h(x) = Ax + (\Delta A)x + m(x) \qquad (6.3.5)$$

where

$$\lim_{x \to 0} \frac{|m(x)|_2}{|x|_2} = 0.$$

Let $D_{(6.3.1)} v$ denote the derivative of v with respect to t along the solutions of (6.3.1). For all $x \in U$, we have

$$\begin{aligned}
D_{(6.3.1)} v(x) &= x^T P \dot{x} + \dot{x}^T P x \\
&= x^T P(f(x) + h(x)) + (f(x) + h(x))^T P x \\
&= x^T P(A + \Delta A)x + x^T P m(x) + x^T (A + \Delta A)^T P x \\
&\quad + m(x)^T P x \\
&= x^T (PA + A^T P)x + x^T [P(\Delta A) + (\Delta A)^T P] x \\
&\quad + 2 x^T P m(x) \\
&= -x^T x + x^T [P(\Delta A) + (\Delta A)^T P] x + 2 x^T P m(x) \\
&\leq -x^T x + \mu_M x^T x + 2 x^T P m(x)
\end{aligned}$$
$$(6.3.6)$$

where μ_M is the largest eigenvalue of $[P(\Delta A) + (\Delta A)^T P]$ (recall that eigenvalues of symmetric matrices are real). We will show that $\mu_M < 1$.

First, we note that by (6.3.3),

$$\begin{aligned}
\|P(\Delta A) + (\Delta A)^T P\|_\infty &\leq \|P\|_\infty \|\Delta A\|_\infty + \|(\Delta A)^T\|_\infty \|P\|_\infty \\
&= \|P\|_\infty (\|\Delta A\|_\infty + \|\Delta A\|_1) \\
&< 1.
\end{aligned}$$

Therefore, to show that $\mu_M < 1$, it suffices to show that for any matrix W, $|\lambda(W)| \leq \|W\|_\infty$, where $\lambda(W)$ is any eigenvalue of W. In fact, there is a vector $x_0 \neq 0$ such that $W x_0 = \lambda(W) x_0$, and thus, $|W x_0|_\infty = |\lambda(W)| \cdot |x_0|_\infty$. Hence

$$|\lambda(W)| = \frac{|W x_0|_\infty}{|x_0|_\infty} \leq \|W\|_\infty.$$

6.3. SYSTEMS WITH FIXED EQUILIBRIA

It follows that $\mu_M < 1$.

Now let $\mu_M = 1 - 3\varepsilon$, $\varepsilon > 0$. Then, by (6.3.6),

$$D_{(6.3.1)}v(x) \leq -3\varepsilon x^T x + 2x^T Pm(x) \tag{6.3.7}$$

for all $x \in U$.

We will show that there is a neighborhood of the origin, $V \subset U$, such that

$$D_{(6.3.1)}v(x) \leq -\varepsilon x^T x \tag{6.3.8}$$

In using (6.3.7) to prove (6.3.8), it suffices to show that

$$x^T Pm(x) \leq \varepsilon x^T x$$

for all $x \in V$. Since

$$\lim_{x \to 0} \frac{|m(x)|_2}{|x|_2} = 0$$

we can choose $V \subset U$ in such a manner that for all $x \in V$,

$$\frac{|m(x)|_2}{|x|_2} \leq \frac{\varepsilon}{\|P\|_2}.$$

By the Schwarz inequality we thus have

$$x^T Pm(x) \leq |x|_2 \, |m(x)|_2 \, \|P\|_2 \leq \varepsilon |x|_2^2 = \varepsilon x^T x \tag{6.3.9}$$

for all $x \in V$. Therefore, by (6.3.9) and (6.3.7), (6.3.8) is true. Therefore, since $P = P^T$ is positive definite, there are positive constants $c_1 = \lambda_{\min}(P)$, $c_2 = \lambda_{\max}(P)$, and $c_3 = \varepsilon$, such that $c_1|x|_2^2 \leq v(x) \leq c_2|x|_2^2$ and $D_{(6.3.1)}v(x) \leq -c_3|x|_2^2$ for all $x \in V$. Hence, the trivial solution of (6.3.1) is exponentially stable (see Section 5.2, Lemma 5.2.1). ∎

Remark 6.3.1

1) Since $\|\Delta A\|_1 \leq n\|\Delta A\|_\infty$, (6.3.3) in Proposition 6.3.1 is guaranteed by the condition

$$\|\Delta A\|_\infty \leq \frac{1}{(n+1)\|P\|_\infty}.$$

2) Proposition 6.3.1 was proved for the equilibrium $x = 0$. It is true for an arbitrary equilibrium. ∎

We will also make use of models for systems with uncertainties and perturbations which are of the form (see Section 6.5)

$$\dot{x} = (A + \Delta A)x + m(x) \qquad (6.3.10)$$

where A and ΔA are constant matrices and where $m \in C(U, \Re^n)$ satisfies the condition

$$\lim_{x \to 0} \frac{|m(x)|_2}{|x|_2} = 0 \qquad (6.3.11)$$

where $U \subset \Re^n$ is a neighborhood of the origin.

Our next result provides sufficient conditions for the exponential stability of the trivial solution of systems represented by (6.3.10).

Proposition 6.3.2 For system (6.3.10), in addition to condition (6.3.11), we assume that

1) A is Hurwitz stable, and

2) $\|\Delta A\|_\infty + \|\Delta A\|_1 < 1/\|P\|_\infty$, where $P = P^T$ is a positive definite matrix determined by the matrix equation

$$PA + A^T P = -E$$

where $E \in \Re^{n \times n}$ denotes the identity matrix.

Then the trivial solution $x = 0$ of (6.3.10) is *exponentially stable*.

Proof: The proof of this result is similar to the proof of Proposition 6.3.1. We omit the details. ∎

6.4 Robust Stability: Perturbed Systems with Perturbed Equilibria

In general, system perturbations may give rise to changes (or even the disappearance) of equilibria in a dynamical system. (A specific example is given in the next section.) In the present section, we address robust stability issues under conditions that allow an equilibrium point of the unperturbed system to change locations under system perturbations. Specifically, for systems under perturbations, we will establish conditions that ensure the *existence* and the *exponential stability* of perturbed equilibria, and we will provide *estimates* of the *distance* between a given equilibrium of the unperturbed system and the corresponding equilibrium of the perturbed system.

As before, we let

$$\dot{x} = f(x) + h(x) \tag{6.4.1}$$

represent a perturbation of the system given by

$$\dot{x} = f(x) \tag{6.4.2}$$

where $f, h \in C(U, \Re^n)$, $U \subset \Re^n$ is an open neighborhood of x_e, and x_e is an equilibrium of (6.4.2).

If system (6.4.1) constitutes a "small" perturbation of (6.4.2), then the *existence* of an equilibrium $\tilde{x}_e$ for (6.4.1) that is "near" x_e can be established by the use of the implicit function theorem. Such an approach, however, will not yield error estimates (e.g., $|x_e - \tilde{x}_e|_\infty$) introduced by the perturbations.

In the main result of the present section, Theorem 6.4.1, we establish the existence of $\tilde{x}_e$ and we determine an estimate for the error $|x_e - \tilde{x}_e|_\infty$. In the proof of Theorem 6.4.1, we require some preliminary results which we give first.

Lemma 6.4.1 Let $q \in C^2(\overline{U}, \Re^n)$, where $U \subset \Re^n$ is a convex open set and $\overline{U}$ denotes the closure of U. Then there exists a $Q \in C^1(U \times U, \Re^{n \times n})$ satisfying the following properties for all $x, y \in U$:

1) $q(x) - q(y) = Q(x, y)(x - y)$

2) $Q(x,y) = Q(y,x)$

3) $Q(x,x) = (Dq)(x)$, where $(Dq)(x) = \partial q(x)/\partial x$ denotes the Jacobian matrix

4) $\|Q(x,y) - Q(z,y)\|_\infty \leq \alpha |x-z|_\infty$

for all x, y, $z \in U$, where $\alpha > 0$ is a constant depending only on q and U.

Proof: Let

$$Q(x,y) = \left(\int_0^1 Dq(x+t(y-x))dt\right)^T.$$

Then Parts 2 and 3 are clearly true. Part 1 can be proved by using the following formula from the calculus:

$$g(x) - g(y) = \left(\int_0^1 \nabla g(x+t(y-x))dt\right)^T (x-y)$$

where $g \in C^1(U, \Re)$ and

$$\nabla g = \left(\frac{\partial g}{\partial x_1}, \cdots, \frac{\partial g}{\partial x_n}\right)^T.$$

Finally, Part 4 is true if we choose α such that

$$\|Dq(x) - Dq(y)\|_\infty \leq \alpha |x-y|_\infty$$

for all x, $y \in U$. The existence of such α is guaranteed since $q \in C^2(\overline{U}, \Re^n)$. ∎

Note that as a consequence of Lemma 6.4.1, for any x, x_e, $\tilde{x}_e \in U$, we have that

$$\|Q(x,x_e) - (Dq)(x_e)\|_\infty \leq \alpha |x - x_e|_\infty \qquad (6.4.3)$$

and that

$$\|Q(x,\tilde{x}_e) - (Dq)(x_e)\|_\infty \leq \alpha \left(|x - x_e|_\infty + |\tilde{x}_e - x_e|_\infty\right). \qquad (6.4.4)$$

6.4. SYSTEMS WITH PERTURBED EQUILIBRIA

To see (6.4.4), we give the following more general inequality, which is a consequence of Lemma 6.4.1:

$$\|Q(x,y) - Q(z,w)\|_\infty \leq \alpha(|x-z|_\infty + |y-w|_\infty)$$

for all $x, y, z, w \in U$.

The above inequalities will be used in the proof of our main result.

Lemma 6.4.2 For the equation

$$x + G(x) = 0$$

where $x \in \Re^n$, $G \in C(\Re^n, \Re^n)$, we assume that $|G(x)|_\infty < \varepsilon$ for all $|x|_\infty \leq \varepsilon$. Then there exists an x_0 such that $|x_0|_\infty < \varepsilon$ and

$$x_0 + G(x_0) = 0.$$

Proof: By assumption, $(-G)$ is a continuous map from $[-\varepsilon, \varepsilon]^n$ to $[-\varepsilon, \varepsilon]^n$. By Brouwer's fixed point theorem (see, e.g., [5]), there exists a fixed point $x_0 \in [-\varepsilon, \varepsilon]^n$ such that $(-G)(x_0) = x_0$, i.e., $x_0 + G(x_0) = 0$.

Finally, we note that $|x_0|_\infty = |G(x_0)|_\infty < \varepsilon$, since $|x_0|_\infty \leq \varepsilon$. This concludes the proof of the lemma. ∎

Lemma 6.4.3 Let A and ΔA be two $n \times n$ matrices. Assume that A^{-1} exists, and that $\|\Delta A\| < 1/\|A^{-1}\|$. Then $(A + \Delta A)^{-1}$ exists and

$$\|(A + \Delta A)^{-1}\| \leq \frac{\|A^{-1}\|}{1 - \|\Delta A\| \cdot \|A^{-1}\|}$$

where $\|\cdot\|$ is any matrix norm. ∎

Proof: By the Gastinel-Kahan Theorem (see, e.g., [3], Fact 13), we know that $\|\Delta A\| < 1/\|A^{-1}\|$ guarantees the existence of $(A + \Delta A)^{-1}$.

Let $G \triangleq (A + \Delta A)^{-1}$. Then

$$G(A + \Delta A) = E$$

where E is the identity matrix. Then

$$GA = E - G(\Delta A),$$

$$G = A^{-1} - G(\Delta A)A^{-1},$$

and

$$\|G\| \leq \|A^{-1}\| + \|G\| \cdot \|\Delta A\| \cdot \|A^{-1}\|.$$

Therefore

$$\|G\| \leq \frac{\|A^{-1}\|}{1 - \|\Delta A\| \cdot \|A^{-1}\|}$$

where $1 - \|\Delta A\| \cdot \|A^{-1}\| > 0$. ■

In the following assumption, we require that the perturbations in system (6.4.1) [relative to system (6.4.2)] are sufficiently small and that the unperturbed system (6.4.2) has x_e as an equilibrium.

Assumption 6.4.1 Let x_e be an equilibrium of (6.4.2). For (6.4.1), we assume that

1) $f, h \in C^2(U, \Re^n)$, where U is an open neighborhood of x_e.

2) The Jacobian matrix

$$\left.\frac{\partial f}{\partial x}(x)\right|_{x=x_e} \triangleq Df(x_e) \triangleq A$$

is Hurwitz stable and therefore there exists a positive definite matrix $P = P^T$, which is determined by the matrix equation

$$PA + A^T P = -E$$

where $E \in \Re^{n \times n}$ is the identity matrix.

6.4. SYSTEMS WITH PERTURBED EQUILIBRIA

3) The perturbation h satisfies

$$\|Dh(x_e)\|_\infty \leq a \tag{6.4.5}$$

$$|h(x_e)|_\infty \leq \frac{\varepsilon}{2\|A^{-1}\|_\infty} \tag{6.4.6}$$

where $\varepsilon > 0$ satisfies

$$\varepsilon < \frac{a}{\alpha} \tag{6.4.7}$$

and $\{x \in \Re^n : |x - x_e|_\infty \leq \varepsilon\} \subset U$, where

$$a \triangleq \frac{1}{4} \min\left\{\|A^{-1}\|_\infty^{-1}, \left((n+1)\|P\|_\infty\right)^{-1}\right\}$$

and α is specified in Lemma 6.4.1 for $q = f + h$. ∎

We are now in a position to state and prove the main result of the present section.

Theorem 6.4.1 If Assumption 6.4.1 is satisfied, then the following statements are true:

1) there exists an equilibrium $\tilde{x}_e$ of system (6.4.1) such that $|\tilde{x}_e - x_e| < \varepsilon$ where x_e is the given equilibrium of (6.4.2) and ε is given in Assumption 6.4.1;

2) the equilibrium $\tilde{x}_e$ of (6.4.1) is exponentially stable; and

3) the following estimate holds,

$$|\tilde{x}_e - x_e|_\infty < 2\|A^{-1}\|_\infty |h(x_e)|_\infty \tag{6.4.8}$$

where $A \triangleq Df(x_e)$.

Proof: Part 1: We will apply Lemma 6.4.2 to prove that there exists an $\tilde{x}_e$ such that $|\tilde{x}_e - x_e| < \varepsilon$ and $\tilde{x}_e$ is an equilibrium of system (6.4.1), where x_e is a given equilibrium for system (6.4.2). To accomplish this, we first rewrite the right-hand side of (6.4.1) as

$$\begin{aligned} f(x) + h(x) &= f(x) + h(x) - (f(x_e) + h(x_e)) + h(x_e) \\ &= Q(x, x_e)(x - x_e) + h(x_e) \end{aligned} \tag{6.4.9}$$

where $Q(x, x_e) = F(x, x_e) + H(x, x_e)$, and F, H and $Q \in C^1(U \times U, \Re^{n \times n})$ satisfy the properties of Lemma 6.4.1 with respect to $q = f$, h and $f + h$, respectively.

Let $A \triangleq Df(x_e)$ and let $\Delta A \triangleq Q(x, x_e) - A$. Then

$$\begin{aligned}\Delta A &= Q(x, x_e) - A \\ &= Q(x, x_e) - Df(x_e) \\ &= Q(x, x_e) - Df(x_e) - Dh(x_e) + Dh(x_e) \\ &= Q(x, x_e) - D(f + h)(x_e) + Dh(x_e).\end{aligned}$$

Therefore, by Lemma 6.4.1,

$$\begin{aligned}\|\Delta A\|_\infty &\leq \|Q(x, x_e) - D(f + h)(x_e)\|_\infty + \|Dh(x_e)\|_\infty \\ &\leq \alpha |x - x_e|_\infty + \|Dh(x_e)\|_\infty.\end{aligned} \quad (6.4.10)$$

In order to apply Lemma 6.4.2, we first utilize Lemma 6.4.3 to show that $(A + \Delta A)^{-1}$ exists whenever $|x - x_e|_\infty \leq \varepsilon$. That is, we show that

$$\|\Delta A\|_\infty < \frac{1}{2\|A^{-1}\|_\infty} \quad (6.4.11)$$

whenever $|x - x_e|_\infty \leq \varepsilon$.

By (6.4.5), (6.4.7), and (6.4.10), for $|x - x_e|_\infty \leq \varepsilon$, we have

$$\|\Delta A\|_\infty \leq \alpha\varepsilon + \|Dh(x_e)\|_\infty < \frac{\|A^{-1}\|_\infty^{-1}}{4} + \frac{\|A^{-1}\|_\infty^{-1}}{4} = \frac{\|A^{-1}\|_\infty^{-1}}{2},$$

i.e., (6.4.11) is true.

Next, (6.4.11) and Lemma 6.4.3 imply that

$$\|(A + \Delta A)^{-1}\|_\infty \leq \frac{\|A^{-1}\|_\infty}{1 - \|\Delta A\|_\infty \|A^{-1}\|_\infty} < 2\|A^{-1}\|_\infty \quad (6.4.12)$$

where we have used (6.4.11) to obtain $1 - \|\Delta A\|_\infty \|A^{-1}\|_\infty > 1/2$.

Next, we let

$$G(x) \triangleq (Q(x, x_e))^{-1} h(x_e) = (A + \Delta A)^{-1} h(x_e). \quad (6.4.13)$$

6.4. SYSTEMS WITH PERTURBED EQUILIBRIA

By (6.4.9), we know that for $|x - x_e|_\infty \leq \varepsilon$

$$f(x) + h(x) = 0 \qquad (6.4.14)$$

if and only if

$$(x - x_e) + G(x) = 0. \qquad (6.4.15)$$

By (6.4.6), (6.4.12), and (6.4.13) we have for $|x - x_e| \leq \varepsilon$

$$\begin{aligned}\|G(x)\|_\infty &\leq \|(A + \Delta A)^{-1}\|_\infty |h(x_e)|_\infty \\ &< 2\|A^{-1}\|_\infty |h(x_e)|_\infty \\ &\leq \varepsilon.\end{aligned} \qquad (6.4.16)$$

In other words, $\|G(x)\|_\infty < \varepsilon$ is true whenever $|x - x_e|_\infty \leq \varepsilon$. By Lemma 6.4.2, there exists an $x = \tilde{x}_e$ that satisfies (6.4.15) and $|\tilde{x}_e - x_e|_\infty < \varepsilon$. Hence, $x = \tilde{x}_e$ satisfies (6.4.14), i.e., $x = \tilde{x}_e$ is an equilibrium of system (6.4.1).

Part 2: We will apply Proposition 6.3.2 to show that the equilibrium $\tilde{x}_e$ of (6.4.1) is exponentially stable. To accomplish this, we rewrite the right-hand side of (6.4.1) as

$$\begin{aligned}f(x) + h(x) &= f(x) + h(x) - (f(\tilde{x}_e) + h(\tilde{x}_e)) \\ &= Q(x, \tilde{x}_e)(x - \tilde{x}_e)\end{aligned} \qquad (6.4.17)$$

where $Q(x, \tilde{x}_e) = F(x, \tilde{x}_e) + H(x, \tilde{x}_e)$ and Q, F and H are the same matrix valued functions as in Part 1 of the present proof. Q, F, and H satisfy the properties 1–4 of Lemma 6.4.1.

By (6.4.17), (6.4.1) is equivalent to the following equation:

$$\dot{x} = Q(x, \tilde{x}_e)(x - \tilde{x}_e). \qquad (6.4.18)$$

Let $A = Df(x_e)$ and $\delta A \triangleq Q(x, \tilde{x}_e) - A$. Then

$$\begin{aligned}\delta A &= Q(x, \tilde{x}_e) - Df(x_e) \\ &= F(x, \tilde{x}_e) - Df(x_e) + H(x, \tilde{x}_e) \\ &= F(x, \tilde{x}_e) - Df(x_e) + H(x, \tilde{x}_e) - Dh(x_e) + Dh(x_e).\end{aligned}$$

By the property (6.4.4), which is a consequence of Lemma 6.4.1, we have for $|x - x_e| < \varepsilon$

$$\begin{aligned}
\|\delta A\|_\infty &< \alpha_1(|x - x_e|_\infty + |\tilde{x}_e - x_e|_\infty) + \alpha_2(|x - x_e|_\infty \\
&\quad + |\tilde{x}_e - x_e|_\infty) + \|Dh(x_e)\|_\infty \\
&< 2\alpha_1\varepsilon + 2\alpha_2\varepsilon + \|Dh(x_e)\|_\infty \\
&= 2\alpha\varepsilon + \|Dh(x_e)\|_\infty \\
&\leq 2a + a \\
&< 4a \\
&\leq \frac{1}{(n+1)\|P\|_\infty}
\end{aligned} \qquad (6.4.19)$$

where a is defined in Assumption 6.4.1 and where we have used (6.4.5) and (6.4.7). Now, (6.4.19) implies

$$\begin{aligned}
\|\delta A\|_\infty + \|\delta A\|_1 &\leq \|\delta A\|_\infty + n\|\delta A\|_\infty \\
&= (n+1)\|\delta A\|_\infty \\
&< \frac{1}{\|P\|_\infty}.
\end{aligned} \qquad (6.4.20)$$

Therefore, by Assumption 6.4.1, (6.4.20), and Proposition 6.3.2, we have proved that $x = \tilde{x}_e$ of

$$\dot{x} = (A + \delta A)(x - \tilde{x}_e) \qquad (6.4.21)$$

is exponentially stable. Since (6.4.18) and (6.4.21) are the same, and are equivalent to (6.4.1), Part 2 of the theorem is proved.

Part 3: Since $x = \tilde{x}_e$ satisfies (6.4.15), we have

$$(\tilde{x}_e - x_e) + G(x_e) = 0. \qquad (6.4.22)$$

Therefore, by (6.4.16) and (6.4.17), we have

$$|\tilde{x}_e - x_e|_\infty = \|G(x_e)\|_\infty < 2\|A^{-1}\|_\infty |h(x_e)|_\infty.$$

Hence, (6.4.8) is proved.

This completes the proof of the theorem. ∎

In the following, we utilize a specific example, to demonstrate the applicability of Theorem 6.4.1. In the next section, we utilize Theorem 6.4.1 in the analysis of Hopfield neural networks.

6.4. SYSTEMS WITH PERTURBED EQUILIBRIA

Example 6.4.1 In (6.4.1) and (6.4.2), let $f(x) = (f_1(x), f_2(x))^T$ and $h(x) = (h_1(x), h_2(x))^T$, where $x = (x_1, x_2)^T$, and where

$$f_1(x) = -2x_1 + \arctan(x_1)$$

$$f_2(x) = -2x_2 + \arctan(x_1 + x_2)$$

$$h_1(x) = \delta_1 \arctan(x_1) + \eta_1$$

and

$$h_2(x) = \delta_2 \arctan(x_1 + x_2) + \eta_2$$

where δ_1, δ_2, η_1 and η_2 are perturbation parameters.

For the equilibrium $x_e = 0$ of (6.4.2), we will use Theorem 6.4.1 to determine bounds for δ_1, δ_2, η_1, and η_2 such that (6.4.1) has an asymptotically stable equilibrium $\tilde{x}_e$ that is near $x_e = 0$, and we determine an estimate for $|\tilde{x}_e|_\infty$.

We have $A = Df(0) = \begin{bmatrix} -1 & 0 \\ 1 & -1 \end{bmatrix}$, which is Hurwitz stable. Also, $PA + A^T P = -E$ with $P = P^T$ yields

$$P = \begin{bmatrix} 3/4 & 1/4 \\ 1/4 & 1/2 \end{bmatrix}.$$

Since $\|A^{-1}\|_\infty = 2$ and $\|P\|_\infty = 1$, we have $a = 1/12$. Then (6.4.5) requires

$$\|Dh(0)\|_\infty = \max\{|\delta_1|, 2\delta_2|\} \leq \frac{1}{12}. \tag{6.4.23}$$

Choose $U = \{x \in \Re^2 : |x|_\infty < 0.1\}$. When (6.4.23) is satisfied, then

$$\|Dh(x) - Dh(y)\|_\infty \leq \max\{0.2(1 + |\delta_1|), 0.8(1 + |\delta_2|)\} \cdot |x - y|_\infty$$
$$\leq \tfrac{5}{3}|x - y|_\infty$$

for $x, y \in U$. Thus, we may choose $\alpha = 5/3$ (see Lemma 6.4.1 and its proof). Then $a/\alpha = 0.05$. By (6.4.7), choose $\varepsilon = 0.04$. Then (6.4.6) becomes

$$|h(0)|_\infty = |\eta_1| + |\eta_2| \leq 0.01. \tag{6.4.24}$$

When both (6.4.23) and (6.4.24) hold, i.e., the perturbation δ_1, δ_2, η_1, and η_2, satisfy parameters

$$\begin{cases} \max\{|\delta_1|, 2|\delta_2|\} \leq 1/12 \\ |\eta_1| + |\eta_2| \leq 0.01, \end{cases} \tag{6.4.25}$$

Assumption 6.4.1 is satisfied. Theorem 6.4.1 implies that (6.4.1) has an exponentially stable equilibrium $\tilde{x}_e$, satisfying $|\tilde{x}_e|_\infty < 4(|\eta_1| + |\eta_2|)$ and in particular [see (6.4.25)], $|\tilde{x}_e| < 0.04$. ∎

6.5 Analysis of Neural Networks with Sigmoidal Activation Functions

In the present section, we consider artificial neural networks described by equations of the form

$$\dot{x} = -Bx + TS(x) + I \tag{S}$$

where $x \in \Re^n$, $B = \text{diag}[b_1, \cdots, b_n]$ with $b_i > 0$, $1 \leq i \leq n$, $T = [T_{ij}]_{n \times n}$ is symmetric, $I \in \Re^n$, and

$$S(x) = (s_1(x_1), \cdots, s_n(x_n))^T \text{ with } s_i \in C^2(\Re, (-1, 1))$$

where s_i is monotonically increasing and $s_i(0) = 0$, $1 \leq i \leq n$. Such systems, called Hopfield neural networks, have been widely studied (see Chapters 2, 3, 5). Since such networks require symmetry in the interconnecting structure, robustness issues in the qualitative analysis of (S) are of paramount importance.

For system (S), we consider the perturbation model

$$\dot{x} = -\tilde{B}x + \tilde{T}\tilde{S}(x) + \tilde{I} \tag{$\tilde{\text{S}}$}$$

where $\tilde{B} = B + \Delta B$, $\Delta B = \text{diag}[\Delta b_1, \cdots, \Delta b_n]$, $\tilde{T} = T + \Delta T$ ($\Delta T \in \Re^{n \times n}$ need not be symmetric), $\tilde{I} = I + \Delta I \in \Re^n$, $\tilde{S}(x) = S(x) + \Delta S(x)$, and

$$\Delta S(x) = (\Delta s_1(x_1), \cdots, \Delta s_n(x_n))^T$$

with $\Delta s_i \in C^2(\Re, (-1, 1))$, $1 \leq i \leq n$.

In the following, we make precise the meaning of *robustness* for system (S).

6.5. SIGMOIDAL ACTIVATION FUNCTIONS

Definition 6.5.1 The system (S) is said to be *robust* if for every asymptotically stable equilibrium x_e of (S), and for every $\varepsilon > 0$, there is a $\delta > 0$, such that for any perturbed system $(\tilde{S})$, as long as

$$\max\{\|\Delta B\|, \|\Delta T\|, |\Delta I|, |\Delta S(x_e)|, |\Delta S'(x_e)|\} < \delta$$

where

$$\Delta S'(x) = \text{diag}\left[\frac{d(\Delta s_1)}{dx_1}(x_1), \cdots, \frac{d(\Delta s_n)}{dx_n}(x_n)\right]$$

there is an asymptotically stable equilibrium $\tilde{x}_e$ of system $(\tilde{S})$ such that $|x_e - \tilde{x}_e| < \varepsilon$. ∎

Remark 6.5.1 Since all norms in a finite dimensional linear space are equivalent, the above definition is independent of the particular choice of vector norm $|\cdot|$ and induced matrix norm $\|\cdot\|$. ∎

Roughly speaking, robustness in the present context means that system (S) is not overly sensitive to small perturbations. In synthesis procedures of associative memories for (S), robustness ensures that small errors encountered in implementations will not adversely affect the accuracy of the desired stored memories. (I.e., robustness ensures that small errors encountered in implementations will not adversely affect the locations of the *desired* asymptotically stable equilibria of system (S), which are used as memories for the neural network.) Thus, robustness of (S), in the sense of Definition 6.5.1, is of practical importance in the implementation of such networks.

A natural question to ask is whether system (S) is perhaps *always* robust (in the sense of Definition 6.5.1). To show that this is not the case, consider the scalar equation

$$\dot{x} = -\frac{2}{\pi}x + \frac{2}{\pi}\arctan(x) \tag{6.5.1}$$

which is clearly a special case of (S). For (6.5.1), $x_e = 0$ is an asymptotically stable equilibrium. However, for any fixed $\varepsilon > 0$, the perturbation of (6.5.1) given by

$$\dot{x} = -\frac{2}{\pi}x + (1+\varepsilon)\frac{2}{\pi}\arctan(x)$$

has no asymptotically stable equilibrium in a sufficiently small neighborhood of $x_e = 0$. To see this, recall that

$$\arctan(x) = x - \frac{x^3}{3} + o(x^4).$$

It is easy to construct other examples of neural networks (S) that are not robust in the sense of Definition 6.5.1.

In our next result, we establish sufficient conditions for the robustness of neural networks (S).

Theorem 6.5.1 Assume that for every asymptotically stable equilibrium x_e of (S), the matrix

$$-B + TS'(x_e)$$

is Hurwitz stable, where

$$S'(x) = \text{diag}\left[\frac{ds_1}{dx_1}(x_1), \cdots, \frac{ds_n}{dx_n}(x_n)\right].$$

Then system (S) is robust (in the sense of Definition 6.5.1). ∎

The proof of the above theorem is not straightforward, and will be given after we have established sufficient conditions for the asymptotic stability of equilibria for perturbed neural networks (Theorem 6.5.2) and estimates for the errors of stored memories in perturbed systems (Theorem 6.5.3). In doing so, we make use of the results developed in Section 6.4. The results of Theorems 6.5.2 and 6.5.3 are of practical importance in their own right.

We first consider the special case where an equilibrium x_e of the original system (S) is not changed in the resulting perturbed system (S̃).

We will require the following assumption.

Assumption 6.5.1 For systems (S) and (S̃), we assume that

1) x_e is an equilibrium of both (S) and (S̃);

6.5. SIGMOIDAL ACTIVATION FUNCTIONS

2) $A \triangleq -B + TS'(x_e)$ is Hurwitz stable;

3)
$$\max\{\|\Delta B\|_\infty, \|\Delta T\|_\infty, \|\Delta T\|_1, |\Delta S'(x_e)|_\infty\} < K_0 \quad (6.5.2)$$

where K_0 is given by

$$\frac{1}{K_0} = 2\|P\|_\infty (1 + \|T\|_\infty + |S'(x_e)|_\infty) \quad (6.5.3)$$

and $P = P^T$ is a positive definite matrix which is determined by
$$PA + A^T P = -E$$
where $E \in \Re^{n \times n}$ is the identity matrix and A is defined in Part 2 above. ∎

We note that in Assumption 6.5.1, K_0 is a positive number that is determined by system (S) and is independent of the system perturbations [see (6.5.3)]. The following result shows that K_0 is an admissible bound for robust stability.

Proposition 6.5.1 Under Assumption 6.5.1, the equilibrium $x = x_e$ of system ($\tilde{S}$) is *exponentially stable*.

Proof: Let
$$f(x) = -Bx + TS(x) + I$$
and
$$h(x) = -(\Delta B)x + (\Delta T)S(x) + T(\Delta S(x)) + \Delta I.$$
Then ($\tilde{S}$) can be expressed as
$$\dot{x} = f(x) + h(x).$$
We have that
$$Df(x_e) = -B + TS'(x_e)$$
and
$$Dh(x_e) = -\Delta B + (\Delta T)S'(x_e) + T(\Delta S'(x_e)).$$

254   CHAPTER 6. PARAMETER PERTURBATIONS

To show that $x = x_e$ of $(\tilde{S})$ is exponentially stable, we invoke Proposition 6.3.1 and Remark 6.3.1. By Part 2 of Assumption 6.5.1, $-B + TS'(x_e)$ is Hurwitz stable. Therefore, Assumption 1 of Proposition 6.3.1 is satisfied. To show that Assumption 2 of Proposition 6.3.1 is also satisfied, it suffices to show that

$$\|Dh(x_e)\|_\infty < \frac{1}{2\|P\|_\infty}, \quad \|Dh(x_e)\|_1 < \frac{1}{2\|P\|_\infty}. \tag{6.5.4}$$

Using (6.5.2) and (6.5.3), we have

$$\begin{aligned}
\|Dh(x_e)\|_\infty &= \| - \Delta B + (\Delta T)S'(x_e) + T(\Delta S'(x_e))\|_\infty \\
&\leq \|\Delta B\|_\infty + \|\Delta T\|_\infty |S'(x_e)|_\infty + \|T\|_\infty |\Delta S'(x_e)|_\infty \\
&\leq \max\{\|\Delta B\|_\infty, \|\Delta T\|_\infty, |\Delta S'(x_e)|_\infty\} \\
&\quad \cdot (1 + |S'(x_e)|_\infty + \|T\|_\infty) \\
&\leq K_0 \cdot \frac{1}{2\|P\|_\infty K_0} \\
&= \frac{1}{2\|P\|_\infty}.
\end{aligned}$$

The proof that

$$\|Dh(x_e)\|_1 \leq \frac{1}{2\|P\|_\infty}$$

proceeds similarly [noting that $\|\Delta B\|_\infty = \|\Delta B\|_1$ and $|\Delta S'(x_e)|_\infty = |\Delta S'(x_e)|_1$, since ΔB and $\Delta S'(x_e)$ are diagonal matrices, and noting that $\|T\|_\infty = \|T\|_1$, since T is symmetric]. ∎

Next, we consider the more general case, which includes equilibrium changes in the perturbed system $(\tilde{S})$.

Let x_e be an equilibrium of system $(\tilde{S})$, and let R_0, L_1, and L_2 denote real numbers satisfying

$$R_0 \geq |x_e|_\infty \tag{6.5.5}$$

and

$$\begin{cases} L_1 \geq \sup_{|x - x_e|_\infty \leq \varepsilon_0} |\tilde{S}'(x)|_\infty \\ L_2 \geq \sup_{|x - x_e|_\infty \leq \varepsilon_0} |\tilde{S}''(x)|_\infty \end{cases} \tag{6.5.6}$$

where ε_0 is a fixed positive number, and

$$\begin{cases} \tilde{S}'(x) \triangleq \operatorname{diag}[d\tilde{s}_1(x_1)/dx_1, \cdots, d\tilde{s}_n(x_n)/dx_n] \\ \tilde{S}''(x) \triangleq \operatorname{diag}[d^2\tilde{s}_1(x_1)/dx_1^2, \cdots, d^2\tilde{s}_n(x_n)/dx_n^2]. \end{cases} \tag{6.5.7}$$

6.5. SIGMOIDAL ACTIVATION FUNCTIONS

In practice, L_1 and L_2 can frequently be chosen independently of x_e and ε_0. For example, if

$$\tilde{s}_j(x_j) = \arctan(\tilde{\lambda}_j x_j)$$

with $\tilde{\lambda}_j > 0$, $1 \leq j \leq n$, then for all $x \in \Re^n$ we have

$$|\tilde{S}'(x)|_\infty \leq \max_{1 \leq j \leq n} \tilde{\lambda}_j$$

and

$$|\tilde{S}''(x)|_\infty \leq \max_{1 \leq j \leq n} \tilde{\lambda}_j^2.$$

Therefore, in the present example, we may choose

$$L_1 = \max_{1 \leq j \leq n} \tilde{\lambda}_j$$

and

$$L_2 = \max_{1 \leq j \leq n} \tilde{\lambda}_j^2.$$

We now require the following hypothesis.

Assumption 6.5.2 Let x_e and $\tilde{x}_e$ denote equilibria for system (S) and ($\tilde{\text{S}}$), respectively. Assume that

1) $A \triangleq -B + TS'(x_e)$ is Hurwitz stable and that $P = P^T$ is a positive definite matrix which is determined by the matrix equation
$$PA + A^T P = -E$$
where $E \in \Re^{n \times n}$ is the identity matrix;

2)
$$\max\{\|\Delta B\|_\infty, \|\Delta T\|_\infty, \|\Delta T\|_1, |\Delta S'(x_e)|_\infty\} < K \quad (6.5.8)$$

where K is given by

$$\frac{1}{K} = 4\|P\|_\infty (1 + L_1 + \|T\|_\infty); \quad (6.5.9)$$

and

256   CHAPTER 6. PARAMETER PERTURBATIONS

3)
$$|\tilde{x}_e - x_e|_1 < \min\{\varepsilon_0, \varepsilon_1\} \qquad (6.5.10)$$

where ε_0 is the same as in (6.5.6), and

$$\varepsilon_1 = \frac{1}{4L_2\|T\|_\infty \|P\|_\infty}. \qquad \blacksquare$$

Theorem 6.5.2 If Assumption 6.5.2 is true, then the equilibrium $\tilde{x}_e$ of system $(\tilde{S})$ is *exponentially stable*.

Proof: First, we express system $(\tilde{S})$ in the following equivalent form:

$$\dot{x} = [-B - \Delta B + (T + \Delta T)\tilde{S}'(\tilde{x}_e)](x - x_e) + m(x - x_e) \qquad (6.5.11)$$

where m satisfies (6.3.5). We now denote

$$\begin{aligned}
\Delta A &\triangleq -B - \Delta B + (T + \Delta T)\tilde{S}'(\tilde{x}_e) - A \\
&= -\Delta B + T\tilde{S}'(\tilde{x}_e) - TS'(x_e) + (\Delta T)\tilde{S}'(\tilde{x}_e) \\
&= -\Delta B + T\tilde{S}''(x')\Lambda(\tilde{x}_e - x_e) + T(\Delta S'(x_e)) + (\Delta T)\tilde{S}'(\tilde{x}_e)
\end{aligned} \qquad (6.5.12)$$

where $\Lambda(x) = \text{diag}[x_1, \cdots, x_n]$ for any $x = (x_1, \cdots, x_n)^T$, $\tilde{S}'$ and $\tilde{S}''$ are defined in (6.5.7), $|x' - x_e|_\infty < |\tilde{x}_e - x_e|_\infty$, and where we have made use of the Mean Value Theorem. Then

$$\begin{aligned}
\|\Delta A\|_\infty &\leq \|\Delta B\|_\infty + L_2\|T\|_\infty |\tilde{x}_e - x_e|_\infty \\
&\quad + \|T\|_\infty |\Delta S'(x_e)| + L_1\|\Delta T\|_\infty \\
&\leq \max\{\|\Delta B\|_\infty, |\Delta S'(x_e)|_\infty\} \\
&\quad \times (1 + L_1 + \|T\|_\infty) + L_2\|T\|_\infty |\tilde{x}_e - x_e|_\infty \\
&< K(1 + L_1 + \|T\|_\infty) + \frac{|\tilde{x}_e - x_e|_\infty}{4\varepsilon_1 \|P\|_\infty} \qquad (6.5.13) \\
&\leq \left(\frac{1}{4} + \frac{1}{4}\right) \frac{1}{\|P\|_\infty} \\
&= \frac{1}{2\|P\|_\infty}
\end{aligned}$$

where we have made use of (6.5.8), (6.5.9), and (6.5.10). [In particular, note that (6.5.10) implies that $|x' - x_e|_\infty \leq |\tilde{x}_e - x_e|_\infty \leq |\tilde{x}_e - x_e|_1 \leq \varepsilon_0$, which allows application of the bounds L_1 and L_2, using (6.5.6).]

6.5. SIGMOIDAL ACTIVATION FUNCTIONS

Similarly as in (6.5.13), we obtain by using (6.5.12) and Assumption 6.5.2

$$\|\Delta A\|_1 < \frac{1}{2\|P\|_\infty}. \tag{6.5.14}$$

Inequalities (6.5.13) and (6.5.14), in turn, imply that

$$\|\Delta A\|_\infty + \|\Delta A\|_1 < \frac{1}{\|P\|_\infty}. \tag{6.5.15}$$

From Part 1 of Assumption 6.5.2, and from (6.5.15) and Proposition 6.3.2, it now follows that the equilibrium $\tilde{x}_e$ of system (6.5.11), which is equivalent to system $(\tilde{S})$, is exponentially stable. ■

Note that in Assumption 6.5.2, we hypothesize the existence of an equilibrium of the perturbed system $(\tilde{S})$, which is not far away from the corresponding equilibrium of the unperturbed system (S). It is reasonable to expect that when the perturbations of the system in question are sufficiently small, such assumptions will be satisfied. In the next assumption, we will remove the above requirement. Specifically, we will address the *existence*, the *exponential stability*, and *error estimates* of an equilibrium $\tilde{x}_e$ of the perturbed system $(\tilde{S})$ [corresponding to an equilibrium x_e of the unperturbed system (S)].

The following assumption requires that the perturbations of system $(\tilde{S})$ [relative to system (S)] are sufficiently small and that the unperturbed system (S) has x_e as an equilibrium.

Assumption 6.5.3 Let x_e be an equilibrium of (S). For (S) and $(\tilde{S})$ assume that:

1) $A \triangleq -B + TS'(x_e)$ is Hurwitz stable and that $P = P^T$ is a positive definite matrix which is determined by the matrix equation

$$PA + A^T P = -E$$

where $E \in \Re^{n \times n}$ is the identity matrix; and

2) $\max\{\|\Delta B\|_\infty, \|\Delta T\|_\infty, \|\Delta T\|_1, |\Delta S(x_e)|_\infty, |\Delta S'(x_e)|_\infty, |\Delta I|_\infty\}$
$\leq M$, where

$$M = \frac{\varepsilon}{2\|A^{-1}\|_\infty(2 + R_0 + \|T\|_\infty)}$$

where R_0 is specified by (6.5.5), and $\varepsilon > 0$ satisfies

$$\varepsilon < \min\{\varepsilon_0, \varepsilon_2, \varepsilon_3\} \qquad (6.5.16)$$

where

$$\varepsilon_2 = \frac{1}{4L_2\|T\|_\infty} \min\left\{\frac{1}{\|P\|_\infty}, \frac{1}{\|A^{-1}\|_\infty}\right\}$$

$$\varepsilon_3 = \frac{\|A^{-1}\|_\infty(2 + R_0 + \|T\|_\infty)}{(1 + L_1 + \|T\|_\infty)} \min\left\{\frac{1}{\|P\|_\infty}, \frac{1}{\|A^{-1}\|_\infty}\right\}$$

where ε_0, L_1, and L_2 are given in (6.5.6) and P is specified in Part 1 of Assumption 6.5.2. ∎

The following result is a consequence of Theorem 6.4.1 in Section 6.4.

Theorem 6.5.3 If Assumption 6.5.3 is satisfied, then the following statements are true:

1) there exists and equilibrium $\tilde{x}_e$ of system ($\tilde{S}$) such that $|\tilde{x}_e - x_e|_\infty < \varepsilon$, where x_e is the given equilibrium of (S) and ε is given in Assumption 6.5.3;

2) the equilibrium $\tilde{x}_e$ of ($\tilde{S}$) is exponentially stable; and

3) the following estimates hold:

$$|\tilde{x}_e - x_e|_\infty \leq c \max\{\|\Delta B\|_\infty, \|\Delta T\|_\infty, |\Delta I|_\infty, |\Delta S(x_e)|_\infty\} \qquad (6.5.17)$$

where $c = 2(2 + R_0 + \|T\|_\infty)\|A^{-1}\|_\infty$, $R_0 \geq |x_e|_\infty$, and

$$A \stackrel{\triangle}{=} -B + TS'(x_e).$$ ∎

6.6. HARD LIMITER ACTIVATION FUNCTIONS

Theorem 6.5.3 may have applications in practice. For example, assuming that $c \approx 1$, and assuming that the desired memory accuracy ($|x_e - \tilde{x}_e|_\infty$) is of the order 10^{-1}, then by (6.5.17) in Theorem 6.5.3 it suffices that the accuracy of the parameters of system (S) be of order 10^{-1}.

Finally, we now show that Theorem 6.5.1 is actually a consequence of Theorem 6.5.3.

Proof of Theorem 6.5.1: For each exponentially stable equilibrium x_e of system (S), we need to show that Definition 6.5.1 is satisfied.

Without loss of generality, we may assume that $\varepsilon > 0$ is sufficiently small so that (6.5.16) is satisfied. Let $\delta = \varepsilon/(2c)$, where c is given in (6.5.17). Then by (6.5.17),

$$|\tilde{x}_e - x_e|_\infty \leq c\delta < 2c\delta = \varepsilon.$$

Therefore, Definition 6.5.1 is satisfied. ∎

6.6 Analysis of Neural Networks with Hard Limiter Activation Functions

Returning to Section 6.1, we now consider neural networks (S) with hard limiter activation functions $S(x) = [\text{sat}(x_1), \cdots, \text{sat}(x_n)]^T$ where $\text{sat}(\cdot)$ denotes the saturation function given by

$$\text{sat}(x_i) = \begin{cases} 1, & x_i > 1 \\ x_i, & -1 \leq x_i \leq 1 \\ -1, & x_i < -1. \end{cases}$$

In this case, system (S) assumes the form

$$\begin{cases} \dot{x} = -Bx + T\text{sat}(x) + I \\ y = \text{sat}(x) \end{cases} \quad (6.6.1)$$

where as before, $x \in \Re^n$, $\dot{x}$ denotes the derivative of x with respect to time t, $B = \text{diag}[b_1, \cdots, b_n]$ with $b_i > 0$, $i = 1, \cdots, n$, $T = [T_{ij}] \in$

$\Re^{n\times n}$ and $I = (I_1,\cdots,I_n)^T \in \Re^n$. Note that the *output vector* $y \in D^n = \{x \in \Re^n: -1 \leq x_i \leq 1,\ i = 1,\cdots,n\}$. We will always assume that the initial states for (6.6.1) satisfy $|x_i(0)| \leq 1,\ i = 1,\cdots,n$.

In Chapter 5, we established results which locate all equilibria of system (6.6.1) and ascertain their qualitative properties. In the present section, we will investigate some of the qualitative limitations incurred during the implementation process of system (6.6.1) which are due to parameter inaccuracies.

To fix ideas, we address in particular the implementation of associative memories via neural networks modeled by (6.6.1). In practice, for the present case, the desired memory patterns are usually represented by bipolar vectors (or by binary vectors). We will call a vector $\alpha \in \Re^n$ a *memory vector* (or simply, a *memory*) of system (6.6.1), if $\alpha = \text{sat}(\beta)$ and if $\beta \in \Re^n$ is an asymptotically stable equilibrium of system (6.6.1). We will conduct in the present section a robustness analysis of the stability properties of bipolar type memory vectors for neural network (6.6.1). Specifically, we will assume that $\alpha^1,\cdots,\alpha^m \in B^n = \{x \in \Re^n:\ x_i = 1 \text{ or } -1,\ i = 1,\cdots,n\}$ are the desired memory vectors and we will investigate under what conditions $\alpha^1,\cdots,\alpha^m$ are also memory vectors of the *perturbed system* described by

$$\begin{cases} \dot{x} = -(B + \Delta B)x + (T + \Delta T)\text{sat}(x) + (I + \Delta I) \\ y = \text{sat}(x). \end{cases} \quad (6.6.2)$$

System (6.6.2) is of course the same as the perturbed model $(\tilde{S})$ given in Section 6.1, corresponding to the unperturbed system (S), represented by (6.6.1). As in Section 6.1, for $(\tilde{S})$, we assume that $\Delta B = \text{diag}[\Delta b_1,\cdots,\Delta b_n]$ with $b_i + \Delta b_i > 0,\ i = 1,\cdots,n,\ \Delta T = [\Delta T_{ij}] \in \Re^{n\times n}$, and $\Delta I = (\Delta I_1,\cdots,\Delta I_n)^T \in \Re^n$. As pointed out earlier in Section 6.1, we assume in the present case that there are no perturbations in $S(x)$, i.e., $\Delta S(x) = 0$.

The problem posed above is of great interest from a practical point of view, especially in VLSI implementations of system (6.6.1), since one cannot realize *precisely* a set of (synthesized) parameters $\{B,T,I\}$. In what follows, we will establish upper bounds for the per-

6.6. HARD LIMITER ACTIVATION FUNCTIONS

missible perturbations ΔB, ΔT and ΔI, phrased in terms of bounds of expressions of the form $\|B^{-1}\Delta B\|_\infty + \|B^{-1}\Delta T\|_\infty + |B^{-1}\Delta I|_\infty$. These results will be employed in Chapters 8 and 9 as the basis of a synthesis algorithm for associative memories, involving system (6.6.1) satisfying prespecified interconnecting structures (interconnection constraints).

In the sequel, we will make use of the notation

$$\delta(x) = \min_{1\leq i \leq n} \{|x_i|\} \text{ for } x \in \Re^n$$

and

$$F(\alpha) = \{x \in \Re^n : x_i\alpha_i > 1, \ i = 1, \cdots, n\}$$

for $\alpha \in B^n = \{x \in \Re^n : x_i = 1 \text{ or } -1, \ i = 1, \cdots, n\}$. Also, we will make use of the following result, which is a direct consequence of Case III of Theorem 5.7.1.

Lemma 6.6.1 Let $\alpha \in B^n$. If

$$\beta = B^{-1}(T\alpha + I) \in F(\alpha)$$

then (α, β) is a pair of stable memory vector and asymptotically stable equilibrium point, respectively, for system (6.6.1).

Proof: Assume that $\alpha \in B^n$. For all $x \in F(\alpha)$, we have sat$(x) = \alpha$. For $\alpha \in B^n$ and $x \in F(\alpha)$, the first equation of (6.6.1) can be written as

$$\dot{x} = -Bx + T\alpha + I. \tag{6.6.3}$$

System (6.6.3) has a unique equilibrium at $x_e = B^{-1}(T\alpha + I)$ and $x_e = \beta \in F(\alpha)$ by assumption. Clearly, this equilibrium is also asymptotically stable, since in system (6.6.3) all eigenvalues $\lambda_i(-B)$ of $-B$ are negative [since $\lambda_i(B) = b_i > 0$]. ∎

We are now in a position to state and prove the main result of the present section.

Theorem 6.6.1 Suppose that $\alpha^1, \cdots, \alpha^m \in B^n$ are desired memory vectors of system (6.6.1), and suppose that $\beta^1, \cdots, \beta^m$ are asymptotically stable equilibrium points of system (6.6.1) corresponding to $\alpha^1, \cdots, \alpha^m$, respectively. Let

$$\nu = \min_{1 \leq l \leq m} \{\delta(\beta^l)\}. \tag{6.6.4}$$

Then $\alpha^1, \cdots, \alpha^m$ are also memory vectors of system (6.6.2), provided that

$$\|B^{-1}\Delta B\|_\infty + \|B^{-1}\Delta T\|_\infty + |B^{-1}\Delta I|_\infty < \nu - 1. \tag{6.6.5}$$

Proof: From Lemma 6.6.1, we see that for $l = 1, \cdots, m$, $\beta^l = B^{-1}(T\alpha^l + I)$, or equivalently, $b_i^{-1}(T_i\alpha^l + I_i) = \beta_i^l$, $i = 1, \cdots, n$, where b_i is the ith diagonal element of matrix B, T_i represents the ith row of matrix T, and I_i and β_i^l are the ith elements of I and β^l, respectively. In the rest of the proof, we assume that

$$\|B^{-1}\Delta T\|_\infty + |B^{-1}\Delta I|_\infty \leq \eta \tag{6.6.6}$$

and

$$\|B^{-1}\Delta B\|_\infty < \nu - \eta - 1, \tag{6.6.7}$$

i.e., (6.6.5) is satisfied. We will show that $\alpha^1, \cdots \alpha^m$ are also memory vectors of (6.6.2).

For $l = 1, \cdots, m$, compute $\Delta T\alpha^l + \Delta I$ and apply (6.6.6) to obtain

$$\begin{aligned} |b_i^{-1}\Delta T_i\alpha^l + b_i^{-1}\Delta I_i| &\leq \sum_{j=1}^n |b_i^{-1}\Delta T_{ij}| + \max_{1 \leq i \leq n} |b_i^{-1}\Delta I_i| \\ &\leq \|B^{-1}\Delta T\|_\infty + |B^{-1}\Delta I|_\infty \\ &\leq \eta \end{aligned} \tag{6.6.8}$$

where $\Delta T_i = [\Delta T_{i1}, \cdots, \Delta T_{in}]$ represents the ith row of ΔT and ΔI_i is the ith component of ΔI.

We now compute

$$\begin{aligned} \bar{\beta}_i^l &\triangleq (b_i + \Delta b_i)^{-1}[(T_i + \Delta T_i)\alpha^l + I_i + \Delta I_i] \\ &= \frac{b_i}{b_i + \Delta b_i}[b_i^{-1}(T_i\alpha^l + I_i) + b_i^{-1}\Delta T_i\alpha^l + b_i^{-1}\Delta I_i] \\ &= \frac{b_i}{b_i + \Delta b_i}(\beta_i^l + b_i^{-1}\Delta T_i\alpha^l + b_i^{-1}\Delta I_i). \end{aligned}$$

6.6. HARD LIMITER ACTIVATION FUNCTIONS

From (6.6.4) and (6.6.8), when $\beta_i^l > 1$ ($\alpha_i^l = 1$), we have

$$\begin{aligned}\bar{\beta}_i^l &\geq \frac{b_i}{b_i + \Delta b_i}(\beta_i^l - |b_i^{-1}\Delta T_i \alpha^l + b_i^{-1}\Delta I_i|) \\ &\geq \frac{b_i}{b_i + \Delta b_i}(\nu - \eta) > 1.\end{aligned} \quad (6.6.9)$$

Also, when $\beta_i^l < -1$ ($\alpha_i^l = -1$), we have

$$\begin{aligned}\bar{\beta}_i^l &\leq \frac{b_i}{b_i + \Delta b_i}(\beta_i^l + |b_i^{-1}\Delta T_i \alpha^l + b_i^{-1}\Delta I_i|) \\ &\leq \frac{b_i}{b_i + \Delta b_i}(-\nu + \eta) < -1.\end{aligned} \quad (6.6.10)$$

Relations (6.6.9) and (6.6.10) are true since (6.6.7) implies that

$$1 + \frac{\Delta b_i}{b_i} \leq 1 + \left|\frac{\Delta b_i}{b_i}\right| < \nu - \eta$$

which is equivalent to

$$\frac{b_i}{b_i + \Delta b_i}(\nu - \eta) > 1.$$

Inequalities (6.6.9) and (6.6.10) in turn imply that

$$\bar{\beta}^l = (B + \Delta B)^{-1}[(T + \Delta T)\alpha^l + (I + \Delta I)] \in F(\alpha^l),$$

$l = 1, \cdots, m$. From Lemma 6.6.1, we now see that $\alpha^1, \cdots, \alpha^m$ are also memory vectors for system (6.6.2). ∎

In the following, we give a geometric interpretation of Theorem 6.6.1 in $\Re^2$. Suppose that $\alpha \in \Re^2$ is a (desired) memory of system (6.6.1) and its corresponding asymptotically stable equilibrium point is β. Then, $\beta = B^{-1}(T\alpha + I)$ *must* be in the region $F(\alpha)$ (cf. the crosshatched region in Fig. 6.6.1), since we have $\nu > 1$ in Theorem 6.6.1.

When we have perturbations ΔB, ΔT, and ΔI as in system (6.6.2), the vector β will be displaced from its original location to, say, $\bar{\beta}$. In order for α to remain as a memory vector for system (6.6.1) after perturbation [i.e., for α to be a memory vector for system (6.6.2)], we require that $\bar{\beta}$ also be in $F(\alpha)$. It is clear from Lemma 6.6.1 that

264   CHAPTER 6. PARAMETER PERTURBATIONS

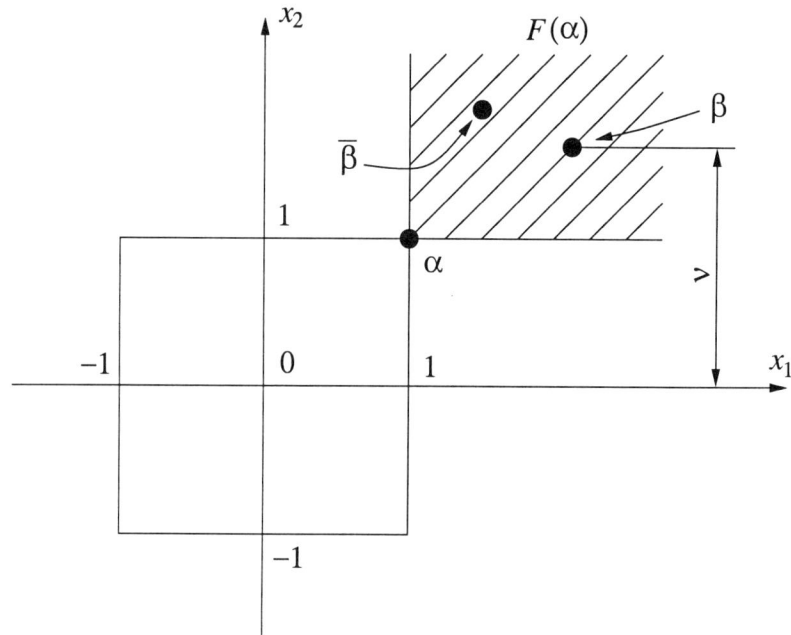

Figure 6.6.1: A geometric interpretation of Theorem 6.6.1

6.7. SUMMARY

as long as $\bar{\beta}$ is in $F(\alpha)$, α will be a memory vector of the perturbed system (6.6.2). Theorem 6.6.1 gives one of the *possible* upper bounds for the perturbations, specified by

$$\|B^{-1}\Delta B\|_\infty + \|B^{-1}\Delta T\|_\infty + |B^{-1}\Delta I|_\infty,$$

which will ensure that the perturbed vector $\bar{\beta}$ and the original vector β are within the same region given by $F(\alpha)$. This upper bound is given by $\nu - 1$ [if ν satisfies condition (6.6.4)].

Remark 6.6.1 In system (6.6.2), we have to require that $b_i + \Delta b_i > 0$ for each i. From Lemma 6.6.1, we see that a perturbation ΔB with $\Delta b_i < 0$ for $i = 1, \cdots, n$ will not change the desired memory vectors $\alpha^1, \cdots, \alpha^m \in B^n$ of system (6.6.1). ■

Remark 6.6.2 When considering perturbations due to an implementation process, the focus is usually on the interconnection matrix T and not on the parameters B and I. Assuming $\Delta B = 0$ and $\Delta I = 0$, system (6.6.2) takes the form

$$\begin{cases} \dot{x} = -Bx + (T + \Delta T)\text{sat}(x) + I \\ y = \text{sat}(x) \end{cases} \quad (6.6.11)$$

and condition (6.6.5) assumes the form

$$\|B^{-1}\Delta T\|_\infty < \nu - 1. \quad (6.6.12)$$

■

6.7 Summary

In the present chapter, we investigated the effects of parameter perturbations on a class of neural networks that can be described by equations of the form

$$\dot{x} = -Bx + TS(x) + I. \quad (S)$$

Such parameter errors may include perturbations ΔT, ΔB, ΔS, and ΔI, resulting in a perturbation model which we assumed to be of the form

$$\dot{x} = -(B + \Delta B)x + (T + \Delta T)[S(x) + \Delta S(x)] + (I + \Delta I). \quad (\tilde{S})$$

We assumed in (S) and ($\tilde{S}$) that the activation functions are either sigmoidal functions or hard limiters (in the form of saturation functions).

We considered first *systems with sigmoidal functions* as activation functions. We defined such systems as being *robust* if for every asymptotically stable equilibrium x_e of system (S), there is an asymptotically stable equilibrium $\tilde{x}_e$ of ($\tilde{S}$) which is near x_e and the distance between x_e and $\tilde{x}_e$, given by $|x_e - \tilde{x}_e|$, can be made as small as desired by requiring that $\max\{\|\Delta B\|, \|\Delta T\|, |\Delta I|, |\Delta S(x_e)|, |\Delta S'(x_e)|\}$ be sufficiently small. Roughly speaking, in the present context, robustness means that system (S) is not overly sensitive to small parameter perturbations. In synthesis procedures of associative memories for system (S), robustness ensures that small errors in parameters encountered in the implementation process will not adversely affect the accuracy of the desired stored memories. Clearly, robustness of system (S), as defined above, is of great practical importance in the implementations of such networks.

We have shown in the present chapter that (S) is robust if for every asymptotically stable equilibrium x_e of (S), x_e is asymptotically stable with respect to the linearization of system (S). This condition can be verified by testing the Hurwitz stability of the coefficient matrix

$$-B + TS'(x_e)$$

for each asymptotically stable equilibrium x_e.

When the above condition is satisfied [i.e., when system (S) is robust], Brouwer's fixed-point theorem was used to obtain the following estimate of the distance between the equilibrium x_e of (S) and the corresponding perturbed equilibrium $\tilde{x}_e$ of system ($\tilde{S}$),

$$|x_e - \tilde{x}_e|_\infty \leq c \cdot \max\{\|\Delta B\|_\infty, \|\Delta T\|_\infty, |\Delta S(x_e)|_\infty, |\Delta I|_\infty\} \quad (6.7.1)$$

6.7. SUMMARY

when in the right-hand side of inequality (6.7.1), the maximal number is sufficiently small. In (6.7.1), $c = 2(2 + R_0 + \|T\|_\infty)\|A^{-1}\|_\infty$ with $R_0 \geq |x_e|_\infty$ and $A = -B + TS'(x_e)$.

A more complete statement of the above result is as follows. Assume that x_e is an asymptotically stable equilibrium with respect to the linearization of system (S) near x_e [i.e., the matrix $A = -B + TS'(x_e)$ is Hurwitz stable which implies that x_e is an asymptotically stable equilibrium with respect to system (S)]. Then there is a constant $M > 0$ (which can be expressed explicitly) such that if

$$\max\{\|\Delta B\|_\infty, \|\Delta T\|_\infty, |\Delta S(x_e)|_\infty, |\Delta S'(x_e)|_\infty, |\Delta I|_\infty\} < M,$$

then there exists a vector $\tilde{x}_e$ which is an asymptotically stable equilibrium of the perturbed system ($\tilde{S}$) and $\tilde{x}_e$ satisfies the estimate (6.7.1).

Summarizing then, we showed in the present chapter that when the neural network (S) is robust and when the implementation errors for (S) are reasonably small, then

1) for every desired memory, there exists a corresponding actual stored memory; and

2) the errors in the memories are less or equal to the parameter errors, multiplied by a computable positive constant [see (6.7.1)].

Next, we considered systems with *hard limiters* (saturation functions) as activation functions under the assumption that $\Delta S(x) = 0$ and that only bipolar vectors (i.e., vectors belonging to B^n) are considered as candidates for desired stable memories.

For $x \in \Re^n$, let

$$\delta(x) = \min_{1 \leq i \leq n} \{|x_i|\}$$

and for $\alpha = (\alpha_1, \cdots, \alpha_n)^T \in B^n$, let $F(\alpha) = \{x \in \Re^n : x_i\alpha_i > 1\}$. Suppose that $\alpha^1, \cdots, \alpha^m$ are desired stable memories of system (S) corresponding to the asymptotically stable equilibria $\beta^1, \cdots, \beta^m$, respectively [i.e., $\alpha^j = \text{sat}(\beta^j)$, $j = 1, \cdots, m$]. Let

$$\nu = \min_{1 \leq j \leq m} |\delta(\beta^j)| > 1. \qquad (6.7.2)$$

We have shown in the present chapter that $\alpha^1, \cdots, \alpha^m$ are also stable memory vectors of system (S̃) provided that

$$\|B^{-1}\Delta B\|_\infty + \|B^{-1}\Delta T\|_\infty + |B^{-1}\Delta I|_\infty < \nu - 1. \qquad (6.7.3)$$

This robustness criterion was proved by using a result (a consequence of results in Chapter 5) which states that if $\alpha \in B^n$ and if $\beta = B^{-1}(T\alpha + I) \in F(\alpha)$, then α is a stable memory and β is a corresponding asymptotically stable equilibrium [i.e., $\alpha = \text{sat}(\beta)$] for system (S).

Now suppose that α is a stable memory and β is a corresponding asymptotically stable equilibrium for system (S). After perturbation, the new asymptotically stable equilibrium point $\overline{\beta}$ is given by

$$\overline{\beta} = (B + \Delta B)^{-1}[(T + \Delta T)\alpha + (I + \Delta I)]. \qquad (6.7.4)$$

When condition (6.7.3) is satisfied, we have shown in the present chapter that $\overline{\beta} \in F(\alpha)$, which implies that α is still a stable memory of system (S̃) (refer to Fig. 6.6.1).

The perturbations ΔB, ΔT, and ΔI give rise to a displacement of the equilibrium β [of system (S)] to a new equilibrium $\overline{\beta}$ [of system (S̃)]. In order for α to remain an invariant stable memory for system (S) after perturbation [i.e., in order for α to be a stable memory for system (S̃)], we require that $\overline{\beta}$ also be in $F(\alpha)$. It is clear that as long as $\overline{\beta}$ remains in $F(\alpha)$, α will be a stable memory of the perturbed system (S̃). This robustness result provides one of the *possible* upper bounds for the perturbations, specified by

$$\|B^{-1}\Delta B\|_\infty + \|B^{-1}\Delta T\|_\infty + |B^{-1}\Delta I|_\infty$$

which will ensure that the perturbed equilibrium $\overline{\beta}$ and the original equilibrium β are within the same region $F(\alpha)$. This upper bound is given by $\nu - 1$, where ν is given in (6.7.2).

For system $(\tilde{S})$, we required that $b_i + \Delta b_i > 0$ for each i. It is clear, however, that a perturbation ΔB with some or all $\Delta b_i < 0$ will not change the desired memory vectors $\alpha^1, \cdots, \alpha^m \in B^n$ of system (S) [refer to (6.7.4)].

When considering perturbations due to an implementation process, the focus is usually on the interconnection matrix T and not on the parameters B and I. When the latter can be ignored (i.e., when we can assume that $\Delta B = 0$ and $\Delta I = 0$), then condition (6.7.3) assumes the simple form

$$\|B^{-1}\Delta T\|_\infty < \nu - 1.$$

In closing, we observe that the concept of robustness introduced in the present chapter for system (S) with sigmoidal activation function is applicable to system (S) with saturation nonlinearities for activation functions as well. We conclude from (6.7.3) that under the present assumptions [that $\Delta S(x) = 0$ and that the desired stored memories be bipolar vectors], system (S) will *always* be robust (in the sense of the present context). Not surprisingly, this tells us that for applications of the type considered herein (e.g., associative memories with bipolar memory vectors), system (S) with saturation nonlinearities for activation functions will in general be less sensitive with respect to parameter perturbations than system (S) with sigmoidal nonlinearities for activation functions.

6.8 Notes and References

In Sections 6.1 and 6.7, we relied on material contained in the survey paper [4]. Sections 6.3, 6.4, and 6.5 are based on material presented in [6] and [7], while Section 6.6 is based on [2]. For a statement and proof of Brouwer's fixed-point theorem (as well as several other fixed-point theorems), refer to [5]. A source for the Gastinel-Kahan Theorem is [3] (see Fact 13 in [3]).

We conclude by emphasizing that the methodology employed in the present chapter in analyzing the qualitative effects of parameter perturbations of neural networks is sufficiently broad to be adapted to classes of recurrent artificial neural networks not considered herein. A case in point is the work reported in [1], where a class of synchronous discrete time neural networks is analyzed, using results which are in the spirit of those presented in Sections 6.3, 6.4, and 6.5.

Bibliography

[1] Z Feng, AN Michel. Robustness analysis and design of a class of discrete-time recurrent neural networks under perturbation. Proceedings of the 1998 American Control Conference, Philadelphia, PA, 1998, pp 53–57.

[2] D Liu, AN Michel. Robustness analysis and design of a class of neural networks with sparse interconnecting structure. Neurocomputing 12:59–76, 1996.

[3] M Mansour. Robust stability of interval matrices. Proceedings of the 28th IEEE Conference on Decision and Control, Tampa, FL, 1989, pp 46–51.

[4] AN Michel, K Wang, D Liu, H Ye. Qualitative limitations incurred in implementations of recurrent neural networks. IEEE Control Systems Magazine 15:52–65, 1995.

[5] MJ Todd. The Computation of Fixed Points and Applications. New York, NY: Springer-Verlag, 1976.

[6] K Wang, AN Michel. Robustness and perturbation analysis of a class of nonlinear systems with applications to neural networks. IEEE Transactions on Circuits and Systems-I: Fundamental Theory and Applications 41:24–32, 1994.

[7] K Wang, AN Michel. Robustness and perturbation analysis of a class of artificial neural networks. Neural Networks 7:251–259, 1994.

Chapter 7

Qualitative Effects of Time Delays

7.1 Introduction

A recurrent neural network is a network that performs computational tasks (recognition, association, and so forth) on a given pattern via interaction between a number of interconnected units characterized by simple functions. One class of neural networks which has received a great deal of attention in the literature, and which we have addressed extensively in the preceding chapters, is described by equations of the form

$$\dot{x}(t) = -Cx(t) + TS(x(t)) + I \qquad (7.1.1)$$

where x is a real n-vector (which denotes the state variables associated with the neurons), I is a real n-vector (representing bias terms), C is a real $n \times n$ diagonal matrix (representing self-feedback terms), T is a real $n \times n$ matrix (representing neuron interconnections), and $S(x)$ is a real n-vector valued function (whose components are sigmoidal nonlinearities representing the neurons).

During the implementation process of artificial neural networks (e.g., by VLSI), time delays may unavoidably be introduced. To account for such delays, the neural network model (7.1.1) has to be modified. Neural networks with time delays which have received attention and which we will address in the present chapter are described by delay equations of the form

$$\dot{x}(t) = -Cx(t) + T_0 S(x(t)) + T_1 S(x(t-\tau)) + I \qquad (7.1.2)$$

where $T \triangleq T_0 + T_1$ and C, S, T and I are defined similarly as in (7.1.1) and $\tau > 0$ denotes transportation delay.

In (7.1.2) the delays associated with the various neurons are of the same size τ. A generalization of (7.1.2) which has been considered in the literature are recurrent neural networks with *multiple delays* described by equations of the form

$$\dot{x}(t) = -Cx(t) + T_0 S(x(t)) + \sum_{i=1}^{K} T_i S(x(t-\tau_i)) + I \qquad (7.1.3)$$

where C, $S(\cdot)$, and I are the same as in (7.1.1), T_i denotes that part of the interconnecting structure which is associated with delay $\tau_i > 0$, $i = 1, \cdots, K$ and where it is assumed that $T = T_0 + \sum_{i=1}^{K} T_i$ with T defined in (7.1.1). Recall that when T is symmetric, (7.1.1) is called *Hopfield neural network*, and accordingly, we will refer to (7.1.3) as a *Hopfield neural network with multiple delays*.

The class of neural networks represented by (7.1.1) is a special class of networks represented by equations of the form

$$\dot{x}_i(t) = -a_i(x_i(t)) \left[b_i(x_i(t)) - \sum_{j=1}^{n} t_{ij} s_j(x_j(t)) \right], \quad i = 1, \cdots, n \qquad (7.1.4)$$

where the x_i denotes the state variable associated with the ith neuron, the function $a_i(\cdot)$ represents an *amplification function*, and $b_i(\cdot)$ is an arbitrary function; however, we will require that $b_i(\cdot)$ be sufficiently well behaved to keep the solutions of (7.1.4) bounded. The matrix $T \triangleq [t_{ij}]$ is a real $n \times n$ matrix and represents the neuron interconnections and the real function $s_i(\cdot)$ is a sigmoidal nonlinearity representing the ith neuron. Letting $x = (x_1, \cdots, x_n)^T$,

7.1. INTRODUCTION

$A(x) = \text{diag}[a_1(x_1), \cdots, a_n(x_n)]$, $B(x) = [b_1(x_1), \cdots, b_n(x_n)]^T$, and $S(x) = [s_1(x_1), \cdots, s_n(x_n)]^T$, (7.1.4) can be rewritten as

$$\dot{x} = -A(x)[B(x) - TS(x)]. \qquad (7.1.5)$$

We recall that when T is symmetric, (7.1.5) constitutes the *Cohen-Grossberg recurrent neural network model* (refer to Section 2.4).

When multiple delays are present, we need to modify the Cohen-Grossberg network model as

$$\begin{aligned}\dot{x}_i(t) = -a_i(x_i(t))\Big[&b_i(x_i(t)) - \sum_{j=1}^n t_{ij}^{(0)} s_j(x_j(t)) \\ &- \sum_{k=1}^K \sum_{j=1}^n t_{ij}^{(k)} s_j(x_j(t-\tau_k))\Big], \quad i=1,\cdots,n\end{aligned} \qquad (7.1.6)$$

where the $t_{ij}^{(k)}$, $k = 1, \cdots, K$, denote the interconnections which are associated with delay τ_k, τ_k denotes the kth time delay for $k = 0, 1, \cdots, K$ such that $0 = \tau_0 < \tau_1 < \cdots < \tau_K$, and x_i, $a_i(\cdot)$, $b_i(\cdot)$, and $s_i(\cdot)$ are the same as the corresponding quantities in (7.1.4). System (7.1.6) can be rewritten as

$$\dot{x}(t) = -A(x(t))\left[B(x(t)) - T_0 S(x(t)) - \sum_{k=1}^K T_k S(x(t-\tau_k))\right] \qquad (7.1.7)$$

where the x, $A(\cdot)$, $B(\cdot)$ and $S(\cdot)$ are defined similarly as in (7.1.5) and where the T_k makes up the interconnections associated with delay τ_k, $k = 0, 1, \cdots, K$ so that $T = T_0 + T_1 + \cdots + T_K$.

In the present chapter, we first study neural networks with *symmetric interconnecting structure* (i.e., Hopfield neural networks and Cohen-Grossberg neural networks) and *with delays*. We first prove that when the delay τ in (7.1.2) is smaller than a computable bound (which depends on the interconnection matrix and on the neuron gains), then the neural network (7.1.2) with delays will have the same *global stability properties* and also the same *local stability properties* as the corresponding neural network (7.1.1) without delays. Recall that neural network (7.1.2) [resp., (7.1.1)] is *globally stable* if all trajectories converge to some equilibrium of the network. As a consequence of this, we can conclude that system (7.1.2) will be globally stable for sufficiently small delays when the corresponding system (7.1.1) is globally stable. In the proof of this result, we make use of an energy functional for system (7.1.2) and we show that this energy functional decreases along the solutions of (7.1.2), ultimately converging to some equilibrium of system (7.1.2). We also show that any asymptotically stable equilibrium of (7.1.2) corresponds to a local minimum of the energy functional. When the delays are smaller than the bound mentioned above, we will prove that the set of all asymptotically stable equilibria of (7.1.2) is identical to the set of all asymptotically stable equilibria of (7.1.1). In other words, not only the global stability of system (7.1.2), but also the local asymptotic stability of various equilibria of (7.1.2) will be unaffected by small delays. Therefore, provided that τ is sufficiently small, all synthesis (learning) methods devised for (7.1.1) (see Chapter 8), are also applicable to (7.1.2) (including the Outer Product Method, the Projection Learning Rule, the Eigenstructure Method, and a method based on the perceptron training algorithm). Moreover, we will establish in the present chapter an effective criterion for determining the asymptotically stable equilibria of system (7.1.2). Next, we also establish results which are in the spirit of the results described above for Cohen-Grossberg neural networks with multiple time delays described by (7.1.6) [resp., (7.1.7)].

In the present chapter we also consider neural networks (7.1.1) and (7.1.2) whose *interconnecting structure need not be symmetric* (and we assume that the networks that we consider may possess more than one equilibrium). Since T is no longer symmetric, such networks are in general no longer globally stable. We will consider network (7.1.2), rather than (7.1.3), only for purposes of simplicity and clarity of presentation. It is not difficult to extend the results that we will present to networks (7.1.3); however, such results are messy and involve a great deal of cumbersome notation and many distracting details.

In analyzing (7.1.2) with T not necessarily symmetric, we first

7.2. HOPFIELD PRELIMINARIES

establish required results for *general* time-delay systems given by

$$\dot{x}(t) = f(x(t), t) + g(x(t - \tau), t - \tau) \tag{7.1.8}$$

where f and g are continuously differentiable functions of appropriate dimensions. System (7.1.2) is clearly a special case of system (7.1.8). Another special case of (7.1.8) of great importance consists of linear systems given by

$$\dot{x}(t) = Ax(t) + Bx(t - \tau) \tag{7.1.9}$$

where A and B are constant matrices of appropriate order.

We will establish two types of sufficient conditions for the asymptotic stability of an equilibrium x_e of system (7.1.8). One type involves *delay dependent results* while the other type *does not involve delays* (i.e., the results hold for *arbitrary delays*). Since all of these are *local results*, we will also present a method for estimating the *domain of attraction* of an asymptotically stable equilibrium x_e for (7.1.8). Finally, we apply the above results [developed for (7.1.8)] in the analysis of neural networks with delays represented by (7.1.2).

In the present chapter we also study the stability properties of an equilibrium x_e of (7.1.8) under the assumption that f and g satisfy certain *sector conditions*. These assumptions enable us to view (7.1.8) as a system endowed with *uncertainties*. This viewpoint, in turn, enables us to consider the *robust stability properties* of an equilibrium x_e of system (7.1.8). Finally, we apply these results in the *robust stability analysis* of an equilibrium of the class of neural networks with delays represented by (7.1.2).

7.2 Preliminaries (Hopfield Neural Networks)

In the present section we first establish some of the notation used throughout this chapter. Next, we provide essential facts from the Lyapunov stability theory relating to differential-difference equations of the type discussed in the preceding section.

A. Notation

Let $\Re$ denote the set of real numbers and let $\Re^n$ denote real n space. If $x \in \Re^n$, then $x^T = (x_1, \cdots, x_n)$ denotes the transpose of x. Let $\Re^{n \times m}$ denote the set of $n \times m$ real matrices. If $B = [b_{ij}] \in \Re^{n \times n}$, then B^T denotes the transpose of B, and $\det(B)$ denotes the determinant of B. For $x \in \Re^n$, let $|x|$ denote the Euclidean vector norm, $|x| = (x^T x)^{1/2}$, and for $A \in \Re^{n \times n}$, let $\|A\|$ denote the norm of A induced by the Euclidean vector norm, i.e., $\|A\| = \sqrt{\lambda_{\max}(A^T A)}$. E denotes the $n \times n$ identity matrix.

Let $\Re^+$ denote the set of non-negative real numbers, i.e., $\Re^+ = [0, +\infty)$. Let X be a subset of $\Re^n$ and let Y be a subset of $\Re^m$. We denote by $C(X, Y)$ the set of all continuous functions from X to Y, and we denote by $C^k(X, Y)$ the set of all functions from X to Y which have continuous derivatives up to order k. Let $\tau > 0$, $x \in C([-\tau, +\infty), \Re^n)$, and $t > 0$. We define $x_t \in C([-\tau, 0], \Re^n)$ as $x_t(s) = x(t+s)$ for $s \in [-\tau, 0]$. For any $\varphi \in C([-\tau, 0], \Re^n)$, the norm of φ, denoted by $\|\varphi\|$, is defined as $\|\varphi\| = \max\{|\varphi(t)| : t \in [-\tau, 0]\}$.

B. Some Background Material

The differential-difference equations of the type discussed in the preceding section are special cases of *functional differential equations* (of the retarded type), given by

$$\dot{x}(t) = F(t, x_t) \qquad (F)$$

where $F \in C(\Re^+ \times G, \Re^n)$ and G is an open and connected subset of the set $C_\tau = C([-\tau, 0], \Re^n)$. For essentials concerning functional differential equations, including existence, uniqueness and continuation of solutions, definition of equilibrium, and the principal Lyapunov stability results for (F), refer, e.g., to [10] and [18]. In the following, we cite two of these results which we will require later, implicitly or explicitly. To this end, we assume that $0 \in G$ and that $\varphi_e = 0 \in C_\tau$ is an equilibrium of (F). ($\varphi_e = 0$ means that $\varphi_e(s) \equiv 0$, $s \in [-\tau, 0]$.) We let $B(r) = \{\varphi \in C_\tau : \|\varphi\| < r\}$ for some $r > 0$. Recall that a function $\psi \in C(\Re^+, \Re^+)$ is said to belong to *class* $\mathcal{K}$ (i.e., $\psi \in \mathcal{K}$) if $\psi(0) = 0$ and ψ is monotonically increasing.

7.2. HOPFIELD PRELIMINARIES

Theorem 7.2.1 For (F) we assume that for every bounded set $D \subset C_\tau$, the range of F on $\Re^+ \times D$ is a bounded set in $\Re^n$ and that there exists a function $v \in C(B(r) \times \Re^+, \Re)$, with $r > 0$, $B(r) \subset G$, and two functions $\psi_1, \psi_2 \in \mathcal{K}$, such that

$$\psi_1(|\varphi(0)|) \leq v(\varphi, t) \leq \psi_2(\|\varphi\|)$$

where $|\cdot|$ denotes the Euclidean norm on $\Re^n$, and

$$D_{(\text{F})}v(\varphi, t) \leq 0$$

for all $\varphi \in B(r)$ and $t \in \Re^+$. [$D_{(\text{F})}v(\varphi, t)$ denotes the derivative of v with respect to t along the solutions of (F).] Then the following statements are true:

(a) The equilibrium $\varphi_e = 0$ of (F) is *uniformly stable*.

(b) If in addition to the above conditions there exists a function $\psi_3 \in \mathcal{K}$ such that

$$D_{(\text{F})}v(\varphi, t) \leq -\psi_3(|\varphi(0)|)$$

for all $\varphi \in B(r)$ and $t \in \Re^+$, then the equilibrium $\varphi_e = 0$ of (F) is *uniformly asymptotically stable*. ∎

As in the case of generalized Hopfield neural networks [system (L)] without delays, we will employ results from the *Invariance Theory* [for functional differential equations (resp., differential-difference equations)] in establishing global stability results for neural networks with delays. Such results are applicable to autonomous functional differential equations given by

$$\dot{x}(t) = F(x_t) \tag{FA}$$

where $F \in C(G, \Re^n)$ and G is an open connected subset of C_τ.

Theorem 7.2.2 For (FA) we assume that F is completely continuous [i.e., F is continuous and for any bounded closed set $D \subset G$, the closure of $F(D) = \{F(x): x \in D\}$ is compact]. Assume that there exists a $v \in C(G, \Re)$ such that $D_{(\text{FA})}v(\varphi) \leq 0$ for all $\varphi \in G$.

Let M be the largest invariant set with respect to (FA) in the set $Z = \{x \in G : D_{(FA)}v(x) = 0\}$. Then every bounded solution φ of (FA) approaches M as $t \to \infty$. ∎

We recall that M is invariant with respect to (FA) if for every solution of (FA) starting in M, it is true that the solution will remain in M for all time thereafter. For the material presented in this subsection, refer, e.g., to Chapter 6, Theorems 6.3.9 and 6.4.1 in [18], and Chapter 4, Lemmas 1.4 and 2.1 in [10].

7.3 Global Stability of Hopfield Neural Networks with Delays

In the present section, we consider Hopfield neural networks with delays described by the retarded type differential-difference equation (7.1.2), given by

$$\dot{x}(t) = -Cx(t) + T_0 S(x(t)) + T_1 S(x(t-\tau)) + I \qquad (7.3.1)$$

where $C = \text{diag}[c_1, \cdots, c_n]$ with $c_i > 0$ for $i = 1, \cdots, n$, $T = T_0 + T_1$ is a symmetric matrix, $I \in \Re^n$, $\tau > 0$, and $S(x) = [s_1(x_1), \cdots, s_n(x_n)]^T$ is a sigmoidal vector function such that $s_i(\cdot) \in C^1(\Re, \Re)$, $s_i(0) = 0$, $s'_i(\rho) \triangleq ds_i(\rho)/d\rho > 0$, $\lim_{\rho \to \infty} s_i(\rho) = 1$, $\lim_{\rho \to -\infty} s_i(\rho) = -1$, and $\lim_{|\rho| \to \infty} s'_i(\rho) = 0$, $i = 1, \cdots, n$. In order to establish our main results, we need to present some preliminary properties for system (7.3.1).

Lemma 7.3.1 Any solution of system (7.3.1) is bounded. ∎

The proof of Lemma 7.3.1 is identical to the proof when $\tau = 0$, noticing that the c_i's are positive and the $s_i(x_i)$'s are bounded, $i = 1, \cdots, n$. (Refer to the proof of Fact 7.6.1 in Section 7.6; or refer to [5].)

Assumption 7.3.1 For any equilibrium x_e of system (7.3.1) [i.e., for any x_e such that $-Cx_e + TS(x_e) + I = 0$ with $T = T_0 + T_1$], the

7.3. HOPFIELD GLOBAL STABILITY

matrix $J(x_e)$ is nonsingular, where

$$J(x) = -T + \text{diag}\left[c_1\left(s_1'(x_1)\right)^{-1}, \cdots, c_n\left(s_n'(x_n)\right)^{-1}\right]. \quad (7.3.2)$$

■

Lemma 7.3.2 For almost all $I \in \Re^n$ (except a set with Lebesgue measure zero), system (7.3.1) satisfies Assumption 7.3.1 ■

Lemma 7.3.2 can easily be proved by using Sard's Theorem [refer to the proof of Lemma 3.3.3 concerning system (L)].

Lemma 7.3.3 When system (7.3.1) satisfies Assumption 7.3.1, the set of equilibria of system (7.3.1) is a discrete set. ■

Lemma 7.3.3 can be proved by the Inverse Function Theorem (see Remark 3.3.2).

Throughout this chapter, we will assume that system (7.3.1) satisfies Assumption 7.3.1. We note that this assumption is also required in the global stability results of artificial neural networks without delays, which we proved in Chapter 3 for system (L) (see also [5] and [16]). In fact, Assumption 7.3.1 is very mild, since by Lemma 7.3.2 this assumption is satisfied for almost all $I \in \Re^n$.

We now state and prove the principal result of the present section.

Theorem 7.3.1 Suppose that Assumption 7.3.1 is satisfied for system (7.3.1), and suppose that

$$\tau\beta\|T_1\| < 1 \quad (7.3.3)$$

where $\beta = \max_{x \in \Re^n}\|D(x)\|$, where $D(x) = \text{diag}[s_1'(x_1), \cdots, s_n'(x_n)]$. Then system (7.3.1) is *globally stable*.

Proof: Let $y = S(x)$ and suppose x_t is a function in $C([-\tau, 0], \Re^n)$. Then $y_t = S(x_t)$ is also in $C([-\tau, 0], \Re^n)$. We define an energy functional $E(x_t)$ associated with (7.3.1) by

$$E(x_t) = -y_t(0)^T T y_t(0) + 2 \sum_{i=1}^{n} \int_0^{(y_t(0))_i} c_i s_i^{-1}(\sigma) d\sigma$$
$$- 2y_t(0)^T I \qquad (7.3.4)$$
$$+ \int_{-\tau}^{0} [y_t(\theta) - y_t(0)]^T T_1^T f(\theta) T_1 [y_t(\theta) - y_t(0)] d\theta$$

where $f(\theta) \in C^1([-\tau, 0], \Re^+)$ which will be specified later. After changing integration variables, (7.3.4) can be represented by

$$E(x_t) = -y(t)^T T y(t) + 2 \sum_{i=1}^{n} \int_0^{y_i(t)} c_i s_i^{-1}(\sigma) d\sigma - 2y(t)^T I$$
$$+ \int_{t-\tau}^{t} [y(w) - y(t)]^T T_1^T f(w-t) T_1 [y(w) - y(t)] dw. \qquad (7.3.5)$$

The derivative of $E(x_t)$ with respect to t along any solution of (7.3.1) can be calculated as

$$\begin{aligned}
dE(x_t)/dt &= -2y(t)^T T D(x(t))[-Cx(t) + T_0 y(t) + T_1 y(t-\tau) + I]\\
&\quad + 2x(t)^T C D(x(t))[-Cx(t) + T_0 y(t) + T_1 y(t-\tau) + I]\\
&\quad -2[-Cx(t) + T_0 y(t) + T_1 y(t-\tau) + I]^T D(x(t))\\
&\quad -[y(t-\tau) - y(t)]^T T_1^T f(-\tau) T_1 [y(t-\tau) - y(t)]\\
&\quad -\int_{t-\tau}^{t} [y(w) - y(t)]^T T_1^T f'(w-t) T_1 [y(w) - y(t)] dw\\
&\quad -\int_{t-\tau}^{t} [-Cx(t) + T_0 y(t) + T_1 y(t-\tau) + I]^T D(x(t))\\
&\quad \times T_1^T f(w-t) T_1 [y(w) - y(t)] dw\\
&\quad -\int_{t-\tau}^{t} [y(w) - y(t)]^T T_1^T f(w-t) T_1 D(x(t))[-Cx(t)\\
&\quad + T_0 y(t) + T_1 y(t-\tau) + I] dw\\
&= -2[-Cx(t) + T_0 y(t) + T_1 y(t-\tau) + I]^T D(x(t))[-Cx(t)\\
&\quad + T_0 y(t) + T_1 y(t-\tau) + I] + 2[-Cx(t) + T_0 y(t)\\
&\quad + T_1 y(t-\tau) + I]^T D(x(t)) T_1 [y(t-\tau) - y(t)]\\
&\quad -[y(t-\tau) - y(t)]^T T_1^T f(-\tau) T_1 [y(t-\tau) - y(t)]\\
&\quad -\int_{t-\tau}^{t} [y(w) - y(t)]^T T_1^T f'(w-t) T_1 [y(w) - y(t)] dw
\end{aligned}$$

7.3. HOPFIELD GLOBAL STABILITY

$$-\int_{t-\tau}^{t} [-Cx(t) + T_0 y(t) + T_1 y(t-\tau) + I]^T D(x(t))$$
$$\times T_1^T f(w-t) T_1 [y(w) - y(t)] dw$$
$$-\int_{t-\tau}^{t} [y(w) - y(t)]^T T_1^T f(w-t) T_1 D(x(t)) [-Cx(t)$$
$$+ T_0 y(t) + T_1 y(t-\tau) + I] dw$$
$$= -\int_{-\tau}^{0} \alpha(x_t, \theta)^T M(x_t, \theta) \alpha(x_t, \theta) d\theta$$
(7.3.6)

where $f'(\theta) = df(\theta)/d\theta$ and $\alpha(x_t, \theta) = [\alpha_1^T, \alpha_2^T, \alpha_3^T]$ such that

$$\alpha_1 = -Cx(t) + T_0 y(t) + T_1 y(t-\tau) + I \quad (7.3.7)$$

$$\alpha_2 = T_1[y(t-\tau) - y(t)] \quad (7.3.8)$$

$$\alpha_3 = T_1[y(t+\theta) - y(t)] \quad (7.3.9)$$

and

$$M(x_t, \theta) = \begin{bmatrix} 2D(x(t))/\tau & -D(x(t))/\tau & D(x(t))T_1^T f(\theta) \\ -D(x(t))/\tau & f(-\tau)E/\tau & 0 \\ f(\theta)T_1 D(x(t)) & 0 & f'(\theta)E \end{bmatrix}$$
(7.3.10)

where E denotes the $n \times n$ identity matrix. To obtain the last equation in (7.3.6), we changed the integration variables from w back to θ. We will show that if the hypotheses of Theorem 7.3.1 are satisfied, then $M(x_t, \theta)$ is positive definite for all $\theta \in [-\tau, 0]$ and all x_t which satisfy (7.3.1). In doing so, we let $U = U_3 U_2 U_1$, where

$$U_1 = \begin{bmatrix} E & 0 & 0 \\ -E/2 & E & 0 \\ 0 & 0 & E \end{bmatrix}, \quad U_2 = \begin{bmatrix} E & 0 & 0 \\ 0 & E & 0 \\ -\tau f(\theta) T_1/2 & 0 & E \end{bmatrix},$$

and

$$U_3 = \begin{bmatrix} E & 0 & 0 \\ 0 & E & 0 \\ 0 & -(1/2)f(\theta)T_1 D(x(t))[f(-\tau)E/\tau - D(x(t))/(2\tau)]^{-1} & E \end{bmatrix}.$$

It is not difficult to verify that $\tilde{M} = U M(x_t, \theta) U^T$ is a diagonal matrix. In fact,

$$\tilde{M} = \text{diag}[M_1, M_2, M_3] \quad (7.3.11)$$

where
$$M_1 = \frac{2D(x(t))}{\tau} \quad (7.3.12)$$

$$M_2 = \frac{f(-\tau)}{\tau}E - \frac{D(x(t))}{2\tau} \quad (7.3.13)$$

and

$$M_3 = f'(\theta)E - \frac{f(\theta)T_1 D(x(t))}{2}\left[\left[\frac{f(-\tau)}{\tau}E - \frac{D(x(t))}{2\tau}\right]^{-1}\right.$$

$$\left. + 2\tau D^{-1}(x(t))\right]\frac{D(x(t))T_1^T f(\theta)}{2}. \quad (7.3.14)$$

It follows that $M(x_t, \theta)$ is positive definite if and only if $\tilde{M}$ is positive definite, and if and only if M_1, M_2, and M_3 are all positive definite.

We now show that if the condition $\tau\beta\|T_1\| < 1$ is satisfied, where $\beta = \max_{x \in \Re}\|D(x)\|$, then we can always find a suitable

$$f(\theta) \in C([-\tau, 0], \Re^+)$$

such that M_1, M_2, and M_3 are positive definite for all x_t which satisfy (7.3.1) and for all θ. From this it follows that $M(x_t, \theta)$ is positive definite and, therefore, $dE(x_t)/dt \leq 0$ along any solution x_t of (7.3.1).

By the assumption that $s_i'(\rho) > 0$ for all $\rho \in \Re$, the matrix M_1 is automatically positive definite. The matrix M_2 will always be positive definite if condition

$$2f(-\tau) - \beta > 0 \quad (7.3.15)$$

is satisfied. For M_3, it is easily shown that if

$$f'(\theta) > \frac{1}{4}f^2(\theta)\|T_1\|^2 \left\|D(x(t))\left[\left(\frac{f(-\tau)}{\tau}E - \frac{D(x(t))}{2\tau}\right)^{-1}\right.\right.$$

$$\left.\left. + 2\tau D^{-1}(x(t))\right]D(x(t))\right\| \quad (7.3.16)$$

7.3. HOPFIELD GLOBAL STABILITY

is true, then M_3 is also positive definite. Notice that the matrix

$$H \triangleq D(x(t)) \left[\left(\frac{f(-\tau)}{\tau} E - \frac{D(x(t))}{2\tau} \right)^{-1} + 2\tau D^{-1}(x(t)) \right] D(x(t))$$

is a diagonal matrix, i.e., $H = \text{diag}[h_1, \cdots, h_n]$. It is easy to show that

$$h_i = \frac{4f(-\tau)s_i'(x_i(t))\tau}{2f(-\tau) - s_i'(x_i(t))}$$

for $i = 1, \cdots, n$. Since $s_i'(x_i(t)) < \beta$ by the definition of β, we have, in view of (7.3.15), that

$$h_i \leq \frac{4f(-\tau)\beta\tau}{2f(-\tau) - \beta}.$$

Therefore, we obtain

$$\|H\| \leq \frac{4f(-\tau)\beta\tau}{2f(-\tau) - \beta}$$

and furthermore, condition (7.3.16) will be satisfied if (7.3.15) is satisfied and

$$f'(\theta) > \frac{1}{4} f^2(\theta) \|T_1\|^2 \frac{4f(-\tau)\beta\tau}{2f(-\tau) - \beta} \quad (7.3.17)$$

is satisfied.

Next, we need to show that there is an $f \in C^1([-\tau, 0], \Re)$ such that conditions (7.3.15) and (7.3.17) are satisfied. We choose

$$f(-\tau) = \left(\beta \tau^2 \|T_2\|^2 \right)^{-1}. \quad (7.3.18)$$

Condition (7.3.15) is satisfied by the choice (7.3.18). Furthermore,

$$\left[f(-\tau)\tau\|T_1\| - \frac{1}{\beta\tau\|T_1\|} \right]^2 + 1 - \frac{1}{\beta^2\tau^2\|T_1\|^2} = 1 - \frac{1}{\beta^2\tau^2\|T_1\|^2} < 0$$

is true because $\beta\tau\|T_1\| < 1$. It follows that

$$kf(-\tau)\tau < 1 \quad (7.3.19)$$

where
$$k = \frac{\|T_1\|^2 f(-\tau)\beta\tau}{2f(-\tau) - \beta}. \tag{7.3.20}$$

Since $kf(-\tau)\tau < 1$, we can always find an l, such that $0 < l < 1$ and $kf(-\tau)\tau < l$. Therefore, we will always have $\gamma > 0$ where γ is given by
$$\gamma = \frac{l}{kf(-\tau)} - \tau. \tag{7.3.21}$$

We now choose $f(\theta)$ on $[-\tau, 0]$ as
$$f(\theta) = \frac{l}{k(\gamma - \theta)}. \tag{7.3.22}$$

It is easily verified that this choice is consistent with (7.3.18). Clearly, $f \in C([-\tau, 0], \Re^+)$ since $\gamma > 0$. The derivative of $f(\theta)$ is given by
$$f'(\theta) = \frac{1}{k(\gamma - \theta)^2} = \frac{k}{l} f^2(\theta) > kf^2(\theta) \tag{7.3.23}$$

since $0 < l < 1$. Combining (7.3.20) and (7.3.23), we can verify that $f(\theta)$ satisfies condition (7.3.17).

Therefore, we have shown that if $\beta\tau\|T_1\| < 1$, then there exists an $f(\theta)$ [given by (7.3.22), where $f(-\tau)$, k, and γ are given by (7.3.18), (7.3.20), and (7.3.21), respectively] such that conditions (7.3.15) and (7.3.17) are satisfied. Thus $M(x_t, \theta)$ is positive definite for all x_t satisfying (7.3.1) and all $\theta \in [-\tau, 0]$. Therefore, we have in fact shown that
$$\frac{dE(x_t)}{dt} \leq 0 \tag{7.3.24}$$

along any solution x_t of (7.3.1), where $E(x_t)$ is the energy functional given by (7.3.4).

We know that if $dE(x_t)/dt = 0$ for some x_t satisfying (7.3.1), then $\alpha_1 = 0$, $\alpha_2 = 0$, and $\alpha_3 = 0$ for all $\theta \in [-\tau, 0]$, where the $\alpha_i's$ are given by (7.3.7)–(7.3.9).

Since for any x_t satisfying Eq. (7.3.1), x_t is bounded (see Lemma 7.3.1), and since $dE(x_t)/dt \leq 0$, it follows from the invariance theory (see Chapter 4, Lemmas 1.4 and 2.1 in [10]; or Chapter 6, Theorem 6.4.1 in [18]; or Section 7.2B), that the limit set of x_t as $t \to \infty$ is a connected subset of the set of all equilibria of system (7.3.1). By Assumption 7.3.1, this set is a discrete set (Lemma 7.3.3). Thus we have proved that x_t approaches some equilibrium of system (7.3.1) as $t \to \infty$. Specifically, we have shown that

$$\lim_{t \to \infty} x(t)$$

exists. ∎

7.4 Local Stability Results for Hopfield Neural Networks with Delays

In the preceding section we showed that when $\tau\beta\|T_1\| < 1$, Hopfield neural networks with delays described by (7.3.1) are globally stable, i.e., any solution of (7.3.1) will converge to *some* equilibrium of (7.3.1). Since in the implementation of Hopfield neural networks as associative memories, information is stored in specific asymptotically stable equilibria (called stable memories), good criteria which ensure the asymptotic stability of an equilibrium of (7.3.1) are of great interest. We address this issue in the present section.

At the present time, there are no known general results which provide necessary and sufficient conditions for the asymptotic stability of an equilibrium for Hopfield neural networks with delays [given by (7.3.1)]. However, several results have been reported which provide sufficient conditions for the asymptotic stability of an equilibrium for (7.3.1). These results are frequently obtained by linearizing (7.3.1) about an equilibrium of interest (see, e.g., [17]). Other results, which make use of sector conditions for nonlinearities, have been obtained by Lyapunov's Second Method (see, e.g., [28]). It should be emphasized that in the case of delay equations, even for linear systems given by

$$\dot{x}(t) = Ax(t) + Bx(t - \tau) \qquad (7.4.1)$$

there are no known general results which constitute necessary and sufficient conditions for the asymptotic stability of the equilibrium $x = 0$. [In (7.4.1), $A \in \Re^{n \times n}$, $B \in \Re^{n \times n}$, $\tau > 0$, and $x \in \Re^n$.] However, many sufficient conditions for the asymptotic stability of the equilibrium $x = 0$ of (7.4.1) have been established (see, e.g., [3], [13], [15]). In th present section we will show that if the conditions of Theorem 7.3.1 are satisfied, then the asymptotic stability of any equilibrium of system (7.3.1) can be deduced from the asymptotic stability of the same equilibrium of system (7.1.1). In other words, if $\tau\beta\|T_1\| < 1$ then (as shown in the preceding section), Hopfield neural networks (7.1.1) and Hopfield neural networks with delays (7.3.1) are both globally stable, and furthermore (as will be shown in the present section), both have the same local stability properties at any equilibrium. This enables us to verify the asymptotic stability of the equilibria of system (7.3.1) by ascertaining the asymptotic stability of corresponding equilibria of system (7.1.1).

In order to proceed further, we require the following.

Definition 7.4.1 An element $\varphi \in C([-\tau, 0], \Re^n)$ is called a *local minimum* of the energy functional E defined by (7.3.4) if there exists a $\delta > 0$, such that for any $\tilde{\varphi} \in C([-\tau, 0], \Re^n)$, $E(\varphi) \leq E(\tilde{\varphi})$ whenever $\|\varphi - \tilde{\varphi}\| < \delta$. ∎

We are now able to establish the following results.

Theorem 7.4.1 Suppose that the conditions of Theorem 7.3.1 are satisfied. If x_e is an equilibrium of (7.3.1) (defined in Assumption 7.3.1), then the following statements are equivalent:

1) x_e is a stable equilibrium of (7.3.1);

2) x_e is an asymptotically stable equilibrium of (7.3.1);

3) φ_{x_e} is a local minimum of the energy functional E given by (7.3.4), where $\varphi_{x_e} \in C([-\tau, 0], \Re^n)$ such that $\varphi_{x_e} \equiv x_e$;

4) $J(x_e)$ is positive definite, where $J(x)$ is given in (7.3.2).

7.4. HOPFIELD LOCAL STABILITY

Proof: (a) 1) $\Longrightarrow$ 2). Since Assumption 7.3.1 is satisfied, the set of equilibria of system (7.3.1) is a discrete set by Lemma 7.3.3. Therefore, when $\varepsilon > 0$ is sufficiently small, there is no other equilibrium in $U(x_e, \varepsilon)$, a neighborhood of x_e, given by

$$U(x_e, \varepsilon) \triangleq \{x \in \Re^n : |x - x_e| < \varepsilon\}. \tag{7.4.2}$$

Since x_e is a stable equilibrium of (7.3.1), there exists an $\eta > 0$ such that for any $\varphi \in C([-\tau, 0], \Re^n)$ satisfying $\|\varphi - x_e\| < \eta$, $\|x_t - x_e\| < \varepsilon$ for all $t > 0$, where x_t is the solution of (7.3.1) with initial condition φ. Thus $x_t \in C([-\tau, 0], U(x_e, \varepsilon))$ for all t. In view of Theorem 7.3.1, x_t will converge to some equilibrium of system (7.3.1). Since x_e is the only equilibrium of (7.3.1) in $U(x_e, \varepsilon)$, it follows that x_t converges to x_e. Thus, we have shown that x_e is an attractive equilibrium of system (7.3.1). Therefore the stable equilibrium x_e of (7.3.1) is an asymptotically stable equilibrium of system (7.3.1).

(b) 2) $\Longrightarrow$ 3). Since x_e is an asymptotically stable equilibrium of system (7.3.1), there exists an $\eta > 0$ such that for any $\varphi \in C([-\tau, 0], \Re^n)$ satisfying $\|\varphi - x_e\| < \eta$, x_t converges to x_e, where x_t is the solution of (7.3.1) with initial condition φ. Therefore $E(\varphi_{x_e}) \leq E(x_t) \leq E(\varphi)$ for any $\varphi \in C([-\tau, 0], \Re^n)$ satisfying $\|\varphi - x_e\| < \eta$. Therefore φ_{x_e} is a local minimum of the energy functional E.

(c) 3) $\Longrightarrow$ 4). Let $\tilde{E}$ be a function from $\Re^n$ to $\Re$ defined by

$$\tilde{E}(x) \triangleq -y^T T y + 2 \sum_{i=1}^{n} \int_0^{y_i} c_i s_i^{-1}(\sigma) d\sigma - 2 y^T I \tag{7.4.3}$$

where $y = S(x)$. Comparing E with $\tilde{E}$, we note that $\tilde{E}$ is a function defined on $\Re^n$ while E is a functional defined on $C([-\tau, 0], \Re^n)$. Since φ_{x_e} is a local minimum of E, x_e must be a local minimum of $\tilde{E}$. For otherwise, there would exist a sequence $\{x_n\} \subset \Re^n$ such that $x_n \to x_e$ as $n \to \infty$ and $\tilde{E}(x_n) < \tilde{E}(x_e)$. Let φ_{x_n} denote the constant function $\varphi_{x_n} \equiv x_n$ in $C([-\tau, 0], \Re^n)$. Then $\|\varphi_{x_n} - \varphi_{x_e}\| \to 0$ as $n \to \infty$, and

$$E(\varphi_{x_n}) = \tilde{E}(x_n) < \tilde{E}(x_e) = E(\varphi_{x_e}).$$

This contradicts the fact that φ_{x_e} is a local minimum of E. Therefore, x_e is a local minimum of $\tilde{E}$. Hence, $\tilde{J}(x_e)$ is positive semidefinite (see, e.g., Theorem 3.6 in [9]), where $\tilde{J}(x)$ is the Hessian matrix of $\tilde{E}$ given by

$$\tilde{J}(x) = \left[\frac{\partial^2 \tilde{E}}{\partial x_i \partial x_j}\right]_{n \times n}. \qquad (7.4.4)$$

It can be shown that

$$\tilde{J}(x) = 2D(x)J(x)D(x)$$

where $D(x) = \text{diag}[s'_1(x_1), \cdots, s'_n(x_n)]$, and $J(x)$ is given by (7.3.2). Therefore, $J(x_e)$ is also positive semidefinite. By Assumption 7.3.1, $J(x_e)$ is a nonsingular matrix. Thus we have shown that $J(x_e)$ is positive definite.

(d) 4) $\Longrightarrow$ 1). We need to prove that x_e is a stable equilibrium of system (7.3.1), i.e., for any $\varepsilon > 0$, there exists a $\delta > 0$, such that for any $\varphi \in C([-\tau, 0], \Re^n)$, if $\|\varphi - x_e\| < \delta$, then $\|x_t - x_e\| < \varepsilon$ where x_t is the solution of (7.3.1) with initial condition φ.

Since $J(x_e)$ is positive definite, then $\tilde{J}(x_e)$ must also be positive definite where $\tilde{J}(x)$ is the Hessian matrix of $\tilde{E}$ given by (7.4.4). Furthermore,

$$\nabla_x \tilde{E}(x) = 2(-Ty + Cx - I)D(x)$$

where $D(x)$ is given in Part (b). Therefore, $\nabla_x \tilde{E}(x_e) = 0$ since x_e is an equilibrium of (7.3.1). It follows (by Theorem 3.6 in [9]) that x_e is a local minimum of $\tilde{E}$, i.e., there exists a $\delta_1 > 0$, $\delta_1 < \varepsilon$, such that whenever $0 < |x - x_e| \leq \delta_1$, $\tilde{E}(x_e) < \tilde{E}(x)$. Let $r = \min\{\tilde{E}(x): |x - x_e| = \delta_1\}$. Then it is true that $r > \tilde{E}(x_e)$. Since $E(\varphi_{x_e}) = \tilde{E}(x_e)$, it follows that $r > E(\varphi_{x_e})$. Note that E is a continuous functional. Therefore, there exists a $\delta > 0$, $\delta < \delta_1$ such that whenever $\|\varphi - x_e\| < \delta$, where $\varphi \in C([-\tau, 0], \Re^n)$, we have $E(\varphi) < r$. Suppose x_t is any solution of (7.3.1) with the initial condition φ such that $\|\varphi - x_e\| < \delta$. We will show that $\|x_t - x_e\| < \delta_1 < \varepsilon$. Otherwise, there would exist a $t_0 > 0$ such that $|x_{t_0}(0) - x_e| = \delta_1$, i.e., $|x(t_0) - x_e| = \delta_1$. By the definition of E and $\tilde{E}$, we have $E(x_{t_0}) \geq \tilde{E}(x(t_0)) \geq r$.

7.5. HOPFIELD NEURAL NETWORK EXAMPLE

Therefore, we obtain $E(x_{t_0}) > E(\varphi)$ which contradicts the fact that E is monotonically decreasing along any solution of (7.3.1). Thus, we have shown that x_e is an asymptotically stable equilibrium of system (7.3.1). ∎

We note that statement 4) in Theorem 7.4.1 is independent of the delay τ. Therefore, if system (7.3.1) satisfies Assumption 7.3.1, and if the condition $\tau\beta\|T_1\| < 1$ is satisfied, then the locations of the (asymptotically) stable equilibria of system (7.3.1) will not depend on the delay τ. This is true if in particular $\tau = 0$. Therefore, if $\tau\beta\|T_1\| < 1$, then system (7.3.1) and system (7.1.1) [obtained by letting $\tau = 0$ in (7.3.1)] will have identical (asymptotically) stable equilibria. We state this in the form of a corollary.

Corollary 7.4.1 Under the conditions of Theorem 7.3.1, x_e is an (asymptotically) stable equilibrium of system (7.3.1) if and only if x_e is an (asymptotically) stable equilibrium of system (7.1.1). This is true if and only if $J(x_e)$ is positive definite, where $J(x)$ is given in Eq. (7.3.2). ∎

Corollary 7.4.1 provides an effective criterion for testing the (asymptotic) stability of any equilibrium of Hopfield neural networks with delays described by (7.3.1). This criterion constitutes necessary and sufficient conditions, as long as $\tau\beta\|T_1\| < 1$.

7.5 An Example for the Hopfield Neural Networks

To illustrate the applicability of some of the preceding results, we consider the system

$$\dot{x}(t) = -Cx(t) + TS(x(t-\tau)) \quad (7.5.1)$$

where $x \in \Re^2$, $C = \text{diag}[1.1, 1.2]$, and $S(x) = [s_1(x_1), s_2(x_2)]^T$ such that

$$s_1(x_1) = \frac{2}{\pi}\tan^{-1}\left(\frac{1.4\pi}{2}x_1\right)$$

and
$$s_2(x_2) = \frac{2}{\pi}\tan^{-1}\left(\frac{1.5\pi}{2}x_2\right)$$
where T is a symmetric matrix given by
$$T = \begin{bmatrix} -0.2 & 1 \\ 1 & -0.1 \end{bmatrix}.$$

System (7.5.1) has three equilibria given by $x_{e_0} = (0, 0)^T$, $x_{e_1} = (0.2140, 0.2091)^T$, and $x_{e_2} = (-0.2140, -0.2091)^T$. The classical method of analyzing the stability of (7.5.1) is to linearize (7.5.1) about each of its equilibria. For example, the linearization of (7.5.1) at the equilibrium x_{e_1} is given by

$$\dot{y}(t) = -Cy(t) + TS_0 y(t - \tau) \qquad (7.5.2)$$

where $y = x - x_{e_1}$, C and T are the same as in (7.5.1), and

$$S_0 = \begin{bmatrix} 1.1462 & 0 \\ 0 & 1.2071 \end{bmatrix}.$$

However, as mentioned earlier, there are no effective existing results for testing the stability of system (7.5.2). For example, the results in [17] cannot be applied in the present case, since system (7.5.2) cannot be decomposed into two one-dimensional subsystems which is essential to the derivation of the results in [17].

Although there exist in the literature some sufficient conditions for the asymptotic stability of linear time-delay systems given by

$$\dot{x}(t) = Ax(t) + Bx(t - \tau) \qquad (7.5.3)$$

where A, B are constant $n \times n$ matrices, these results are in general very restrictive when applied to system (7.5.2). For example, the results of [13] yield

$$2\tau(\|A\| + \|B\|)\sqrt{\frac{\lambda_{\max}(P)}{\lambda_{\min}(P)}}\|PB\| < 1 \qquad (7.5.4)$$

as a condition for the asymptotic stability of the equilibrium $x = 0$ of system (7.5.3), where P is the positive definite matrix such that

$(A+B)^T P + P(A+B) = -E$, and E is the identity matrix. When the bound given in (7.5.4) is applied to system (7.5.2), we obtain that the equilibrium $y = 0$ (or $x = x_{e_1}$) is asymptotically stable if the delay $\tau < 0.014$. Thus, by the classical method of linearization, we know that the equilibrium x_{e_1} of system (7.5.1) is asymptotically stable if $\tau < 0.014$.

If we apply Corollary 7.4.1 to system (7.5.1), it is easily shown that $J(x_{e_1})$ and $J(x_{e_2})$ are positive definite, and $J(x_{e_0})$ is not positive definite, where $J(x)$ is defined by (7.3.2). Thus, we know by Corollary 7.4.1 that when $\tau < 0.579$, x_{e_1} and x_{e_2} are (asymptotically) stable equilibria of system (7.5.1) while x_{e_0} is not (asymptotically) stable. Therefore, for the present example, Corollary 7.4.1 provides stability conditions which are significantly less restrictive than other existing results discussed above. Additionally, Theorem 7.3.1 shows that system (7.5.1) is globally stable when $\tau < 0.579$.

7.6 Preliminaries (Cohen-Grossberg Neural Networks)

In the present chapter, we assume that the Cohen-Grossberg neural networks (7.1.4), given by

$$\dot{x}_i = -a_i(x_i) \left[b_i(x_i) - \sum_{j=1}^{n} t_{ij} s_j(x_j) \right], \quad i = 1, \cdots, n \quad (7.6.1)$$

and the Cohen-Grossberg neural networks with delays (7.1.6), given by

$$\dot{x}_i(t) = -a_i(x_i(t)) \left[b_i(x_i(t)) - \sum_{j=1}^{n} t_{ij}^{(0)} s_j(x_j(t)) \right. \\ \left. - \sum_{k=1}^{K} \sum_{j=1}^{n} t_{ij}^{(k)} s_j(x_j(t - \tau_k)) \right] \quad (7.6.2)$$

satisfy the following assumptions.

Assumption 7.6.1

1) The function a_i is bounded, positive, and continuous;

2) the function b_i is continuous;

3) $T \triangleq [t_{ij}]$ is a symmetric matrix;

4) $s_j \in C^1(\Re, \Re)$ is a sigmoidal function [so that $s_j(0) = 0$, $s'_j(x_j) \triangleq ds_j(x_j)/dx_j > 0$, $\lim_{x_j \to \infty} s_j(x_j) = 1$, $\lim_{x_j \to -\infty} s_j(x_j) = -1$, and $\lim_{|x_j| \to \infty} s'_j(x_j) = 0$]; and

5) $\lim_{x_i \to +\infty} b_i(x_i) = +\infty$ and $\lim_{x_i \to -\infty} b_i(x_i) = -\infty$. ∎

Assumption 7.6.1 is hypothesized in many references dealing with artificial feedback neural networks without delays (see, e.g., [14]). We note in particular that Part 5) of Assumption 7.6.1 ensures the boundedness of the solutions of the neural network (7.6.1) (*without delays*). In the following, we show in Fact 7.6.1 that Part 5) of Assumption 7.6.1 ensures also the boundedness of the solutions of the neural network (7.6.2) (*with delays*).

More generally, we could replace Part 5) of Assumption 7.6.1 by some other hypothesis which ensures the boundedness of solutions of (7.6.2). For example, it can be shown that parts (e) and (f) of Theorem 1 in [5] ensure the boundedness of the solutions of neural network (7.6.1) and also of neural network (7.6.2). ∎

Fact 7.6.1 If Assumption 7.6.1 is satisfied for systems (7.6.1) and (7.6.2), then any solutions of (7.6.1) and (7.6.2) are bounded.

Proof: We only need to consider system (7.6.2) since (7.6.1) is a special case of (7.6.2). We know by Assumption 7.6.1 that the terms $s_j(x_j(t))$ and $s_j(x_j(t - \tau_k))$ are bounded for all $j = 1, \cdots, n$. Furthermore, since $\lim_{x_i \to +\infty} b_i(x_i) = +\infty$ and $\lim_{x_i \to -\infty} b_i(x_i) = -\infty$,

7.6. COHEN-GROSSBERG PRELIMINARIES

there must exist an $M > 0$ such that

$$b_i(x_i(t)) - \sum_{j=1}^{n} t_{ij}^{(0)} s_j(x_j(t)) - \sum_{k=1}^{K} \sum_{j=1}^{n} t_{ij}^{(k)} s_j(x_j(t - \tau_k)) > 0$$

whenever $x_i(t) \geq M$ and

$$b_i(x_i(t)) - \sum_{j=1}^{n} t_{ij}^{(0)} s_j(x_j(t)) - \sum_{k=1}^{K} \sum_{j=1}^{n} t_{ij}^{(k)} s_j(x_j(t - \tau_k)) < 0$$

whenever $x_i(t) \leq -M$ for all $i = 1, \cdots, n$. Since $a_i(x_i(t))$ is positive by Assumption 7.6.1, it can be concluded that, for any solution $x(t)$ of (7.6.2), $\dot{x}_i(t) < 0$ whenever $x_i(t) \geq M$ and $\dot{x}_i(t) > 0$ whenever $x_i(t) \leq -M$ for all $i = 1, \cdots, n$. We may assume that for the initial condition $x_0(\cdot)$ (x_0 is a function), $\|x_0\| < M$, for otherwise we just pick a larger M. Thus we can conclude that $|x_i(t)| < M$ for all $t \geq 0$ and all $i = 1, \cdots, n$. ∎

If we let $x = (x_1, \cdots, x_n)^T \in \Re^n$,

$$A(x) = \text{diag}[a_1(x_1), \cdots, a_n(x_n)] \in \Re^{n \times n},$$

$B(x) = (b_1(x_1), \cdots, b_n(x_n))^T \in \Re^n$, $T = [t_{ij}]$, and

$$S(x) = (s_1(x_1), \cdots, s_n(x_n))^T,$$

then (7.6.1) can be rewritten as

$$\dot{x} = -A(x)[B(x) - TS(x)]. \tag{7.6.3}$$

When delays are present in the Cohen-Grossberg neural networks, we need to modify (7.6.3) as

$$\dot{x}(t) = -A(x(t))\left[B(x(t)) - T_0 S(x(t)) - \sum_{k=1}^{K} T_k S(x(t - \tau_k))\right] \tag{7.6.4}$$

where the T_k make up the interconnections associated with delay τ_k, $k = 0, 1, \cdots, K$, so that $T = T_0 + T_1 + \cdots + T_K$, $0 = \tau_0 < \tau_1 < \cdots <$

τ_K, and $A(x)$, $B(x)$, T, and $S(x)$ are the same as in (7.6.3). Clearly, (7.6.4) is equivalent to (7.6.2).

In order to ensure that the Cohen-Grossberg neural networks (7.6.3) [or equivalently (7.6.1)] possess global stability, we require [similarly as in Chapter 3 for system (L)] that the set of all equilibria of (7.6.3) be a discrete set. To this end, we will require throughout this chapter, the following hypothesis.

Assumption 7.6.2 For any equilibrium x_e of (7.6.3), the matrix $J(x_e)$ is nonsingular, where

$$J(x) = -T + \mathrm{diag}\left[\frac{b'_1(x_1)}{s'_1(x_1)}, \cdots, \frac{b'_n(x_n)}{s'_n(x_n)}\right] \qquad (7.6.5)$$

and $b'_i(x_i) \triangleq db_i(x_i)/dx_i$ for $i = 1, \cdots, n$. ∎

It can be proved, using Sard's Theorem [similarly as for system (L) in Chapter 3] that the following result is true (see also [16]).

Lemma 7.6.1 For almost all $T \in \Re^{n \times n}$ (except a set with Lebesgue measure zero), system (7.6.3) satisfies Assumption 7.6.2. ∎

Furthermore, by using the inverse function theorem (see Remark 3.4 in [16] or Chapter 3), we can establish the following result.

Lemma 7.6.2 When system (7.6.3) satisfies Assumption 7.6.2, the set of equilibria of system (7.6.3) is a discrete set. ∎

7.7 Global Stability of Cohen-Grossberg Neural Networks with Multiple Delays

In the present section, we address the global stability properties of Cohen-Grossberg neural networks with multiple delays described by the retarded type differential-difference equation (7.6.4), or equivalently by (7.6.2). To establish the main result of the present section, we require the following properties of system (7.6.4).

7.7. COHEN-GROSSBERG GLOBAL STABILITY

Lemma 7.7.1 If system (7.6.4) satisfies Assumption 7.6.2, then the set of equilibria of system (7.6.4) is a discrete set. [I.e., if system (7.6.4) satisfies Assumption 7.6.2 (with $T = T_0 + \sum_{k=1}^{K} T_k$), then the set of points x_e such that $B(x_e) - TS(x_e) = 0$ is discrete.] Furthermore, system (7.6.4) satisfies Assumption 7.6.2 for almost all $T \in R^{n \times n}$ (except on a set of Lebesgue measure zero). ∎

Lemma 7.7.1 follows from Lemma 7.6.2 and from Lemma 7.6.1.

We are now in a position to establish the main result of this section.

Theorem 7.7.1 Suppose that for system (7.6.4), Assumptions 7.6.1 and 7.6.2 are satisfied, and suppose that

$$\sum_{k=1}^{K} (\tau_k \beta \|T_k\|) < 1 \tag{7.7.1}$$

where $\beta = \max_{x \in \Re^n} \|A(x)S'(x)\|$ and $S'(x) \triangleq \text{diag}[s'_1(x_1), \cdots, s'_n(x_n)]$. Then system (7.6.4) is *globally stable*.

Proof: Since inequality (7.7.1) is satisfied, there must exist a sequence of positive numbers $(\alpha_1, \cdots, \alpha_K)$, such that

$$\sum_{k=1}^{K} \alpha_k = 1, \quad \tau_k \beta \|T_k\| < \alpha_k \quad \text{for } k = 1, \cdots, K. \tag{7.7.2}$$

To prove the present result, we define for any $x_t \in C([-\tau_K, 0], \Re^n)$ an energy functional $E(x_t)$ associated with (7.6.4) by

$$\begin{aligned} E(x_t) = &-S^T(x_t(0))TS(x_t(0)) \\ &+ 2\sum_{i=1}^{n} \int_{0}^{[x_t(0)]_i} b_i(\sigma) s'_i(\sigma) d\sigma \\ &+ \sum_{k=1}^{K} \frac{1}{\alpha_k} \int_{-\tau_k}^{0} [S(x_t(\theta)) - S(x_t(0))]^T T_k^T f_k(\theta) \\ &\times T_k [S(x_t(\theta)) - S(x_t(0))] d\theta \end{aligned} \tag{7.7.3}$$

where $(\alpha_1, \cdots, \alpha_K)$ is a sequence of positive numbers such that condition (7.7.2) is satisfied and $f_k(\theta) \in C^1([-\tau_k, 0], \Re^n)$, $k = 1, \cdots, K$, will be specified later. After changing integration variables, (7.7.3) can be written as

$$E(x_t) = -S^T(x(t))TS(x(t)) + 2\sum_{i=1}^{n} \int_0^{x_i(t)} b_i(\sigma)s_i'(\sigma)d\sigma$$
$$+ \sum_{k=1}^{K} \frac{1}{\alpha_k} \int_{t-\tau_k}^{t} [S(x(w)) - S(x(t))]^T T_k^T f_k(w-t) \quad (7.7.4)$$
$$\times T_k[S(x(w)) - S(x(t))]dw.$$

The derivative of $E(x_t)$ with respect to t along any solution of (7.6.4) can be computed as

$$\frac{dE(x_t)}{dt} = -2S^T(x(t))TS'(x(t))A(x(t))\bigg[-B(x(t)) + T_0S(x(t))$$
$$+ \sum_{k=1}^{K} T_k S(x(t-\tau_k))\bigg] + 2x(t)^T B(x(t))S'(x(t))A(x(t))$$
$$\times \bigg[-B(x(t)) + T_0 S(x(t)) + \sum_{k=1}^{K} T_k S(x(t-\tau_k))\bigg]$$
$$- \sum_{k=1}^{K} \frac{1}{\alpha_k} \bigg\{ [S(x(t-\tau_k)) - S(x(t))]^T T_k^T f_k(-\tau_k)T_k$$
$$\times [S(x(t-\tau_k)) - S(x(t))] + \int_{t-\tau_k}^{t} [S(x(w)) - S(x(t))]^T$$
$$\times T_k^T f_k'(w-t)T_k[S(x(w)) - S(x(t))]dw$$
$$+ \int_{t-\tau_k}^{t} \bigg[-B(x(t)) + T_0 S(x(t)) + \sum_{k=1}^{K} T_k S(x(t-\tau_k))\bigg]^T$$
$$\times A(x(t))S'(x(t))T_k^T f_k(w-t)T_k[S(x(w)) - S(x(t))]dw$$
$$+ \int_{t-\tau_k}^{t} [S(x(w)) - S(x(t))]^T T_k^T f_k(w-t)T_k S'(x(t))A(x(t))$$
$$\times \bigg[-B(x(t)) + T_0 S(x(t)) + \sum_{k=1}^{K} T_k S(x(t-\tau_k))\bigg] dw \bigg\}$$
(7.7.5)

where $f'(\theta) = df(\theta)/d\theta$. If we adopt the notation

$$H_0 = -B(x(t)) + T_0 S(x(t)) + \sum_{k=1}^{K} T_k S(x(t-\tau_k)), \quad (7.7.6)$$

$$H_k = T_k[S(x(t-\tau_k)) - S(x(t))], \quad k = 1, \cdots, K, \quad (7.7.7)$$

7.7. COHEN-GROSSBERG GLOBAL STABILITY

$$G_k = T_k[S(x(w)) - S(x(t))], \quad k = 1, \cdots, K, \tag{7.7.8}$$

$$Q = A(x(t))S'(x(t)) = S'(x(t))A(x(t)), \tag{7.7.9}$$

(7.7.5) can be rewritten as

$$\begin{aligned}
\frac{dE(x_t)}{dt} &= -2S^T(x(t))TQH_0 + 2x(t)^T B(x(t))QH_0 \\
&\quad - \sum_{k=1}^{K} \frac{1}{\alpha_k} \Big\{ H_k^T f_k(-\tau_k) H_k + \int_{t-\tau_k}^{t} [G_k^T f_k'(w-t) G_k \\
&\quad + H_0^T Q T_k^T f_k(w-t) G_k + G_k^T f_k(w-t) T_k Q H_0] dw \Big\} \\
&= -2H_0^T Q H_0 + 2 \sum_{k=1}^{K} H_k^T Q H_0 - \sum_{k=1}^{K} \frac{1}{\alpha_k} \Big\{ H_k^T f_k(-\tau_k) H_k \\
&\quad + \int_{t-\tau_k}^{t} [G_k^T f_k'(w-t) G_k + H_0^T Q T_k^T f_k(w-t) G_k \\
&\quad + G_k^T f_k(w-t) T_k Q H_0] dw \Big\} \\
&= \sum_{k=1}^{K} \Big[2H_k^T Q H_0 - \frac{1}{\alpha_k} \Big\{ 2H_0^T Q H_0 + H_k^T f_k(-\tau_k) H_k \\
&\quad + \int_{t-\tau_k}^{t} [G_k^T f_k'(w-t) G_k + H_0^T Q T_k^T f_k(w-t) G_k \\
&\quad + G_k^T f_k(w-t) T_k Q H_0] dw \Big\} \Big] \\
&= - \sum_{k=1}^{K} \int_{-\tau_k}^{0} [\eta_k(x_t, \theta)]^T M_k(x_t, \theta) \eta_k(x_t, \theta) d\theta
\end{aligned} \tag{7.7.10}$$

where $[\eta_k(x_t, \theta)]^T = [H_0^T, H_k^T, \tilde{G}_k^T]^T$ with H_0 and H_k given by (7.7.6) and (7.7.7),

$$\tilde{G}_k = T_k[S(x(t+\theta)) - S(x(t))], \quad k = 1, \cdots, K \tag{7.7.11}$$

$$M_k(x_t, \theta) = \begin{bmatrix} 2\alpha_k Q/\tau_k & -Q/\tau_k & QT_k^T f_k(\theta)/\alpha_k \\ -Q/\tau_k & f_k(-\tau_k)E/(\tau_k \alpha_k) & 0 \\ f_k(\theta)T_k Q/\alpha_k & 0 & f_k'(\theta)E/\alpha_k \end{bmatrix} \tag{7.7.12}$$

and E denotes the $n \times n$ identity matrix. To obtain the last expression of (7.7.10), we changed the integration variables from w to θ.

We will now show that if the hypotheses of Theorem 7.7.1 are satisfied, then $M_k(x_t, \theta)$ is positive definite for all $\theta \in [-\tau_k, 0]$ and all x_t which satisfy (7.6.4), for $k = 1, \cdots, K$. In doing so, we let $U = U_3 U_2 U_1$, where

$$U_1 = \begin{bmatrix} E/\sqrt{\alpha_k} & 0 & 0 \\ E/(2\sqrt{\alpha_k}) & \sqrt{\alpha_k}E & 0 \\ 0 & 0 & \sqrt{\alpha_k}E \end{bmatrix}$$

$$U_2 = \begin{bmatrix} E & 0 & 0 \\ 0 & E & 0 \\ -\tau_k f_k(\theta) T_k/(2\alpha_k) & 0 & E \end{bmatrix}$$

and

$$U_3 = \begin{bmatrix} E & 0 & 0 \\ 0 & E & 0 \\ 0 & f_k(\theta) T_k Q U_4/\alpha_k & E \end{bmatrix}$$

where

$$U_4 = -\frac{1}{2} \left[\frac{f_k(-\tau_k)}{\tau_k} E - \frac{Q}{2\tau_k} \right]^{-1}.$$

It is not difficult to verify that $\tilde{M}_k = U M_k(x_t, \theta) U^T$ is a diagonal matrix. In fact,

$$\tilde{M}_k = \text{diag}[M_{k,1}, M_{k,2}, M_{k,3}] \tag{7.7.13}$$

where

$$M_{k,1} = \frac{2Q}{\tau_k} \tag{7.7.14}$$

$$M_{k,2} = \frac{f_k(-\tau_k)}{\tau_k} E - \frac{Q}{2\tau_k} \tag{7.7.15}$$

and

$$M_{k,3} = f'_k(\theta)E - \frac{f_k(\theta)T_k Q}{2\alpha_k} \left[\left(\frac{f_k(-\tau_k)}{\tau_k} E - \frac{Q}{2\tau_k} \right)^{-1} + 2\tau_k Q^{-1} \right] \frac{Q T_k^T f_k(\theta)}{2\alpha_k}. \tag{7.7.16}$$

It follows that $M_k(x_t, \theta)$ is positive definite if and only if $\tilde{M}_k$ is positive definite and if and only if $M_{k,1}$, $M_{k,2}$, and $M_{k,3}$ are all positive definite.

7.7. COHEN-GROSSBERG GLOBAL STABILITY

We now show that if the condition $\tau_k \beta \|T_k\| < \alpha_k$ is satisfied, where
$$\beta = \max_{x \in \Re} \|A(x)S'(x)\| = \max_{x \in \Re} \|Q\|$$
then we can always find a suitable $f_k(\theta) \in C([-\tau_k, 0], \Re^+)$ such that $M_{k,1}$, $M_{k,2}$, and $M_{k,3}$ are positive definite for all x_t which satisfy (7.6.4) and for all $\theta \in [-\tau_k, 0]$. From this it follows that $M_k(x_t, \theta)$ is positive definite for all $k = 1, \cdots, K$ and therefore $dE(x_t)/dt \leq 0$ along any solution x_t of (7.6.4).

By the assumptions that $s_i'(x_i) > 0$ and $a_i(x_i) > 0$ for all $x_i \in \Re$, the matrix $M_{k,1}$ is automatically positive definite. The matrix $M_{k,2}$ will always be positive definite if condition
$$2f_k(-\tau_k) - \beta > 0 \tag{7.7.17}$$
is satisfied. For $M_{k,3}$, it is easily shown that if

$$\begin{aligned} f_k'(\theta) > {} & \tfrac{1}{4} f_k^2(\theta) \frac{\|T_k\|^2}{\alpha_k^2} \\ & \times \left\| Q \left[\left(\frac{f_k(-\tau_k)}{\tau_k} E - \frac{Q}{2\tau_k} \right)^{-1} + 2\tau_k Q^{-1} \right] Q \right\| \end{aligned} \tag{7.7.18}$$

is true, then $M_{k,3}$ is also positive definite. Notice that the matrix

$$D \triangleq Q \left[\left(\frac{f_k(-\tau_k)}{\tau_k} E - \frac{Q}{2\tau_k} \right)^{-1} + 2\tau_k Q^{-1} \right] Q$$

is a diagonal matrix, i.e., $D = \text{diag}[d_1, \cdots, d_n]$. If we denote $Q = \text{diag}[q_1, \cdots, q_n]$, then it is easy to show that

$$d_i = \frac{4 f_k(-\tau_k) q_i \tau_k}{2 f_k(-\tau_k) - q_i} \quad \text{for } i = 1, \cdots, n.$$

Since $q_i < \beta$ by the definitions of β and Q, we have, in view of (7.7.17), that
$$d_i \leq \frac{4 f_k(-\tau_k) \beta \tau_k}{2 f_k(-\tau_k) - \beta}.$$

Therefore, we obtain
$$\|D\| \leq \frac{4 f_k(-\tau_k) \beta \tau_k}{2 f_k(-\tau_k) - \beta}$$

and, furthermore, condition (7.7.18) will be satisfied if (7.7.17) is satisfied and

$$f'_k(\theta) > \frac{1}{4}f_k^2(\theta)\frac{\|T_k\|^2}{\alpha_k^2}\frac{4f_k(-\tau_k)\beta\tau_k}{2f_k(-\tau_k) - \beta} \qquad (7.7.19)$$

is satisfied.

Next, we need to show that there is an $f_k \in C^1([-\tau_k, 0], \Re)$ such that conditions (7.7.17) and (7.7.19) are satisfied. We choose

$$f_k(-\tau_k) = \left[\beta\tau_k^2\frac{\|T_k\|^2}{\alpha_k^2}\right]^{-1}. \qquad (7.7.20)$$

Condition (7.7.17) is satisfied by the choice (7.7.20). Furthermore,

$$\left[f_k(-\tau_k)\frac{\|T_k\|}{\alpha_k} - \frac{\alpha_k}{\beta\tau_k\|T_k\|}\right]^2 + 1 - \frac{\alpha_k^2}{\beta^2\tau_k^2\|T_k\|^2}$$
$$= 1 - \frac{\alpha_k^2}{\beta^2\tau_k^2\|T_k\|^2} < 0 \qquad (7.7.21)$$

is true because $\beta\tau_k\|T_k\| < a_k$. It follows from (7.7.21) that

$$\delta f_k(-\tau_k)\tau_k < 1 \qquad (7.7.22)$$

where

$$\delta = \frac{\|T_k\|^2 f_k(-\tau_k)\beta\tau_k}{\alpha_k^2[2f_k(-\tau_k) - \beta]}. \qquad (7.7.23)$$

Since $\delta f_k(-\tau_k)\tau_k < 1$, we can always find an l such that $0 < l < 1$, and $\delta f_k(-\tau_k)\tau_k < l$. Therefore, we will always have $\gamma > 0$ where γ is given by

$$\gamma = \frac{l}{\delta f_k(-\tau_k)} - \tau_k. \qquad (7.7.24)$$

We now choose $f_k(\theta)$ on $[-\tau_k, 0]$ as

$$f_k(\theta) = \frac{l}{\delta(\gamma - \theta)}. \qquad (7.7.25)$$

It is easily verified that this choice is consistent with (7.7.20). Clearly, $f_k \in C^1([-\tau_k, 0], \Re^+)$ since $\gamma > 0$. The derivative of $f_k(\theta)$ is given by

$$f'_k(\theta) = \frac{l}{\delta(\gamma - \theta)^2} = \frac{\delta}{l}f_k^2(\theta) > \delta f_k^2(\theta) \qquad (7.7.26)$$

7.7. COHEN-GROSSBERG GLOBAL STABILITY

since $l < 1$. Combining (7.7.23) and (7.7.26), we can verify that $f_k(\theta)$ satisfies condition (7.7.19).

Therefore, we have shown that if $\beta \tau_k \|T_k\| < \alpha_k$, then there exists an $f_k(\theta)$ [given by (7.7.25), where $f_k(-\tau_k)$, δ, and γ are given by (7.7.20), (7.7.23), and (7.7.24), respectively] such that conditions (7.7.17) and (7.7.19) are satisfied. Thus $M_k(x_t, \theta)$ is positive definite for all x_t satisfying Eq. (7.6.4) and all $\theta \in [-\tau_k, 0]$ for $k = 1, \cdots, K$. We have shown that

$$\frac{dE(x_t)}{dt} \leq 0 \quad (7.7.27)$$

along any solution x_t of (7.6.4), where $E(x_t)$ is the energy functional given by (7.7.3).

We know from (7.7.10) that if $dE(x_t)/dt = 0$, then $H_0 = 0$, $H_k = 0$, and $\tilde{G}_k = 0$ for $k = 1, \cdots, K$, where H_0, H_k, and $\tilde{G}_k$ are given by (7.7.6), (7.7.7), and (7.7.11), respectively. For any $\varphi \in C([-\tau_K, 0], \Re^n)$, we denote $\dot{E}_\varphi = 0$ if

$$-B(\varphi(0)) + T_0 S(\varphi(0)) + \sum_{k=1}^{K} T_k S(\varphi(-\tau_k)) = 0 \quad (7.7.28)$$

$$T_k[S(\varphi(-\tau_k)) - S(\varphi(0))] = 0, \quad k = 1, \cdots, K \quad (7.7.29)$$

$$\begin{aligned} T_k[S(\varphi(-\theta)) - S(\varphi(0))] &= 0 \\ \text{for all } \theta \in [-\tau_K, 0], \quad k &= 1, \cdots, K. \end{aligned} \quad (7.7.30)$$

It is obvious that for any solution x_t of (7.6.4), $dE(x_t)/dt = 0$ if and only if $\dot{E}_{x_t} = 0$.

Since for any x_t satisfying (7.6.4), x_t is bounded (Fact 7.6.1) and since $dE(x_t)/dt \leq 0$, it follows from the invariance theory (see Section 7.2B; or see Chapter 4, Lemmas 1.4 and 2.1 in [10]) that the limit set of x_t as $t \to \infty$ is the invariant subset of the set $\Lambda = \{\varphi \in C([-\tau_K, 0], \Re^n): \dot{E}_\varphi = 0\}$. Therefore, we have $|x_t - \varphi| \to 0$ as $t \to \infty$ for some $\varphi \in \Lambda$. In particular, we have $x_t(0) \to \varphi(0)$ and $x_t(-\tau_k) \to \varphi(-\tau_k)$ as $t \to \infty$, $k = 1, \cdots, K$. Combining this with (7.7.28) and (7.7.29), we conclude that

$$-B(x_t(0)) + T_0 S(x_t(0)) + \sum_{k=1}^{K} T_k S(x_t(-\tau_k)) \to 0$$

and
$$T_k[S(x_t(\varphi(-\tau_k))) - S(x_t(0))] \to 0, \quad k = 1, \cdots, K$$
as $t \to \infty$. It follows that
$$-B(x_t(0)) + TS(x_t(0)) \to 0,$$
or
$$-B(x(t)) + TS(x(t)) \to 0,$$
as t approaches ∞. Now since x_t is bounded (Fact 7.6.1), we conclude that any point in the limit set of $x(t)$ as $t \to \infty$ is an equilibrium of system (7.6.4) [or, equivalently, an equilibrium of system (7.6.3)]. Furthermore, since the set of equilibria of system (7.6.4) is a discrete set (Lemma 7.7.1), it follows that $x(t)$ approaches some equilibrium of system (7.6.4) as t tends to ∞. ∎

Consider a special case of (7.6.4), a Hopfield neural network with identical delay τ, described by the equation
$$\dot{x}(t) = -Cx(t) + T_0 S(x(t)) + T_1 S(x(t - \tau)) \tag{7.7.31}$$
where $C = \text{diag}[c_1, \cdots, c_n]$ with $c_i > 0$ for $i = 1, \cdots, n$, and T_0, T_1, and $S(x)$ are the same as in (7.6.4). Applying Theorem 7.7.1, we obtain that system (7.7.31) is globally stable if
$$\tau \beta \|T_1\| < 1 \tag{7.7.32}$$
where β is defined in the same way as in Theorem 7.7.1, noticing, however, that $A(x)$ equals the identity matrix in this case. We see that the bound condition (7.7.32) for the global stability of system (7.7.31) is identical to the result given in Theorem 7.3.1.

7.8 Local Stability Results for Cohen-Grossberg Neural Networks with Multiple Delays

In the preceding section, we showed that if
$$\sum_{k=1}^{K} \tau_k \beta \|T_k\| < 1 \tag{7.8.1}$$

7.8. COHEN-GROSSBERG LOCAL STABILITY

the Cohen-Grossberg neural networks with multiple delays described by

$$\dot{x}(t) = -A(x(t))\Big[B(x(t)) - T_0 S(x(t)) - \sum_{k=1}^{K} T_k S(x(t - \tau_k))\Big] \quad (7.8.2)$$

or equivalently, by

$$\dot{x}_i(t) = -a_i(x_i(t))\Big[b_i(x_i(t)) - \sum_{j=1}^{n} t_{ij}^{(0)} s_j(x_j(t)) - \sum_{k=1}^{K} \sum_{j=1}^{n} t_{ij}^{(k)} s_j(x_j(t - \tau_k))\Big], \quad i = 1, \cdots, n \quad (7.8.3)$$

possess global stability. For similar reasons as in the case of Hopfield neural networks, good criteria which ensure the asymptotic stability of an equilibrium of (7.8.2) are of great interest. We address this issue in the present section.

At the present time, there are no known general results which provide necessary and sufficient conditions for the asymptotic stability of an equilibrium for Cohen-Grossberg neural networks with multiple delays (7.8.2). As pointed out in Section 7.4, even for special cases of (7.8.2), such as Hopfield neural networks with one delay [described by (7.3.1)], there are only results which provide sufficient conditions for the asymptotic stability of an equilibrium. Some of these results are obtained by linearizing (7.8.2) about an equilibrium of interest, while other results, which make use of sector conditions for nonlinearities, have been obtained by Lyapunov's Second Method. In the present section, we will show that if the conditions of Theorem 7.7.1 are satisfied, then the asymptotic stability of an equilibrium of (7.8.2) can be deduced from the asymptotic stability of the same corresponding equilibrium of system

$$\dot{x} = -A(x)[B(x) - TS(x)]. \quad (7.8.4)$$

In other words, if (7.8.1) is true, then (similarly as shown in the preceding section), Cohen-Grossberg neural networks (7.8.4) and Cohen-Grossberg neural networks with multiple delays (7.8.2) are both globally stable, and furthermore, as will be shown in the present section, both have similar local stability properties at an asymptotically stable equilibrium. This enables us to verify the asymptotic stability of the equilibria of system (7.8.2) by ascertaining the asymptotic stability of corresponding equilibria of system (7.8.4).

Similarly as in the case of Hopfield neural networks with delays, we will require the following concept.

Definition 7.8.1 An element $\varphi \in C([-\tau, 0], \Re^n)$ is called a *local minimum* of the energy functional E defined by (7.7.3) if there exists a $\delta > 0$ such that for any $\tilde{\varphi} \in C([-\tau, 0], \Re^n)$, $E(\varphi) \leq E(\tilde{\varphi})$ whenever $\|\varphi - \tilde{\varphi}\| < \delta$. ∎

We are now able to establish the following results.

Theorem 7.8.1 Suppose that the conditions of Theorem 7.7.1 are satisfied. If x_e is an equilibrium of (7.8.2) (defined in Lemma 7.7.1), then the following statements are equivalent:

1) x_e is a stable equilibrium of (7.8.2);

2) x_e is an asymptotically stable equilibrium of (7.8.2);

3) φ_{x_e} is a local minimum of the energy functional E given by (7.7.3), where $\varphi_{x_e} \in C([-\tau, 0], \Re^n)$ such that $\varphi_{x_e} \equiv x_e$; and

4) $J(x_e)$ is positive definite, where $J(x)$ is given in (7.6.5) in Assumption 7.6.2.

Proof: (a) 1) $\Longrightarrow$ 2). Since Assumption 7.6.2 is satisfied, the set of equilibria of system (7.8.2) is a discrete set by Lemma 7.7.1. Therefore, when $\varepsilon > 0$ is sufficiently small, there is no other equilibrium in $U(x_e, \varepsilon)$, a neighborhood of x_e, given by

$$U(x_e, \varepsilon) \triangleq \{x \in \Re^n : |x - x_e| < \varepsilon\}. \tag{7.8.5}$$

Since x_e is a stable equilibrium of (7.8.2), there exists an $\eta > 0$ such that for any $\varphi \in C([-\tau, 0], \Re^n)$ satisfying $\|\varphi - x_e\| < \eta$, $\|x_t - x_e\| < \varepsilon$ for all $t > 0$, where x_t is the solution of (7.8.2) with initial condition φ. Thus $x_t \in C([-\tau, 0], U(x_e, \varepsilon))$ for all t. In view of Theorem 7.7.1

7.8. COHEN-GROSSBERG LOCAL STABILITY

x_t will converge to some equilibrium of system (7.8.2). Since x_e is the only equilibrium of (7.8.2) in $U(x_e, \varepsilon)$, it follows that x_t converges to x_e. Thus we have shown that x_e is an attractive equilibrium of system (7.8.2). Therefore the stable equilibrium x_e of (7.8.2) is an asymptotically stable equilibrium of system (7.8.2).

(b) 2) $\Longrightarrow$ 3). Since x_e is an asymptotically stable equilibrium of system (7.8.2), there exists an $\eta > 0$ such that for any $\varphi \in C([-\tau, 0], \Re^n)$ satisfying $\|\varphi - x_e\| < \eta$, x_t converges to x_e, where x_t is the solution of (7.8.2) with initial condition φ. Therefore $E(\varphi_{x_e}) \leq E(x_t) \leq E(\varphi)$ for any $\varphi \in C([-\tau, 0], \Re^n)$ satisfying $\|\varphi - x_e\| < \eta$. Therefore, φ_{x_e} is a local minimum of the energy functional E.

(c) 3) $\Longrightarrow$ 4). Let $\tilde{E}$ be a function from $\Re^n$ to $\Re$ defined by

$$\tilde{E}(x) \stackrel{\triangle}{=} -S(x)^T T S(x) + 2 \sum_{i=1}^{n} \int_0^{x_i} b_i(\sigma) s_i'(\sigma) d\sigma. \quad (7.8.6)$$

Comparing E with $\tilde{E}$, we note that $\tilde{E}$ is a function defined on $\Re^n$, while E is a functional defined on $C([-\tau, 0], \Re^n)$. Since φ_{x_e} is a local minimum of E, x_e must be a local minimum of $\tilde{E}$. Otherwise there would exist a sequence $\{x_n\} \subset \Re^n$ such that $x_n \to x_e$ as $n \to \infty$ and $\tilde{E}(x_n) < \tilde{E}(x_e)$. Let φ_{x_n} denote the constant function $\varphi_{x_n} \equiv x_n$ in $C([-\tau, 0], \Re^n)$. Then $|\varphi_{x_n} - \varphi_{x_e}| \to 0$ as $n \to \infty$ and

$$E(\varphi_{x_n}) = \tilde{E}(x_n) < \tilde{E}(x_e) = E(\varphi_{x_e}).$$

This contradicts the fact the φ_{x_e} is a local minimum of E. Therefore, x_e is a local minimum of $\tilde{E}$. Hence $\tilde{J}(x_e)$ is positive semidefinite (see, e.g., Theorem 3.6 in [9]), where $\tilde{J}(x)$ is the Hessian matrix of $\tilde{E}$ given by

$$\tilde{J}(x) = \left[\frac{\partial^2 \tilde{E}}{\partial x_i \partial x_j} \right]. \quad (7.8.7)$$

It can be shown that

$$\tilde{J}(x) = 2S'(x) J(x) S'(x) \quad (7.8.8)$$

where $S'(x) = \text{diag}[s_1'(x_1), \cdots, s_n'(x_n)]$ and $J(x)$ is given by (7.6.5) in Assumption 7.6.2. Therefore, $J(x_e)$ is also positive semidefinite.

By Assumption 7.6.2, $J(x_e)$ is a nonsingular matrix. Thus we have shown that $J(x_e)$ is positive definite.

(d) 4) $\Longrightarrow$ 1). We need to prove that x_e is a stable equilibrium of system (7.8.2), i.e., for any $\varepsilon > 0$, there exists a $\delta > 0$ such that for any $\varphi \in C([-\tau, 0], \Re^n)$, if $\|\varphi - x_e\| < \delta$, then $\|x_t - x_e\| < \varepsilon$, where x_t is the solution of (7.8.2) with initial condition φ.

Since $J(x_e)$ is positive definite, then $\tilde{J}(x_e)$ must also be positive definite where $\tilde{J}(x)$ is the Hessian matrix of $\tilde{E}$ given by (7.8.8). Furthermore,

$$\nabla_x \tilde{E}(x) = 2[-TS(x) + B(x)]^T S'(x)$$

where $S'(x)$ is given in Part (c). Therefore, $\nabla_x \tilde{E}(x_e) = 0$ since x_e is an equilibrium of (7.8.2). It follows (by Theorem 3.6 in [9]) that x_e is a local minimum of $\tilde{E}$, i.e., there exists a $\delta_1 > 0$, $\delta_1 < \varepsilon$, such that whenever $0 < |x - x_e| \leq \delta_1$, $\tilde{E}(x_e) < \tilde{E}(x)$. Let $r = \min\{\tilde{E}(x): |x - x_e| = \delta_1\}$. Then it is true that $r > \tilde{E}(x_e)$. Since $E(\varphi_{x_e}) = \tilde{E}(x_e)$, it follows that $r > E(\varphi_{x_e})$. Note that E is a continuous functional. Therefore, there exists a $\delta \in (0, \delta_1)$ such that whenever $\|\varphi - x_e\| < \delta$, where $\varphi \in C([-\tau, 0], \Re^n)$, we have $E(\varphi) < r$. Suppose x_t is any solution of (7.8.2) with the initial condition φ such that $\|\varphi - x_e\| < \delta$. We will show that $\|x_t - x_e\| < \delta_1 < \varepsilon$. Otherwise there would exist a $t_0 > 0$ such that $|x_{t_0}(0) - x_e| = \delta_1$, i.e., $|x(t_0) - x_e| = \delta_1$. By the definition of E and $\tilde{E}$, we have $E(x_{t_0}) \geq \tilde{E}(x(t_0)) \geq r$. Therefore, we obtain $E(x_{t_0}) > E(\varphi)$, which contradicts the fact that E is monotonically decreasing along any solution of (7.8.2). Thus we have shown that x_e is an asymptotically stable equilibrium of system (7.8.2). ∎

We note that statement 4) in Theorem 7.8.1 is independent of the delays τ_k, $k = 1, \cdots, K$. Therefore, if system (7.8.2) satisfies Assumptions 7.6.1 and 7.6.2 and if the condition $\sum_{k=1}^{K} \tau_k \beta \|T_k\| < 1$ is satisfied, then the locations of the (asymptotically) stable equilibria of system (7.8.2) will not depend on the delays τ_k for $k = 1, \cdots, K$. This is true if, in particular, $\tau_k = 0$, $k = 1, \cdots, K$. Therefore, if

7.9. ARBITRARY BOUNDED DELAYS

$\sum_{k=1}^{K} \tau_k \beta \|T_k\| < 1$, then systems (7.8.2) and (7.8.4) [obtained by letting $\tau_k = 0$ for $k = 1, \cdots, K$ in (7.8.2)] will have identical (asymptotically) stable equilibria. We state this in the form of a corollary.

Corollary 7.8.1 Under the conditions of Theorem 7.7.1, x_e is an (asymptotically) stable equilibrium of system (7.8.2) if and only if x_e is an (asymptotically) stable equilibrium of system (7.8.4). This is true if and only if $J(x_e)$ is positive definite, where $J(x)$ is given in (7.6.5) (in Assumption 7.6.2). ∎

Corollary 7.8.1 provides an effective criterion for testing the (asymptotic) stability of any equilibrium of Cohen-Grossberg neural networks with multiple delays described by (7.8.2). This criterion constitutes necessary and sufficient conditions, as long as

$$\sum_{k=1}^{K} \tau_k \beta \|T_k\| < 1.$$

7.9 Nonlinear Systems with Arbitrary Bounded Delays

In the remainder of this chapter, our goal will be to establish local stability results for time-delay neural networks described by equations of the form

$$\dot{x}(t) = -Cx(t) + TS(x(t - \tau)) + I$$

having interconnecting structure (specified by T) which is not necessarily symmetric. In the process of accomplishing this, we establish some preliminary stability results in a much broader context, which are important in their own right. In doing so, we return to system (7.1.8), given by

$$\dot{x}(t) = f(x(t), t) + g(x(t - \tau), t - \tau) \qquad (7.9.1)$$

where $x \in \Omega \subset \Re^n$, and $f, g \in C^1(\Omega \times \Re^+, \Re^n)$. We will assume that $x = 0$ is an equilibrium of (7.9.1). Accordingly, we assume that

$$f(0, t) = 0 \tag{7.9.2}$$

$$g(0, t) = 0 \tag{7.9.3}$$

for all $t \in \Re^+$. Under the assumptions given in (7.9.2) and (7.9.3), (7.9.1) can equivalently be expressed as

$$\dot{x}(t) = A(x(t), t)x(t) + B(x(t-\tau), t-\tau)x(t-\tau) \tag{7.9.4}$$

where $A(x, t) = [a_{ij}(x, t)]$, $B(x, t) = [b_{ij}(x, t)]$, and $a_{ij}(x, t), b_{ij}(x, t) \in C(\Omega \times \Re^+, \Re)$ for $1 \leq i, j \leq n$. The choices for $A(x, t)$ and $B(x, t)$ are not unique. One of these choices is given by

$$A(x, t) = \left[\left(\int_0^1 \nabla_x f_1(sx, t) ds\right)^T, \cdots, \left(\int_0^1 \nabla_x f_n(sx, t) ds\right)^T\right]^T$$

and

$$B(x, t) = \left[\left(\int_0^1 \nabla_x g_1(sx, t) ds\right)^T, \cdots, \left(\int_0^1 \nabla_x g_n(sx, t) ds\right)^T\right]^T$$

where

$$f(x, t) = (f_1(x, t), \cdots, f_n(x, t))^T, \quad g(x, t) = (g_1(x, t), \cdots, g_n(x, t))^T,$$

$$\nabla_x f_i(x, t) = \left[\frac{\partial}{\partial x_1} f_i(x, t), \cdots, \frac{\partial}{\partial x_n} f_i(x, t)\right]^T,$$

and $\nabla_x g_i(x, t)$ is similarly defined, $i = 1, \cdots, n$. Then $f(x, t) = A(x, t)x$ and $g(x, t) = B(x, t)x$. This follows from the fact that for any $h(x, t) \in C^1(\Omega \times \Re^+, \Re)$, we always have

$$h(x, t) - h(y, t) = \left(\int_0^1 \nabla_x h(sx + (1-s)y, t) ds\right)^T (x - y)$$

for any $x, y \in \Omega$.

We assume in (7.9.4) that $\tau = \tau(t) \in C(\Re^+, \Re^+)$, i.e., τ is a continuous and time-varying time-delay, and that τ is bounded. In

7.9. ARBITRARY BOUNDED DELAYS

view of the preceding assumptions, $A(x,t)$ and $B(x,t)$ are continuous functions from $\Omega \times \Re^+$ to $\Re^{n \times n}$. We will henceforth assume that $A(x,t) = [a_{ij}(x,t)]$ and $B(x,t) = [b_{ij}(x,t)]$ satisfy the conditions

$$a_{ij}^m \leq a_{ij}(x,t) \leq a_{ij}^M \tag{7.9.5}$$

$$b_{ij}^m \leq b_{ij}(x,t) \leq b_{ij}^M \tag{7.9.6}$$

for all $1 \leq i,j \leq n$ and $(x,t) \in \Omega \times \Re^+$.

In the present and in the next section, we will establish some sufficient conditions for the asymptotic stability of the equilibrium $x = 0$ of (7.9.4). In this section, we will concentrate on the case when the bound of the delay is arbitrary (i.e., there are no restrictions for the bound of the delay). The asymptotic stability condition which we will establish in this section is a so-called *delay independent condition*, i.e., the condition is applicable for any bounded delay, no matter how large the bound is. In the next section, we consider the case when the bound of the delay is fixed and we obtain some *delay dependent results*.

To arrive at the main results of this section, we require some additional notation. Let J_1, J_2 denote two subsets of $\{1, 2, \cdots, n\}$ (J_1 and J_2 are not necessarily distinct). We define $A_{J_1 J_2} = [a_{kl}^{J_1 J_2}]$ by

$$a_{kl}^{J_1 J_2} = \begin{cases} a_{kl}^M & \text{if } k \in J_1 \text{ and } l \in J_2, \text{ or if } k \notin J_1 \text{ and } l \notin J_2 \\ a_{kl}^m & \text{if } k \in J_1 \text{ and } l \notin J_2, \text{ or if } k \notin J_1 \text{ and } l \in J_2 \end{cases} \tag{7.9.7}$$

where the a_{kl}^m, a_{kl}^M are given in (7.9.5). Let J_3 be a third subset of $\{1, 2, \cdots, n\}$. We define $B_{J_1 J_3} = [b_{kl}^{J_1 J_3}]$ by

$$b_{kl}^{J_1 J_3} = \begin{cases} b_{kl}^M & \text{if } k \in J_1 \text{ and } l \in J_3, \text{ or if } k \notin J_1 \text{ and } l \notin J_3 \\ b_{kl}^m & \text{if } k \in J_1 \text{ and } l \notin J_3, \text{ or if } k \notin J_1 \text{ and } l \in J_3 \end{cases} \tag{7.9.8}$$

where the b_{kl}^m, b_{kl}^M are given in (7.9.6).

With this notation, we are now able to present our first result.

Theorem 7.9.1 The equilibrium $x = 0$ of the system described by (7.9.4)–(7.9.6) is asymptotically stable if there exists a positive definite matrix P, and a matrix $\Lambda = \text{diag}[\lambda_1, \cdots, \lambda_n]$, $\lambda_i > 0$, $i =$

$1, \cdots, n$, such that for all triples of independent subsets J_1, J_2, J_3 of the set $\{1, 2, \cdots, n\}$, the matrix $S(J_1, J_2, J_3)$ is negative definite, where

$$S(J_1, J_2, J_3) = (A_{J_1 J_2})^T P + P(A_{J_1 J_2}) + \Lambda \\ + P(B_{J_1 J_3})\Lambda^{-1}(B_{J_1 J_3})^T P \tag{7.9.9}$$

and $A_{J_1 J_2}$, $B_{J_1 J_3}$ are defined by (7.9.7) and (7.9.8), respectively.

Proof: We use the Lyapunov functional

$$v(x_t) = x(t)^T P x(t) + \int_{-\tau}^{0} x_t(\theta)^T \Lambda x_t(\theta) d\theta.$$

Then,

$$\lambda_{\min}(P)|x_t(0)|^2 \leq v(x_t) \leq (\lambda_{\max}(P) + \tau \lambda_{\max}(\Lambda))\|x_t\|^2. \tag{7.9.10}$$

The time derivative of v along solutions of (7.9.4) is given by

$$\begin{aligned} D_{(7.9.4)} v(x_t) &= \dot{x}(t)^T P x(t) + x(t)^T P \dot{x}(t) + x(t)^T \Lambda x(t) \\ &\quad - x(t-\tau)^T \Lambda x(t-\tau) \\ &= x(t)^T \{A(x(t),t)^T P + PA(x(t),t) + \Lambda \\ &\quad + PB(x(t-\tau), t-\tau)\Lambda^{-1} B(x(t-\tau), t-\tau)^T P\} x(t) \\ &\quad - [\Lambda^{\frac{1}{2}} x(t-\tau) - \Lambda^{-\frac{1}{2}} B(x(t-\tau), t-\tau)^T P x(t)]^T \\ &\quad \times [\Lambda^{\frac{1}{2}} x(t-\tau) - \Lambda^{-\frac{1}{2}} B(x(t-\tau), t-\tau)^T P x(t)] \\ &\leq x(t)^T [A(x(t),t)^T P + PA(x(t),t) + \Lambda \\ &\quad + PB(x(t-\tau), t-\tau)\Lambda^{-1} B(x(t-\tau), t-\tau)^T P] x(t) \\ &= 2 x(t)^T PA(x(t), t) x(t) + x(t)^T \Lambda x(t) \\ &\quad + x(t)^T PB(x(t-\tau), t-\tau)\Lambda^{-1} \\ &\quad \times B(x(t-\tau), t-\tau)^T P x(t). \end{aligned} \tag{7.9.11}$$

Let $y(t) = Px(t)$. In the following, we suppress the explicit dependence on t, when convenient. Let $J_1 = \{k \in \{1, \cdots, n\} : y_k \geq 0\}$, and $J_2 = \{k \in \{1, \cdots, n\} : x_k \geq 0\}$. Define $\tilde{J}_1 = \{1, \cdots, n\} - J_1$, and

7.9. ARBITRARY BOUNDED DELAYS

$\tilde{J}_2 = \{1, \cdots, n\} - J_2$. Then

$$\begin{aligned}
2x^T PA(x,t)x &= 2y^T A(x,t)x \\
&= 2(y_1, \cdots, y_n) A(x,t)(x_1, \cdots, x_n)^T \\
&= 2 \sum_{k,l} y_k a_{kl}(x,t) x_l \\
&= 2 \sum_{k,l \in (J_1 \times J_2) \cup (\tilde{J}_1 \times \tilde{J}_2)} y_k a_{kl}(x,t) x_l \\
&\quad + 2 \sum_{k,l \in (J_1 \times \tilde{J}_2) \cup (\tilde{J}_1 \times J_2)} y_k a_{kl}(x,t) x_l \\
&\leq 2 \sum_{k,l \in (J_1 \times J_2) \cup (\tilde{J}_1 \times \tilde{J}_2)} y_k a_{kl}^M x_l \\
&\quad + 2 \sum_{k,l \in (J_1 \times \tilde{J}_2) \cup (\tilde{J}_1 \times J_2)} y_k a_{kl}^m x_l \\
&= 2 y^T A_{J_1 J_2} x \\
&= 2 x^T P A_{J_1 J_2} x \\
&= x^T \left[(A_{J_1 J_2})^T P + P(A_{J_1 J_2}) \right] x.
\end{aligned} \tag{7.9.12}$$

If we let $w = B(x(t-\tau), t-\tau)^T Px(t) = B(x(t-\tau), t-\tau)^T y$ (suppressing in w the dependence on t and τ), then the third term of (7.9.11) assumes the form

$$x(t)^T PB(x(t-\tau), t-\tau) \Lambda^{-1} B(x(t-\tau), t-\tau)^T Px(t) = w^T \Lambda^{-1} w.$$

We now obtain for $1 \leq l \leq n$,

$$w_l = \sum_{1 \leq k \leq n} y_k b_{kl}(x(t-\tau), t-\tau)$$

$$= \sum_{k \in J_1} y_k b_{kl}(x(t-\tau), t-\tau) + \sum_{k \notin J_1} y_k b_{kl}(x(t-\tau), t-\tau).$$

Hence,

$$\sum_{k \in J_1} y_k b_{kl}^m + \sum_{k \notin J_1} y_k b_{kl}^M \leq w_l \leq \sum_{k \in J_1} y_k b_{kl}^M + \sum_{k \notin J_1} y_k b_{kl}^m$$

and

$$w_l^2 \leq \max \left\{ \left(\sum_{k \in J_1} y_k b_{kl}^m + \sum_{k \notin J_1} y_k b_{kl}^M \right)^2, \left(\sum_{k \in J_1} y_k b_{kl}^M + \sum_{k \notin J_1} y_k b_{kl}^m \right)^2 \right\}.$$

Let

$$J_3 = \left\{ l \in \{1, \cdots, n\} : \left(\sum_{k \in J_1} y_k b_{kl}^m + \sum_{k \notin J_1} y_k b_{kl}^M \right)^2 \leq \left(\sum_{k \in J_1} y_k b_{kl}^M + \sum_{k \notin J_1} y_k b_{kl}^m \right)^2 \right\}.$$

Then,

$$\begin{aligned}
w^T \Lambda^{-1} w &= \sum_{1 \leq l \leq n} \lambda_l^{-1} w_l^2 \\
&\leq \sum_{l \in J_3} \lambda_l^{-1} \left(\sum_{k \in J_1} y_k b_{kl}^M + \sum_{k \notin J_1} y_k b_{kl}^m \right)^2 \\
&\quad + \sum_{l \notin J_3} \lambda_l^{-1} \left(\sum_{k \in J_1} y_k b_{kl}^m + \sum_{k \notin J_1} y_k b_{kl}^M \right)^2 \qquad (7.9.13) \\
&= (y_1, \cdots, y_n)(B_{J_1 J_3})^T \Lambda^{-1} B_{J_1 J_3} (y_1, \cdots, y_n)^T \\
&= x^T P (B_{J_1 J_3})^T \Lambda^{-1} B_{J_1 J_3} P x
\end{aligned}$$

where $B_{J_1 J_3}$ is defined in (7.9.8). Therefore, from (7.9.11), (7.9.12), and (7.9.13), we obtain

$$\begin{aligned}
D_{(7.9.4)} v(x_t) &\leq x^T \Lambda x + x^T \left[(A_{J_1 J_2})^T P + P A_{J_1 J_2} \right] x \\
&\quad + x^T P (B_{J_1 J_3})^T \Lambda^{-1} B_{J_1 J_3} P x \\
&= x^T \Big[\Lambda + (A_{J_1 J_2})^T P + P A_{J_1 J_2} \\
&\quad + P (B_{J_1 J_3})^T \Lambda^{-1} B_{J_1 J_3} P \Big] x \qquad (7.9.14) \\
&= x^T S(J_1, J_2, J_3) x \\
&\leq \max \Big\{ \lambda_{\max}(S(J_1, J_2, J_3)), \\
&\qquad J_k \subset \{1, \cdots, n\}, \ k = 1, 2, 3 \Big\} |x_t(0)|^2.
\end{aligned}$$

By assumption, $S(J_1, J_2, J_3)$ is negative definite for all J_1, J_2, J_3, three independent subsets of $\{1, \cdots, n\}$, which are not necessarily distinct. There are only a finite number of matrices $S(J_1, J_2, J_3)$. Thus $\max\big\{ \lambda_{\max}(S(J_1, J_2, J_3)), \ J_k \subset \{1, \cdots, n\}, \ k = 1, 2, 3 \big\} < 0$. By (7.9.10) and (7.9.14), it now follows from Lyapunov results (see

Theorem 7.2.1; or Theorem 6.3.9 in [18]; or Theorem 5.2.1 in [10]) that the equilibrium $x = 0$ of system (7.9.4)–(7.9.6) is asymptotically stable. ∎

Remark 7.9.1 i) We note that there are a total of 2^n different subsets of $\{1, \cdots, n\}$. Thus, there are a total of 2^{3n} combinations of (J_1, J_2, J_3) such that the J_1, J_2, J_3 are three independent subsets of $\{1, \cdots, n\}$. By the definitions (7.9.7) and (7.9.8), we know that $A_{J_1 J_2} = A_{J_2 J_1}$ and $B_{J_1 J_3} = B_{J_3 J_1}$. Thus $S(J_1, J_2, J_3) = S(J_2, J_1, J_3)$, and $S(J_1, J_2, J_3) = S(J_3, J_2, J_1)$. Therefore, there are a total of $2^{(3n-2)}$ different $S(J_1, J_2, J_3)$ that need to be verified for definiteness.

ii) If $\Omega = \Re^n$, the condition in Theorem 7.9.1 yields asymptotic stability in the large of the equilibrium $x = 0$, since (7.9.10) and (7.9.14) hold for any $x_t \in C\left([-\tau, 0], \Re^n\right)$ (refer to [10] or [18]).

iii) If in (7.9.4), $B(x, t) \equiv 0$, we obtain the system

$$\dot{x}(t) = A(x(t), t)x(t). \tag{7.9.15}$$

Applying Theorem 7.9.1, the equilibrium $x = 0$ of (7.9.15) is asymptotically stable if there exists $\Lambda = \text{diag}[\lambda_1, \cdots, \lambda_n]$ with $\lambda_i > 0$, $i = 1, \cdots, n$, such that $(A_{J_1 J_2})^T P + P A_{J_1 J_2} + \Lambda$ is negative definite for all J_1, J_2, where the $J_1 J_2$ are two independent subsets of $\{1, \cdots, n\}$. The above conclusion implies the known result that the equilibrium $x = 0$ of (7.9.15) is asymptotically stable if the matrix $(A_{J_1 J_2})^T P + P A_{J_1 J_2}$ is negative definite for all J_1, J_2, where the J_1, J_2 are two independent subsets of $\{1, \cdots, n\}$ (see e.g., [25]). This follows, since when $(A_{J_1 J_2})^T P + P A_{J_1 J_2}$ is negative definite for all J_1, J_2, we can always find a $\Lambda = \text{diag}\{\lambda_1, \cdots, \lambda_n\}$ with $\lambda_i > 0$, $i = 1, \cdots, n$, such that $(A_{J_1 J_2})^T P + P A_{J_1 J_2} + \Lambda$ is negative definite for J_1, J_2.

7.10 Nonlinear Systems with Fixed Bounded Delays

In Section 7.9 we presented a sufficient condition for the asymptotic stability of a family of nonlinear systems with arbitrary but bounded time delay. This stability condition does not involve explicitly any time delays and is valid for arbitrary large but bounded delays.

In applications, system delays are frequently fixed and their bounds are known. For such systems, we establish in the present section a sufficient condition for asymptotic stability, provided that the time delay is sufficiently small. This result provides a partial answer to the following question: if the equilibrium $x = 0$ of system (7.9.4) *without delays* (i.e., with $\tau = 0$) is asymptotically stable, then under what conditions is the equilibrium $x = 0$ of (7.9.4), *with delays* (i.e., with $\tau > 0$), still asymptotically stable?

Theorem 7.10.1 The equilibrium $x = 0$ of the system described by (7.9.4)–(7.9.6) is asymptotically stable if there exists a positive definite matrix $P = P^T$, such that

$$\overline{\lambda}[(A+B)^T P + P(A+B)]$$
$$+ 2\tau[l(A) + l(B)]\sqrt{\frac{\lambda_{\max}(P)}{\lambda_{\min}(P)}} l(PB) < 0 \qquad (7.10.1)$$

where $\lambda_{\max}$ and $\lambda_{\min}$ denote the largest and smallest eigenvalues of a matrix, respectively, and

$$\overline{\lambda}\left[(A+B)^T P + P(A+B)\right]$$
$$\triangleq \max\left\{\lambda_{\max}[(A+B)^T_{J_1 J_2} P + P(A+B)_{J_1 J_2}]: \qquad (7.10.2)\right.$$
$$\left. J_1, J_2 \text{ are two independent subsets of } \{1, \cdots, n\}\right\},$$

$$(A+B)_{J_1 J_2} \triangleq A_{J_1 J_2} + B_{J_1 J_2}, \qquad (7.10.3)$$

$$l(A) \triangleq \max\{\|A_{J_1 J_2}\|:$$
$$J_1, J_2 \text{ are two independent subsets of } \{1, \cdots, n\}\}, \qquad (7.10.4)$$

$$l(B) \triangleq \max\{\|B_{J_1 J_2}\|:$$
$$J_1, J_2 \text{ are two independent subsets of } \{1, \cdots, n\}\}, \qquad (7.10.5)$$

$$l(PB) \triangleq \max\{\|PB_{J_1 J_2}\|:$$
$$J_1, J_2 \text{ are two independent subsets of } \{1, \cdots, n\}\}, \qquad (7.10.6)$$

7.10. FIXED BOUNDED DELAYS

and where $A_{J_1 J_2}$ and $B_{J_1 J_2}$ are defined by (7.9.7), (7.9.8).

Proof: We choose a Lyapunov function $v(x) = x^T P x$, where $P = P^T$ is a positive definite matrix satisfying (7.10.1). This function is clearly positive definite and radially unbounded.

The derivative of v along the solutions of (7.9.4) is given by

$$\begin{aligned}
D_{(7.9.4)} v(x(t)) &= \dot{x}(t)^T P x(t) + x(t)^T P \dot{x}(t) \\
&= [A(x(t),t) x(t) + B(x(t-\tau), t-\tau) \\
&\quad \times x(t-\tau)]^T P x(t) + x(t)^T P \\
&\quad \times [A(x(t),t) x(t) + B(x(t-\tau), t-\tau) x(t-\tau)] \\
&= x(t)^T \Big\{ [A(x(t),t) + B(x(t-\tau), t-\tau)]^T P \\
&\quad + P[A(x(t),t) + B(x(t-\tau), t-\tau)] \Big\} x(t) \\
&\quad - [x(t) - x(t-\tau)]^T B(x(t-\tau), t-\tau)^T P x(t) \\
&\quad - x(t)^T P B(x(t-\tau), t-\tau) \\
&\quad \times [x(t) - x(t-\tau)].
\end{aligned}$$
(7.10.7)

Since

$$\begin{aligned}
x(t)^T & \Big\{ [A(x(t),t) + B(x(t-\tau), t-\tau)]^T P + P[A(x(t),t) x(t) \\
&+ B(x(t-\tau), t-\tau) x(t-\tau)] \Big\} x(t) \\
&\leq x(t)^T \Big[((A+B)_{J_1 J_2})^T P + P(A+B)_{J_1 J_2} \Big] x(t)
\end{aligned}$$
(7.10.8)

for certain J_1, J_2, where J_1, J_2 are two independent subsets of $\{1, \cdots, n\}$, we have

$$\begin{aligned}
x(t)^T & \Big\{ [A(x(t),t) + B(x(t-\tau), t-\tau)]^T P + P[A(x(t),t) x(t) \\
&+ B(x(t-\tau), t-\tau) x(t-\tau)] \Big\} x(t) \\
&\leq |x(t)|^2 \lambda_{\max} \Big[((A+B)_{J_1 J_2})^T P + P(A+B)_{J_1 J_2} \Big] \\
&\leq |x(t)|^2 \bar{\lambda} [(A+B)^T P + P(A+B)]
\end{aligned}$$

where $\bar{\lambda}[(A+B)^T P + P(A+B)]$ is defined in (7.10.3). Hence

$$\begin{aligned}
D_{(7.9.4)} v(x(t)) &\leq |x(t)|^2 \bar{\lambda} [(A+B)^T P + P(A+B)] \\
&\quad + 2|x(t)| \cdot \|P B(x(t-\tau), t-\tau)\| \cdot |x(t) - x(t-\tau)|.
\end{aligned}$$

Since $A(x,t)$ and $B(x,t)$ satisfy (7.9.5) and (7.9.6), it follows that

$$\|PB(x(t-\tau), t-\tau)\| \leq l(PB) \qquad (7.10.9)$$

$$\|A(x(t), t)\| \leq l(A) \qquad (7.10.10)$$

$$\|B(x(t-\tau), t-\tau)\| \leq l(B) \qquad (7.10.11)$$

for all $(x(t), t)$ and $(x(t-\tau), (t-\tau)) \in \Omega \times \Re^+$, where $l(PB)$, $l(A)$, and $l(B)$ are defined in (7.10.4)–(7.10.6). Inequalities (7.10.8)–(7.10.11) are not difficult to prove, using similar arguments as in (7.9.12). Thus

$$\begin{aligned}D_{(7.9.4)}v(x(t)) \leq\ &|x(t)|^2 \overline{\lambda}[(A+B)^T P + P(A+B)] \\ &+ 2|x(t)| \cdot |x(t) - x(t-\tau)|l(PB).\end{aligned} \qquad (7.10.12)$$

Claim 1 For any $t > \tau$, we have

$$v(x(t)) < \max\{v(x(s)): s \in [t-2\tau, t]\}. \qquad (7.10.13)$$

Proof: If there exists some $t > \tau$ such that

$$v(x(t)) = \max\{v(x(s)): s \in [t-2\tau, t]\},$$

then

$$D_{(7.9.4)}v(x(t)) \geq 0 \qquad (7.10.14)$$

and

$$\lambda_{\min}(P)|x(s)|^2 \leq v(x(s)) \leq v(x(t)) \leq \lambda_{\max}(P)|x(t)|^2 \qquad (7.10.15)$$

for all $s \in [t-2\tau, t]$. Inequality (7.10.15) implies that

$$\max\{|x(s)|: s \in [t-2\tau, t]\} \leq \sqrt{\frac{\lambda_{\max}(P)}{\lambda_{\min}(P)}}|x(t)|. \qquad (7.10.16)$$

On the other hand,

$$\begin{aligned}|x(t) - x(t-\tau)| &= \left|\int_{t-\tau}^{t} \dot{x}(s)ds\right| \\ &= \Big|\int_{t-\tau}^{t}[A(s, x(s))x(s) \\ &\quad + B(s-\tau, x(s-\tau))x(s-\tau)]ds\Big| \\ &\leq \tau[l(A) + l(B)]\max\{|x(s)|: \\ &\quad s \in [t-2\tau, t]\}\end{aligned} \qquad (7.10.17)$$

7.10. FIXED BOUNDED DELAYS

where $l(A)$, $l(B)$ are defined in (7.10.4)–(7.10.5). In the last inequality, we have used (7.10.10) and (7.10.11).

Combining (7.10.16) and (7.10.17), we have

$$|x(t) - x(t-\tau)| \leq \tau[l(A) + l(B)]\sqrt{\frac{\lambda_{\max}(P)}{\lambda_{\min}(P)}}|x(t)|. \qquad (7.10.18)$$

Applying (7.10.18) to (7.10.12), we have

$$\begin{aligned}D_{(7.9.4)}v(x(t)) &\leq |x(t)|^2 \overline{\lambda}[(A+B)^T P + P(A+B)] \\ &\quad + 2|x(t)|^2 \tau[l(A) + l(B)]\sqrt{\frac{\lambda_{\max}(P)}{\lambda_{\min}(P)}}\, l(PB) \\ &= |x(t)|^2 \Big\{ \overline{\lambda}[(A+B)^T P + P(A+B)] \\ &\quad + 2\tau[l(A) + l(B)]\sqrt{\frac{\lambda_{\max}(P)}{\lambda_{\min}(P)}}\, l(PB) \Big\} \\ &< 0 \end{aligned}$$
$$(7.10.19)$$

since (7.10.1) holds. Thus (7.10.19) contradicts (7.10.14). Therefore, the statement of Claim 1 is true.

We now define

$$y(n) = \max\{v(x(s)) \colon s \in [(2n-1)\tau, (2n+1)\tau]\} \qquad (7.10.20)$$

for all $n = 0, 1, \cdots$. Then, $y(n)$ is strictly monotonically decreasing. For otherwise, we may assume that $y(k) \leq y(k+1)$ for some k. Since

$$y(k+1) = \max\{v(x(s)) \colon s \in [(2k+1)\tau, (2k+3)\tau]\} = v(x(s_0))$$

for some $s_0 \in [(2k+1)\tau, (2k+3)\tau]$, it follows that

$$v(x(s_0)) = \max\{v(x(s)) \colon s \in [s_0 - 2\tau, s_0]\}$$

which is not possible by Claim 1. Therefore, $y(n)$ is monotonically decreasing and converging to a, $a \geq 0$. We will use the next two claims to show that $a = 0$, which is essential to our conclusion.

Claim 2 Assume that $a > 0$. Then there exists a $\delta > 0$ and a positive integer N such that for any $t \geq (2N+1)\tau$, if $v(x(t)) \geq a$ then $D_{(7.9.4)}v(x(t)) < -\delta$.

Proof: Given an $\varepsilon_0 > 0$ (we will specify what this ε_0 is later), since $y(n)$ is monotonically decreasing to a, there exists an integer N, such that when $n \geq N$, $a + \varepsilon_0 \geq y(n) \geq a$. For $t \geq (2N+1)\tau$, if $v(x(t)) \geq a$, then

$$v(x(s)) \leq a + \varepsilon_0 \leq v(x(t)) + \varepsilon_0$$

for $s \geq t - 2\tau$. This implies that

$$|x(s)|^2 \lambda_{\min}(P) \leq |x(t)|^2 \lambda_{\max}(P) + \varepsilon_0$$

for $s \in [t - 2\tau, t]$ (this is actually true for $s \geq t - 2\tau$). Hence,

$$|x(s)|^2 \leq \frac{\lambda_{\max}(P)}{\lambda_{\min}(P)} x(t)^2 + \frac{\varepsilon_0}{\lambda_{\min}(P)}$$
$$\leq \left(\sqrt{\frac{\lambda_{\max}(P)}{\lambda_{\min}(P)}} |x(t)| + \sqrt{\frac{\varepsilon_0}{\lambda_{\min}(P)}} \right)^2$$

for $s \in [t - 2\tau, t]$. Thus,

$$\max\{|x(s)|: s \in [t - 2\tau, t]\}$$
$$\leq \sqrt{\frac{\lambda_{\max}(P)}{\lambda_{\min}(P)}} |x(t)| + \sqrt{\frac{\varepsilon_0}{\lambda_{\min}(P)}}. \quad (7.10.21)$$

Applying (7.10.21) and (7.10.17), we obtain

$$|x(t) - x(t - \tau)| \leq \tau[l(A) + l(B)]\sqrt{\frac{\lambda_{\max}(P)}{\lambda_{\min}(P)}} |x(t)|$$
$$+ \tau[l(A) + l(B)]\sqrt{\frac{\varepsilon_0}{\lambda_{\min}(P)}}. \quad (7.10.22)$$

From (7.10.12) and (7.10.22) it follows that

$$D_{(7.9.4)}v(x(t)) \leq |x(t)|^2 \left\{ \overline{\lambda}[(A+B)^T P + P(A+B)] \right.$$
$$+ 2\tau[l(A) + l(B)]\sqrt{\frac{\lambda_{\max}(P)}{\lambda_{\min}(P)}} l(PB) \right\}$$
$$+ 2|x(t)|\tau[l(A) + l(B)]l(PB)\sqrt{\frac{\varepsilon_0}{\lambda_{\min}(P)}}.$$
$$(7.10.23)$$

7.10. FIXED BOUNDED DELAYS

When $n \geq N$, $y(n) \leq a + \varepsilon_0$. Therefore, we have, by the definition of $y(n)$, that
$$v(x(t)) \leq a + \varepsilon_0$$
for $t \geq (2N+1)\tau$, which implies that
$$|x(t)| \leq \sqrt{\frac{a + \varepsilon_0}{\lambda_{\min}(P)}} \qquad (7.10.24)$$
for $t \geq (2N+1)\tau$. Combining (7.10.23) and (7.10.24), we obtain
$$\begin{aligned} D_{(7.9.4)}v(x(t)) \leq &\frac{a+\varepsilon_0}{\lambda_{\min}(P)}\left\{\overline{\lambda}[(A+B)^T P + P(A+B)]\right. \\ &\left. + 2\tau[l(A) + l(B)]\sqrt{\frac{\lambda_{\max}(P)}{\lambda_{\min}(P)}}l(PB)\right\} \\ &+ 2\sqrt{\frac{a+\varepsilon_0}{\lambda_{\min}(P)}}\tau[l(A)+l(B)]l(PB)\sqrt{\frac{\varepsilon_0}{\lambda_{\min}(P)}}. \end{aligned}$$
$$(7.10.25)$$

Since we assumed that $a > 0$ and since (7.10.1) is true, when we choose ε_0 sufficiently small, it must follow that
$$D_{(7.9.4)}v(x(t)) < -\delta$$
for some $\delta > 0$. Furthermore, ε_0 and δ do not depend on t. This concludes the proof of Claim 2.

Claim 3 Assume that $a > 0$. Then $D_{(7.9.4)}v(x(t)) < 0$ for all $t \geq (2N+1)\tau$, where N is determined in Claim 2.

Proof: The proof is by contradiction. If Claim 3 is not true, then there exists a $t_1 \geq (2N+1)\tau$, such that $D_{(7.9.4)}v(x(t_1)) \geq 0$. By Claim 2, we know that $v(x(t_1)) < a$. We can choose an integer M sufficiently large so that $(2M-1)\tau \geq t_1$. Assume that the maximal value of $v(x(s))$ in the interval $[t_1, (2M+1)\tau]$ is attained at t_2, where $t_2 \in [t_1, (2M+1)\tau]$. Then

i) $v(x(t_2)) \geq y(M) \geq a$,

ii) $t_2 \neq t_1$, since $v(x(t_1)) < a$, and

iii) $t_2 \neq (2M+1)\tau$ because of Claim 1.

Therefore, $t_2 \in (t_1, (2M+1)\tau)$, and

iv) $D_{(7.9.4)}v(x(t_2)) = 0$ since $v(x(t_2))$ attains the maximal value.

Facts i) and iv) lead to a contradiction of Claim 2. Thus the conclusion of Claim 3 has to be true.

Using Claims 2 and 3, we are now able to prove that $a = 0$. If we assume that $a > 0$, then the conclusions in Claims 2 and 3 hold. In Claim 3, we have shown that $D_{(7.9.4)}v(x(t)) < 0$ for $t \geq (2N+1)\tau$. Thus $v(x(t))$ is monotonically decreasing when $t \geq (2N+1)\tau$. Since $y(n) = \max\{v(x(s)): s \in [(2N-1)\tau, (2N+1)\tau]\}$ is monotonically decreasing to a, the $v(x(t))$ is also monotonically decreasing to a when $t \geq (2N+1)\tau$. Hence, it follows that $v(x(t)) \geq a$ when $t \geq (2N+1)\tau$. By Claim 2, we have $D_{(7.9.4)}v(x(t)) < -\delta$ for all $t \geq (2N+1)\tau$, where δ is positive and is independent of t. Thus $v(x(t))$ converges to $-\infty$ as t approaches ∞, which is impossible since $v(x) \geq 0$ by definition. This contradiction is a consequence of the assumption that $a > 0$. Therefore, we have proved that $a = 0$.

The fact that $a = 0$ implies that $y(n)$ converges to 0. By the definition of $y(n)$, we know that $v(x(t))$ converges to 0 as t goes to ∞. Thus $|x(t)|$ will also converge to 0 since $\lambda_{\min}(P)|x(t)|^2 \leq v(x(t))$, no matter what the initial value is. Therefore we have proved that the equilibrium $x = 0$ of (7.9.4) is *attractive*, or *globally attractive* if $\Omega = \Re^n$, assuming that the conditions of Theorem (7.10.1) hold.

To complete the proof of Theorem 7.10.1, we need to show that $x = 0$ is *stable*. We will accomplish this by invoking the definition of stability.

For any $\varepsilon > 0$, there exists any $\eta > 0$, such that

$$\eta(1 + l(B)\tau)\exp(l(A)\tau) < \sqrt{\frac{\lambda_{\min}(P)}{\lambda_{\max}(P)}}\varepsilon. \qquad (7.10.26)$$

We set the initial condition to $|x(t)| \leq \eta$ for $t \in [-\tau, 0]$. When $t \in [0, \tau]$, we have

$$x(t) = x(0) + \int_0^t [A(s, x(s))x(s) + B(s - \tau, x(s - \tau))x(s - \tau)]ds.$$

7.10. FIXED BOUNDED DELAYS

It follows that for $t \in [0, \tau]$

$$|x(t)| \leq \eta + \int_0^t \Big[\|A(s, x(s))\| \cdot |x(s)| + \|B(s - \tau, x(s - \tau))\|\eta\Big] ds$$
$$\leq \eta + \int_0^t [l(A)|x(s)| + l(B)\eta] ds$$

where $l(A)$, $l(B)$ are defined by (7.10.4) and (7.10.5). Using Gronwall's inequality (see, e.g., [18]), we obtain

$$|x(t)| \leq \eta(1 + l(B)\tau)\exp(l(A)\tau) \qquad (7.10.27)$$

for $t \in [0, \tau]$. Inequality (7.10.27) is actually true for all $t \in [-\tau, \tau]$. By (7.10.26), we have

$$|x(t)| < \sqrt{\frac{\lambda_{\min}(P)}{\lambda_{\max}(P)}}\varepsilon,$$

and $v(x(t)) < \lambda_{\min}(P)\varepsilon^2$ for $t \in [-\tau, \tau]$. Thus $y(0) < \lambda_{\min}(P)\varepsilon^2$, and furthermore, $y(n) < \lambda_{\min}(P)\varepsilon^2$ for all n since $y(n)$ is monotonically decreasing, where $y(n)$ is defined by (7.10.20). Thus, $v(x(t)) < \lambda_{\min}(P)\varepsilon^2$, which implies that $|x(t)| < \varepsilon$ for all $t \geq -\tau$. By the definition of stability, we have proved that the equilibrium $x = 0$ is stable. This completes the proof of Theorem 7.10.1. ∎

Remark 7.10.1 i) If $\Omega = \Re^n$, where Ω is the domain of x satisfying (7.9.4), then the equilibrium $x = 0$ of (7.9.4) is asymptotically stable in the large under the conditions of Theorem 7.10.1 ([10], [18]).

ii) When $\tau = 0$, the inequality (7.10.1) reduces to $\overline{\lambda}[(A+B)^T P + P(A+B)] < 0$, a result reported previously [25] in a different but equivalent form, for the case of (7.9.4)–(7.9.6) *without time delays*.

iii) If we apply the criteria in Part ii) of this remark (or the criteria reported in [25]) to verify that the equilibrium of (7.9.4)–(7.9.6) *without delay* is asymptotically stable, i.e., $\overline{\lambda}[(A+B)^T P + P(A+B)] < 0$, then we can always find an upper bound for τ such that the inequality (7.10.1) is satisfied. The equilibrium $x = 0$ will remain asymptotically stable if the delay is less than that bound.

iv) Consider the special case of (7.9.4) given by

$$\dot{x}(t) = Ax(t) + Bx(t-\tau) \qquad (7.10.28)$$

where A, B are two fixed matrices such that $(A+B)$ is Hurwitz stable. In applying Theorem 7.10.1 to system (7.10.28), we choose a matrix P such that $(A+B)^T P + P(A+B) = -E$, where E denotes the identity matrix. Then the equilibrium $x = 0$ of (7.10.28) is asymptotically stable if

$$2\tau(\|A\| + \|B\|)\sqrt{\frac{\lambda_{\max}(P)}{\lambda_{\min}(P)}}\|PB\| < 1. \qquad (7.10.29)$$

The asymptotic stability condition (7.10.29) was also reported (with incomplete proof) in [13].

7.11 Stability Analysis of Time-Delay Neural Networks with Nonsymmetric Interconnecting Structure

The present section consists of two parts.

A. Small Gain Conditions and Sector Conditions

In the previous two sections, we have obtained some sufficient conditions for the asymptotic stability of a family of nonlinear time-delay systems. To verify these conditions, we either need to determine in Theorem 7.9.1 the definiteness of 2^{3n-2} matrices, or we need to compute in Theorem 7.10.1 the norms of 2^{2n+1} matrices. These numbers of computations are acceptable when n is not very large. However, artificial neural networks usually consist of interconnections of large numbers of neurons. In such cases, direct applications of Theorems 7.9.1 or 7.10.1 are not practical. However, because of the special structure of the equations describing neural networks, we are able to reduce the number of computation steps significantly in the applications of these theorems. In this section, we establish some

7.11. NONSYMMETRIC NEURAL NETWORKS

practical sufficient conditions for the asymptotic stability of a family of the neural networks with delays. *These conditions require certain verification involving only one matrix or one inequality.*

In the present section we consider a family of artificial neural networks with delays, described by equations of the form

$$\dot{x}(t) = -Cx(t) + TS(x(t-\tau)) + I \qquad (7.11.1)$$

where $x \in \Omega \subset \Re^n$, $C = \text{diag}[c_1, \cdots, c_n]$ with $c_i > 0$, $1 \le i \le n$, $T = [T_{ij}] \in \Re^{n \times n}$, $I = (I_1, \cdots I_n)^T \in \Re^n$ is a constant vector, and $S(x) = [s_1(x_1), \cdots, s_n(x_n)]^T$ with $s_i \in C^1(\Re, (-1,1))$ where s_i is monotonically increasing, for $i = 1, \cdots, n$. A special case of (7.11.1), when $\tau = 0$ and T is symmetric, has been studied widely and is called the Hopfield neural network. In this section, we consider the asymptotic stability of the equilibrium x_e of (7.11.1). Without loss of generality, we can assume that $x_e = 0$, $S(0) = 0$, and $I = 0$ [for otherwise, we let $\tilde{x} = x - x_e$, and we define $\tilde{S}(\tilde{x}) = S(\tilde{x} + x_e) - S(x_e)$, to obtain the new description of the neural network (7.11.1), $\dot{\tilde{x}} = -C\tilde{x} + T\tilde{S}(\tilde{x}(t-\tau))$, which satisfies our assumption]. We have $s_i(0) = 0$ for $i = 1, \cdots, n$ and we assume that $s_i(x_i)$ satisfies the sector conditions

$$0 \le \sigma_i^m \le \frac{s_i(x_i)}{x_i} \le \sigma_i^M \qquad (7.11.2)$$

$1 \le i \le n$ for $x \in \Omega$. The new form of the neural network is now given by

$$\dot{x}(t) = -Cx(t) + TS(x(t-\tau)) \qquad (7.11.3)$$

where C, T, and S are given in (7.11.1), with the sector condition (7.11.2) satisfied. The time-delay neural network (7.11.3) has been studied in [2] and [17]. In both [2] and [17], it is assumed that C is a diagonal matrix with identical positive elements, i.e., associated with each neuron is the same capacitance and input resistance. The results in [17] rely on the linearization of (7.11.3) and yield local results. We now apply the results of the previous two sections to neural networks with time-delays described by (7.11.3).

Theorem 7.11.1 The equilibrium $x = 0$ of (7.11.3) is asymptotically stable for any arbitrarily bounded delay τ if there exists a positive definite matrix P, and a matrix $\Lambda = \text{diag}[\lambda_1, \cdots, \lambda_n]$, $\lambda_i > 0$, $i = 1, \cdots, n$, such that

$$S^M \triangleq -(C^T P + PC) + \Lambda + PT\Sigma^M \Lambda^{-1} \Sigma^M T^T P \qquad (7.11.4)$$

is negative definite, where $\Sigma^M = \text{diag}[\sigma_1^M, \cdots, \sigma_n^M]$, and σ_i^M are defined by (7.11.2) for $i = 1, \cdots, n$.

Proof: We can rewrite (7.11.3) as

$$\dot{x}(t) = -Cx(t) + T\Sigma(x(t-\tau))x(t-\tau) \qquad (7.11.5)$$

where $\Sigma(x) = \text{diag}[\sigma_1(x_1), \cdots, \sigma_n(x_n)]$, and $\sigma_i(x_i) = s_i(x_i)/x_i$, $i = 1, \cdots, n$. Then $\sigma_i(x_i) \in [\sigma_i^m, \sigma_i^M]$, for $i = 1, \cdots, n$. Using the same Lyapunov functional as in Theorem 7.9.1,

$$v(x_t) = x(t)^T P x(t) + \int_{-\tau}^{0} x_t(\theta)^T \Lambda x_t(\theta) d\theta,$$

we obtain along the solutions of (7.11.3)

$$\begin{aligned} D_{(7.11.3)}v(x_t) &= -x(t)^T(C^T P + PC)x(t) + x(t)^T \Lambda x(t) \\ &\quad + x(t)^T PT\Sigma(x(t-\tau))\Lambda^{-1}\Sigma(x(t-\tau))T^T P x(t) \end{aligned} \qquad (7.11.6)$$

using similar arguments as in the derivation of (7.9.11). If we let $y^T = (y_1, \cdots, y_n) = x(t)^T PT$ (for given t), then the last term of (7.11.6) assumes the form

$$\begin{aligned} y^T \Sigma \Lambda^{-1} \Sigma y &= \sum_{i=1}^{n} y_i^2 \lambda_i^{-1} \sigma_i^2(x_i(t-\tau)) \\ &\leq \sum_{i=1}^{n} y_i^2 \lambda_i^{-1} (\sigma_i^M)^2 \\ &= x(t)^T PT\Sigma^M \Lambda^{-1} \Sigma^M T^T P x(t). \end{aligned} \qquad (7.11.7)$$

Then,

$$\begin{aligned} D_{(7.11.3)}v(x_t) &\leq x(t)^T[-(C^T P + PC) + \Lambda + PT\Sigma^M \Lambda^{-1} \Sigma^M T^T P]x(t) \\ &= x(t)^T S^M x(t). \end{aligned}$$

Therefore, the equilibrium $x = 0$ of (7.11.3) is asymptotically stable if S^M is negative definite. ∎

7.11. NONSYMMETRIC NEURAL NETWORKS

Corollary 7.11.1 The equilibrium $x = 0$ of (7.11.3) is asymptotically stable if

$$\|P_0 T\| < \frac{1}{\bar{\sigma}^M} \qquad (7.11.8)$$

where $P_0 = \text{diag}[1/c_1, \cdots, 1/c_n]$ and $\bar{\sigma}^M = \max\{\sigma_i^M : 1 \leq i \leq n\}$. ∎

If $\Omega = \Re^n$, then the conditions of Theorem 7.11.1 or Corollary 7.11.1 imply that $x = 0$ is the only equilibrium of neural network (7.11.3), and this equilibrium is asymptotically stable in the large ([10], [18]).

Corollary 7.11.1 follows from Theorem 7.11.1 in a straightforward manner by choosing P as P_0, and Λ as the identity matrix. Corollary 7.11.1 yields a kind of *small gain condition*. When the gain $\bar{\sigma}^M$ is sufficiently small, (7.11.8) will be satisfied and the equilibrium $x = 0$ of (7.11.3) will be asymptotically stable for arbitrarily bounded delay.

In [12], the neural network

$$\dot{x} = -x + TS(x) + I \qquad (7.11.9)$$

is considered, where $T = [T_{ij}]$, $I = (I_1, \cdots, I_n)^T$,

$$S(x) = (s_1(x_1), \cdots, s_n(x_n))^T$$

and $0 < s_i'(x_i) \leq 1$, $i = 1, \cdots, n$, where $s_i'(x_i) = ds_i(x_i)/dx_i$. It is shown in [12] that the equilibrium $x = 0$ of (7.11.9) is asymptotically stable if $\|T\| < 1$. This condition can easily be obtained by applying Corollary 7.11.1 (letting $P_0 = E$, the identity matrix, and $\bar{\sigma}^M = 1$). Furthermore, Corollary 7.11.1 shows that the condition $\|T\| < 1$ is so strong that it guarantees not only the asymptotic stability of the equilibrium $x = 0$ of the nondelayed neural network (7.11.9), but also the asymptotic stability of the equilibrium $x = 0$ of system (7.11.9) with an additional arbitrarily bounded delay, given by

$$\dot{x}(t) = -x(t) + TS(x(t-\tau)) + I.$$

Both Theorem 7.11.1 and Corollary 7.11.1 are applicable to neural networks with arbitrary bounded delays. As noted before, the bound of the delays is frequently not very large and is usually known. Under such circumstances, results such as Theorem 7.11.1 and Corollary 7.11.1 will be conservative and therefore, we need to determine criteria which involve only fixed bounded delays. The following results are a consequence of Theorem 7.10.1.

Theorem 7.11.2 The equilibrium $x = 0$ of (7.11.3) is asymptotically stable if there exists a positive definite matrix P, such that

$$\begin{aligned}
2\|PT\|\tilde{\sigma}^M &+ 2\tau[\bar{c} + \|T\|(\tilde{\sigma}^M + \|\Sigma_0\|)] \\
&\times \sqrt{\frac{\lambda_{\max}(P)}{\lambda_{\min}(P)}} \|PT\|(\tilde{\sigma}^M + \|\Sigma_0\|) \\
&< -\lambda_{\max}\Big[(-C + T\Sigma_0)^T P \\
&\quad + P(-C + T\Sigma_0)\Big]
\end{aligned} \qquad (7.11.10)$$

where $\tilde{\sigma}^M = \max\{(\sigma_i^M - \sigma_i^m)/2 : 1 \leq i \leq n\}$,

$$\Sigma_0 = \operatorname{diag}\Big[(\sigma_1^m + \sigma_1^M)/2, \cdots, (\sigma_n^m + \sigma_n^M)/2\Big]$$

and $\bar{c} = \max\{c_i : 1 \leq i \leq n\}$.

Proof: We consider (7.11.5), which is the equivalent of (7.11.3), which in turn is a special case of (7.9.4) with

$$A(x(t), t) \equiv -C$$

and

$$B(x(t - \tau), t - \tau) = T\Sigma(x(t - \tau))$$

where $\Sigma(x) = \operatorname{diag}[\sigma_1(x_1), \cdots, \sigma_n(x_n)]$, and $\sigma_i(x_i) = s_i(x_i)/x_i$, $i = 1, \cdots, n$. The proof of Theorem 7.11.2 is basically the same as the proof of Theorem 7.10.1, except that in place of (7.10.10)–(7.10.13), we need to use (7.11.11)–(7.11.14) given by

$$\begin{aligned}
x(t)^T &[(-C + T\Sigma)^T P + P(-C + T\Sigma)]x(t) \\
&= x(t)^T[(-C + T\Sigma_0)^T P + P(-C + T\Sigma_0)]x(t) \\
&\quad + x(t)^T[T(\Sigma - \Sigma_0)^T P + PT(\Sigma - \Sigma_0)]x(t) \\
&\leq |x(t)|^2 \Big[\lambda_{\max}[(-C + T\Sigma_0)^T P + P(-C + T\Sigma_0)] \\
&\quad + \|PT\|\tilde{\sigma}^M\Big],
\end{aligned} \qquad (7.11.11)$$

7.11. NONSYMMETRIC NEURAL NETWORKS

$$\|PT\Sigma\| \leq \|PT\| \cdot \|\Sigma\| \leq \|PT\|(\tilde{\sigma}^M + \|\Sigma_0\|), \quad (7.11.12)$$

$$\| - C\| \leq \bar{c}, \quad (7.11.13)$$

$$\|T\Sigma\| \leq \|T\| \cdot \|\Sigma\| \leq \|T\|(\tilde{\sigma}^M + \|\Sigma_0\|), \quad (7.11.14)$$

where Σ is the short representation of $\Sigma(x(t - \tau))$. The rest of the proof follows readily, taking into account the above modifications. ∎

The following result is an obvious consequence of Theorem 7.11.2.

Corollary 7.11.2 Assume that $-C + T\Sigma_0$ is Hurwitz stable. Then the equilibrium $x = 0$ of (7.11.3) is asymptotically stable if

$$2\|P_1 T\|\tilde{\sigma}^M + 2\tau[\bar{c} + \|T\|(\tilde{\sigma}^M + \|\Sigma_0\|)] \\ \times \sqrt{\frac{\lambda_{\max}(P_1)}{\lambda_{\min}(P_1)}} \|P_1 T\|(\tilde{\sigma}^M + \|\Sigma_0\|) < 1 \quad (7.11.15)$$

where $P_1 = P_1^T$ is positive definite and $(-C + T\Sigma_0)^T P_1 + P_1(-C + T\Sigma_0) = -E$, and where E is the identity matrix. ∎

Remark 7.11.1 i) If $\Omega = \Re^n$, then the conditions of Theorem 7.11.2 or Corollary 7.11.2 imply that $x = 0$ is the only equilibrium for neural network (7.11.3), and this equilibrium is asymptotically stable in the large ([10], [18]).

ii) From Corollary 7.11.2, we see that instability of $x = 0$ for (7.11.3) may be due to two factors: a large sector $\tilde{\sigma}^M$, and a large gain $\|\Sigma_0\|$. When both $\tilde{\sigma}^M$ and $\|\Sigma_0\|$ are sufficiently small, the condition (7.11.15) is always satisfied and the equilibrium $x = 0$ of (7.11.13) is then asymptotically stable, assuming $-C + T\Sigma_0$ is Hurwitz stable.

iii) When there is no delay, i.e., $\tau \equiv 0$, (7.11.15) reduces to $2\|P_1 T\|\tilde{\sigma}^M < 1$. If this is the case, we only require that the sector $\tilde{\sigma}^M$ be very small, no matter what the gain $\|\Sigma_0\|$ is, as long as $-C + T\Sigma_0$ is Hurwitz stable. However, in the presence of delays, no matter how small, the gain factor is important as well.

iv) In Corollary 7.11.1, we require that $\|P_0 T\| < 1/\bar{\sigma}^M$. Thus $\|P_0 T\| < 1/\|\Sigma_0\|$ since $\bar{\sigma}^M \geq \|\Sigma_0\|$. This means the norm of $\|T\|$

should be fairly small, supposing the gain factor $\|\Sigma_0\|$ is fixed. This is quite a strong restriction for neural networks. The reason for this restriction is that Corollary 7.11.1 is applicable for any arbitrarily bounded delay. To compensate for large delays to maintain stability, we require that the magnitude of the delay term $TS(x(t-\tau))$ decreases. For fixed bounded delays, we do not have this restriction. In Corollary 7.11.2 with the gain factor $\|\Sigma_0\|$ fixed, no matter how large the norm of T is, if the delay is sufficiently small and if the output function $S(x)$ is sufficiently close to becoming a linear function (i.e., the sector $\tilde{\sigma}^M$ is sufficiently small), we will always have that the equilibrium $x = 0$ is asymptotically stable.

v) When (7.11.3) reduces to a linear system, i.e., when $\tilde{\sigma}^M = 0$, then (7.11.14) reduces to

$$2\tau(\bar{c} + \|T\| \cdot \|\Sigma_0\|)\sqrt{\frac{\lambda_{\max}(P_1)}{\lambda_{\min}(P_1)}}\|P_1T\| \cdot \|\Sigma_0\| < 1. \qquad (7.11.16)$$

This condition can also be obtained from the result (7.10.29), which is a sufficient condition for the asymptotic stability for linear systems and was first reported in [13].

B. Linearization and Domain of Attraction

In Part A of the present section, we have given two sufficient conditions, (7.11.8) of Corollary 7.11.1, and (7.11.15) of Corollary 7.11.2, for the asymptotic stability of the equilibrium $x = 0$ of the time-delay neural networks described by (7.11.3). If (7.11.8) [or (7.11.15)] is satisfied, then the equilibrium $x = 0$ of (7.11.3) is asymptotically stable for arbitrarily bounded delays (or fixed bounded delays). However, if (7.11.8) [or (7.11.15)] is not satisfied, then it does not necessarily follow that the equilibrium $x = 0$ is not asymptotically stable.

When the equilibrium $x = 0$ of (7.11.3) is asymptotically stable, but not globally asymptotically stable, then the domain of attraction of the equilibrium is of great interest. In the following, we present a method of estimating the domain of attraction for an asymptotically stable equilibrium of (7.11.3).

7.11. NONSYMMETRIC NEURAL NETWORKS

When (7.11.8), or (7.11.15) is not satisfied, we can deduce the asymptotic stability of the equilibrium $x = 0$ of the nonlinear system (7.11.3) from the linearization of (7.11.3), given by

$$\dot{x}(t) = -Cx(t) + TD(0)x(t - \tau) \qquad (7.11.17)$$

where $D(x) = [s_1'(x_1), \cdots, s_n'(x_n)]^T$ (see, e.g., Theorem 12.9.1 of [10]). To ascertain the asymptotic stability of the equilibrium $x = 0$ of (7.11.17), we use some existing results. For example, by applying the results given in [23], we can show that the equilibrium $x = 0$ of (7.11.17) is asymptotically stable if

$$\|P_0 T\| < \frac{1}{|D(0)|} \qquad (7.11.18)$$

for arbitrary bounded delays, where $P_0 = \text{diag}[1/c_1, \cdots, 1/c_n]$. For the case of fixed bounded delays, using (7.11.16), we know that the equilibrium $x = 0$ of (7.11.17) is asymptotically stable if

$$2\tau(\bar{c} + \|T\| \cdot |D(0)|)\sqrt{\frac{\lambda_{\max}(P_1)}{\lambda_{\min}(P_1)}}\|P_1 T\| \cdot |D(0)| < 1 \qquad (7.11.19)$$

where $\bar{c} = \max\{c_i : i = 1, \cdots, n\}$,

$$P_1(-C + TD(0))^T + (-C + TD(0))P_1 = -E,$$

and E is the identity matrix, assuming that $-C + TD(0)$ is Hurwitz stable [i.e., assuming that the equilibrium $x = 0$ of the linearized system (7.11.17) with $\tau = 0$ is asymptotically stable].

If we verify, by the above criteria, that the equilibrium $x = 0$ of the linearized system (7.11.17) is asymptotically stable, then we know that the equilibrium $x = 0$ of the original system (7.11.3) must be asymptotically stable in a neighborhood of the origin (see, e.g., Theorem 12.9.1 of [10]), i.e., $x = 0$ is a local stable attractor. For practical reasons (e.g., the setting of initial conditions of each neuron), it is necessary to estimate a subset of the domain of attraction which is as large as possible. (In general it is not possible to determine the entire domain of attraction of $x = 0$.) We will demonstrate how we can use Corollaries 7.11.1 and 7.11.2 to accomplish this task.

As in the case of arbitrarily bounded delays, if (7.11.18) is satisfied, then the equilibrium $x = 0$ of the original system (7.11.3) must be locally attractive. For each $i = 1, \cdots, n$, we have $s'_i(0) < 1/\|P_0 T\|$, since (7.11.18) is satisfied. Let $\delta_i \subset \Re$ be the largest open interval containing 0 such that $s_i(x_i)/x_i < 1/\|P_0 T\|$ holds, including infinite intervals. We define $H = \prod_{i=1}^{n} \delta_i$ to be an open hyper-rectangle in $\Re^n$. Thus, for any $x \in H$, we have $s_i(x_i)/x_i < 1/\|P_0 T\|$, $i = 1, \cdots, n$, which implies that the condition (7.11.8) is satisfied if $x \in H \subset \Omega$. When applied to (7.11.3), the Lyapunov function used in the proof of Theorem 7.9.1 is given by

$$v(x_t) = x(t)^T P_0 x(t) + \int_{-\tau}^{0} x_t(\theta)^T x_t(\theta) d\theta.$$

Let $r \geq 0$, and define

$$V_r = \{x_t \in C\left([-\tau, 0], \Omega\right) : v(x_t) = x(t)^T P_0 x(t) + \int_{-\tau}^{0} x_t(\theta)^T x_t(\theta) < r\}.$$

When r is sufficiently small, we have $V_r \subset C\left([-\tau, 0], H\right)$. Let

$$r_0 = \sup\{r \geq 0 \colon V_r \subset C\left([-\tau, 0], H\right])\}.$$

Then a subset of the domain of attraction for the equilibrium $x = 0$ of (7.11.3) is V_{r_0}. The above method applies for any bounded delay. Note that V_{r_0} depends on the bound of the delay, and furthermore, note that as the bound of the delay increases, the domain of attraction V_{r_0} decreases.

For the case of fixed delays, if the neural network (7.11.3) satisfies (7.11.19) (i.e., the equilibrium $x = 0$ of the linearized systems is asymptotically stable), then the equilibrium $x = 0$ of (7.11.3) is locally attractive. In this case, the equation

$$2\|P_1 T\| w + 2\tau[\bar{c} + \|T\|(w + |D(0)|)]$$

$$\times \sqrt{\frac{\lambda_{\max}(P_1)}{\lambda_{\min}(P_1)}} \|P_1 T\|(w + |D(0)|) = 1 \quad (7.11.20)$$

7.12. ROBUST STABILITY ANALYSIS

will have only one positive solution, w_0. Consider each $s_i(x_i)$ for $i = 1, \cdots, n$. Let $\delta_i \subset \Re$ be the largest open interval containing 0, including infinite intervals, such that

$$s'_i(0) - w_0 < s_i(x_i)/x_i < s'_i(0) + w_0$$

is satisfied. We define $H = \prod_{i=1}^{n} \delta_i$ to be an open hyper-rectangle in $\Re^n$. Then (7.11.15) is satisfied for $x \in H \subset \Omega$. Let $r > 0$, and define

$$B_r = \{x \in \Re^n : |x|^2 < r/\|P_1\|\}.$$

When r is sufficiently small, we have $B_r \subset H$. Define $r_0 = \sup\{r > 0 : B_r \subset H\}$. Then a subset of the domain of attraction for the equilibrium $x = 0$ of (7.11.3) is $C([-\tau, 0], B_{r_0})$.

We conclude the present subsection by pointing out that as in the case of dynamical systems described by ordinary differential equations (see, e.g., [20]), the methodology employed herein of determining estimates for the domain of attraction of an asymptotically stable equilibrium of dynamical systems determined by delay equations [such as (7.11.3)] is among the most effective in terms of generality and quality of estimates.

7.12 Robust Stability Analysis of Time-Delay Neural Networks

In the previous section, we discussed the stability of time-delay neural networks

$$\dot{x} = -Cx + TS(x(t - \tau))$$

and we established some sufficient conditions under which the equilibrium $x = 0$ of such networks is asymptotically stable. In our analyses, we assumed that the matrices C and T are precisely known. However, in the implementations of artificial neural networks by circuits, parameter uncertainties will always be present. Accordingly, perturbation analyses of neural network models are essential. In the present section we consider a perturbation model of (7.11.3) given by the equation

$$\dot{x} = -(C + \Delta C)x + (T + \Delta T)S(x(t - \tau)) \tag{7.12.1}$$

where $C = \text{diag}[c_1, \cdots, c_n]$ with $c_i > 0$, $i = 1, \cdots, n$, $\Delta C = \text{diag}[\Delta c_1, \cdots, \Delta c_n]$, T, $\Delta T \in \Re^{n \times n}$, and $S(x) = [s_1(x_1), \cdots, s_n(x_n)]^T$ with $0 \leq \sigma_i^m \leq s_i(x_i)/x_i \leq \sigma_i^M$ for $i = 1, \cdots, n$.

Proposition 7.12.1 The equilibrium $x = 0$ of neural network (7.12.1) is asymptotically stable for any arbitrary bounded delay if

$$2\|P_0\| \cdot \|\Delta C\| + \|P_0T\|^2(\overline{\sigma}^M)^2 + \|P_0\|^2\|\Delta T\|^2(\overline{\sigma}^M)^2 \tag{7.12.2}$$

$$+ 2\|P_0T\| \cdot \|\Delta T\|\overline{\sigma}^M < 1$$

where $P_0 = \text{diag}[1/c_1, \cdots, 1/c_n]$, and $\overline{\sigma}^M = \max\{\sigma_i^M : 1 \leq i \leq n\}$. ∎

This result is a consequence of Theorem 7.11.1. In the interests of brevity, we omit the details of the proof. The next result which we also state without proof is a consequence of Theorem 7.11.2.

Proposition 7.12.2 The equilibrium $x = 0$ of neural network (7.12.1) is asymptotically stable if

$$\begin{aligned}
2(\|P_1T\| + \|P_1\| \cdot \|\Delta T\|)\tilde{\sigma}^M &+ 2\tau[(\|C\| + \|\Delta C\|) \\
+ (\|T\| + \|\Delta T\|)(\tilde{\sigma}^M + \|\Sigma_0\|)]&\sqrt{\frac{\lambda_{\max}(P)}{\lambda_{\min}(P)}} \\
\times (\|P_1T\| + \|P_1\| \cdot \|\Delta T\|)(\tilde{\sigma}^M &+ \|\Sigma_0\|) \\
+ 2(\|\Delta C\| + \|\Delta T\| \cdot \|\Sigma_0\|)\|P_1\| &< 1
\end{aligned} \tag{7.12.3}$$

where P_1 is positive definite, $P_1(-C + T\Sigma_0)^T + (-C + T\Sigma_0)P_1 = -E$, E denotes the identity matrix,

$$\Sigma_0 = \text{diag}\left[(\sigma_1^m + \sigma_1^M)/2, \cdots, (\sigma_n^m + \sigma_n^M)/2\right],$$

and $\tilde{\sigma}^M = \max\{(\sigma_i^M - \sigma_i^m)/2 : i = 1, \cdots, n\}$, and where we assume that $-C + T\Sigma_0$ is Hurwitz stable. ∎

7.13. EXAMPLES

Propositions 7.12.1 and 7.12.2 provide us with methods of testing the asymptotic stability of the equilibrium $x = 0$ of the perturbed neural network model (7.12.1), with arbitrary bounded delay or fixed bounded delay, respectively. Furthermore, when the perturbation norms $\|\Delta C\|$ and $\|\Delta T\|$ are known *a priori*, we can employ Propositions 7.12.1 and 7.12.2 to estimate the domain of attraction of the equilibrium, similarly as was done in Part B of Section 7.11.

7.13 Examples

To demonstrate the applicability of some of the preceding results, we now consider some specific examples.

Example 7.13.1 Consider a neural network

$$\dot{x}(t) = -Cx(t) + TS(x(t-\tau)) \quad (7.13.1)$$

where $x \in \Re^{10}$,

$$C = \text{diag}[3.5, 1.8, 3.6, 3.6, 1.49, 1.95, 1.74, 1.55, 2.89, 3.62] \quad (7.13.2)$$

$S(x) = (s_1(x_1), \cdots, s_n(x_{10}))^T$ with

$$s_i(x_i) = \frac{2}{\pi} \tan^{-1}(x_i) \quad (7.13.3)$$

for $i = 1, \cdots, 10$, and $T = T_0/2$, where

$$T_0 = \begin{bmatrix} 0.1 & 0.5 & 0.5 & 0.5 & 0.5 & 0.5 & -0.5 & 0.5 & 0.5 & 0.5 \\ 0.5 & -3.6 & 0.5 & -0.5 & 0.5 & 0.5 & 0.5 & 0.5 & 0.5 & 0.5 \\ 0.5 & 0.5 & 0.8 & 0.5 & 0.5 & -0.5 & 0.5 & 0.5 & 0.5 & -0.5 \\ 0.5 & 0.5 & 0.5 & 0.2 & 0.5 & 0.5 & 0.5 & 0.5 & -0.5 & 0.5 \\ -0.5 & 0.5 & -0.5 & 0.5 & -2.65 & 0.5 & 0.5 & -0.5 & 0.5 & 0.5 \\ 0.5 & 0.5 & 0.5 & 0.5 & -0.5 & -2.45 & 0.5 & 0.5 & 0.5 & -0.5 \\ 0.5 & 0.5 & -0.5 & 0.5 & 0.5 & 0.5 & -2.35 & 0.5 & 0.5 & -0.5 \\ 0.5 & 0.5 & 0.5 & -0.5 & 0.5 & 0.5 & 0.5 & -2.9 & 0.5 & 0.5 \\ -0.5 & 0.5 & 0.5 & 0.5 & 0.5 & -0.5 & 0.5 & 0.5 & -3.55 & 0.5 \\ 0.5 & 0.5 & 0.5 & 0.5 & 0.5 & 0.5 & -0.5 & 0.5 & 0.5 & -2.5 \end{bmatrix}$$

$$(7.13.4)$$

This system satisfies the condition $\|P_0T\| < 1/\overline{\sigma}^M$, since $P_0 = C^{-1}$, $\|P_0T\| = 1.19$, $\overline{\sigma}^M = \max\{s_i'(x_i)\} = 0.6366$, and $1/\overline{\sigma}^M = 1.5708$. In view of Corollary 7.11.1, the equilibrium $x = 0$ of (7.13.1) is the only equilibrium of system (7.13.1) and it is asymptotically stable in the large for any arbitrarily bounded delay τ. ∎

Example 7.13.2 We consider system (7.13.1) once more, where C and S are given by (7.13.2) and (7.13.3), and where $T = T_0$ is given by (7.13.4).

It is easily verified that the system no longer satisfies the condition $\|P_0T\| < 1/\overline{\sigma}^M$ of Corollary 7.11.1. Thus we are unable to ascertain the asymptotic stability of the equilibrium $x = 0$ of this system for any arbitrarily bounded delay. However, if we assume that we know that the bound of the delay is 0.05 units, i.e., $\tau = \tau(t) \le 0.05$, then we are able to apply Corollary 7.11.2 to determine that the equilibrium $x = 0$ of (7.13.1) is asymptotically stable. Furthermore, we can determine that $C\left([-\tau, 0], B_r\right)$ is a subset of the domain of attraction, where $B_r = \{x \in \Re^{10} : |x| < 1.72\}$.

We note that a result in [2] (Theorem 3) is not applicable in the present example. In general, for small delays, Theorem 7.11.2 is much less conservative than existing results. ∎

Example 7.13.3 We consider the robustness problem of neural networks represented by the equation

$$\dot{x}(t) = -(C + \Delta C)x(t) + (T + \Delta T)S(x(t - \tau)) \qquad (7.13.5)$$

where C and S are given by (7.13.2) and (7.13.3), $T = T_0$ is given by (7.13.4), and $\tau = \tau(t) \le 0.05$. We assume that it is known that $\|\Delta C\| \le 0.1$ and $\|\Delta T\| \le 0.1$.

Using Proposition 7.12.2, we conclude that the equilibrium $x = 0$ of the perturbed neural network (7.13.5) is asymptotically stable and that a subset of the domain of attraction is $C\left([-\tau, 0], B_{r_1}\right)$, where $B_{r_1} = \{x \in \Re^{10} : |x| < 1.25\}$. ∎

7.14 Summary

In the implementation process of artificial feedback neural networks (especially by VLSI), transmission delays may unavoidably be introduced. It is known that in globally stable feedback neural networks without time delays, oscillations can occur after the introduction of delays (see, e.g., [1], [6], [17]). It is therefore important to take the effects of time delays into account in the qualitative analysis of such networks.

In the present chapter we first presented global and local stability results for Hopfield neural networks with identical delays, described by equations of the form

$$\dot{x}(t) = -Cx(t) + T_0 S(x(t)) + T_1 S(x(t-\tau)) + I \quad (7.14.1)$$

and for Cohen-Grossberg neural networks with multiple delays described by equations of the form

$$\dot{x}(t) = -A(x(t))\left[B(x(t)) - T_0 S(x(t)) - \sum_{k=1}^{K} T_k S(x(t-\tau_k))\right]. \quad (7.14.2)$$

Recall that both of these networks are endowed with symmetric interconnecting structure. Specifically, we showed that for a given set of parameters, Hopfield neural networks described by

$$\dot{x}(t) = -Cx(t) + TS(x(t)) + I \quad (7.14.3)$$

with $T = T_0 + T_1$ and neural networks described by (7.14.1) will possess similar global and local qualitative behavior, provided that the time delays are sufficiently small. Similarly, we showed that for a given set of parameters, Cohen-Grossberg neural networks described by

$$\dot{x}(t) = -A(x(t))[B(x(t)) - TS(x(t))] \quad (7.14.4)$$

with $T = T_0 + \sum_{k=1}^{K} T_k$ and neural networks described by (7.14.2) will possess similar global and local qualitative behavior, provided that the time delays are sufficiently small.

In the present chapter we also presented local stability results for neural networks described by equations of the form

$$\dot{x}(t) = -Cx(t) + TS(x(t-\tau)) + I \qquad (7.14.5)$$

under the assumption that the interconnecting structure (specified by T) need not be symmetric. These results include small gain, sector, and linearization results for stability, estimates for the domain of attraction of an equilibrium, and robust stability results.

A. Global Stability Results

We assumed in (7.14.1) that the activation functions s_i are sigmoidal functions and we assumed that the matrix $T = T_0 + T_1$ is symmetric. In applying the Invariance Theory to establish global stability of system (7.14.1), we associated with this system the energy functional given by

$$\begin{aligned}E(x_t) =& -y_t(0)^T T y_t(0) + 2 \sum_{i=1}^n \int_0^{(y_t(0))_i} c_i s_i^{-1}(\sigma) d\sigma \\ & -2y_t(0)^T I \\ & + \int_{-\tau}^0 [y_t(\theta) - y_t(0)]^T T_1^T f(\theta) T_1 [y_t(\theta) - y_t(0)] d\theta\end{aligned} \qquad (7.14.6)$$

where $x_t(\cdot)$ denotes a continuous function on $[-\tau, 0]$ defined by $x_t(s) = x(t+s)$ for all $s \in [-\tau, 0]$, $y(t) \triangleq S(x(t))$, and f is a continuously differentiable, non-negative, scalar valued function defined on $[-\tau, 0]$. We showed that there exists an $f(\cdot)$ such that the time derivative of E along the solutions of system (7.14.1) is a non-positive valued function provided that

$$\tau \beta \|T_1\| < 1 \qquad (7.14.7)$$

where $\tau > 0$ denotes the time delay in system (7.14.1),

$$\beta \triangleq \max_{x \in \Re^n} \|S'(x)\|, \quad S'(x) = \mathrm{diag}\left[\frac{ds_1}{dx_1}(x_1), \cdots, \frac{ds_n}{dx_n}(x_n)\right]$$

and $\|\cdot\|$ denotes the matrix norm induced by the Euclidean vector norm.

7.14. SUMMARY

Next, we showed that every solution of system (7.14.1) is bounded and for almost all $I \in \Re^n$ (except a set with Lebesgue measure zero), the set of equilibria of system (7.14.1) is a discrete set. These facts enabled us to conclude, by invoking the Invariance Theory, that when $T = T_0 + T_1$ is symmetric and when (7.14.7) is satisfied for almost every $I \in \Re^n$, the system (7.14.1) is globally stable.

Using a refinement to the functional given in (7.14.6) involving the various delays for system (7.14.2), we invoked the Invariance Theory once more to establish the sufficient condition for the global stability of (7.14.2) given by

$$\sum_{k=1}^{K} \tau_k \beta \|T_k\| < 1 \qquad (7.14.8)$$

where $\tau_k > 0$, $k = 1, \cdots, K$ denote the time delays in system (7.14.2),

$$\beta \triangleq \max_{x \in \Re^n} \|A(x) S'(x)\|, \quad S'(x) = \text{diag}\left[\frac{ds_1}{dx_1}(x_1), \cdots, \frac{ds_n}{dx_n}(x_n)\right]$$

and $\|\cdot\|$ denotes the matrix norm induced by the Euclidean vector norm.

B. Local Stability Results

As mentioned on several occasions, in the application of artificial neural networks to associative memories, as well as in other applications, the aim is to store information in stable memories which correspond to specific asymptotically stable equilibria. Good criteria which ensure such (local) stability properties are therefore very important. We addressed this question in the present chapter for systems (7.14.1) and (7.14.2).

We first pointed out that even for the case of *linear* delay equations given by

$$\dot{x}(t) = Ax(t) + Bx(t - \tau) \qquad (7.14.9)$$

where A and B are real $n \times n$ matrices and $\tau > 0$ is a delay, there are no known general results which constitute necessary and sufficient conditions for the asymptotic stability of the equilibrium $x_e = 0$. Accordingly, the problem of determining the local stability properties of an equilibrium of a delay differential equation is non-trivial, even in the case of linear systems. However, by utilizing the special structure of Hopfield (or Cohen-Grossberg) neural networks with time delays, we showed in the present chapter that under the conditions of global stability given in the preceding subsection, the asymptotic stability of an equilibrium of system (7.14.1) [or of system (7.14.2)] can be deduced from the asymptotic stability of the corresponding equilibrium of system (7.14.3) [or of system (7.14.4)]. In other words, if (7.14.7) is satisfied for system (7.14.1) [or if (7.14.8) is satisfied for system (7.14.2)], then the Hopfield neural network (7.14.3) without delays and the Hopfield neural network with delay (7.14.1) [or the Cohen-Grossberg neural network (7.14.4) without delays and the Cohen-Grossberg neural network with delays (7.14.2)] are globally stable (for almost every $I \in \Re^n$), and furthermore, both system (7.14.3) and system (7.14.5) [or both system (7.14.4) and system (7.14.2)] have identical equilibria with the same local stability properties at each equilibrium.

We summarize the above results in the following *more general* and precise equivalent statements, given here for system (7.14.1). When system (7.14.1) satisfies (7.14.7) [and thus, (7.14.1) is globally stable], then the following statements are equivalent:

1) x_e is a stable equilibrium of (7.14.1);

2) x_e is an asymptotically stable equilibrium of (7.14.1);

3) φ_{x_e} is a local minimum of the energy functional given by (7.14.6), where $\varphi_{x_e} \in C([-\tau, 0], \Re^n)$ such that $\varphi_{x_e} \equiv x_e$; and

4) $J(x_e)$ is positive definite, where $J(x)$ is given in (7.3.2).

The above results show that when the time delay τ is sufficiently small (i.e., when $\tau \beta \|T_1\| < 1$), then a study of the stability properties of the equilibria of a Hopfield neural network with delays [system (7.14.1)] can be reduced to a study of the stability properties of the

7.14. SUMMARY

equilibria of a corresponding Hopfield neural network without delays [system (7.14.3)].

All of the preceding statements apply also to Cohen-Grossberg neural networks with multiple delays, (7.14.2), with condition (7.14.7) replaced by condition (7.14.8).

C. Systems with Non-Symmetric Interconnecting Structure

When the interconnecting structure in neural networks described by equations of the form

$$\dot{x}(t) = -Cx(t) + TS(x(t-\tau)) + I \qquad (7.14.10)$$

is not symmetric, the network will in general be no longer globally stable. In such cases, the local stability properties of the individual equilibria are of great interest.

In the present chapter we established conditions for asymptotic stability of an equilibrium of (7.14.10), assuming (without loss of generality) that $I = 0$, so that (7.14.10) assumes the form

$$\dot{x}(t) = -Cx(t) + TS(x(t-\tau)) \qquad (7.14.11)$$

and assuming that the sigmoidal functions $S(\cdot) = [s_1(\cdot), \cdots, s_n(\cdot)]^T$ satisfy the *sector conditions* $(i = 1, \cdots, n)$,

$$0 \leq \sigma_i^m \leq \frac{s_i(x_i)}{x_i} \leq \sigma_i^M. \qquad (7.14.12)$$

For system (7.14.11) we first established in the present chapter the following result: The equilibrium $x_e = 0$ of system (7.14.11) is asymptotically stable *for any arbitrary bounded delay* τ if there exists a positive definite matrix P, and a matrix $\Lambda = \text{diag}[\lambda_1, \cdots, \lambda_n]$, $\lambda_i > 0$, $i = 1, \cdots, n$, such that

$$S^M \triangleq -(C^T P + PC) + \Lambda + PT\Sigma^M \Lambda^{-1} \Sigma^M TP \qquad (7.14.13)$$

is negative definite, where $\Sigma^M = \text{diag}[\sigma_1^M, \cdots, \sigma_n^M]$, and σ_i^M are defined by (7.14.12) for $i = 1, \cdots, n$.

A direct consequence of the above result is the following: The equilibrium $x_e = 0$ of (7.14.11) is asymptotically stable if

$$\|P_0 T\| < \frac{1}{\overline{\sigma}_M} \qquad (7.14.14)$$

where $P_0 = \text{diag}[1/c_1, \cdots, 1/c_n]$ and $\overline{\sigma}^M = \max\{\sigma_i^M : 1 \leq i \leq n\}$.

Both of the above results are applicable to neural networks with arbitrary bounded delays. As noted before, the bounds of delays are frequently not very large and are often known. In these cases, results such as the ones given above will usually be conservative, and therefore, we need to determine results which involve *fixed bounded delays*. To this end, we established the following results in the present chapter: The equilibrium $x_e = 0$ of system (7.14.11) is asymptotically stable if there exists a positive definite matrix P such that

$$\begin{aligned} 2\|PT\|\tilde{\sigma}^M &+ 2\tau[\overline{c} + \|T\|(\tilde{\sigma}^M + \|\Sigma_0\|)] \\ &\times \sqrt{\frac{\lambda_{\max}(P)}{\lambda_{\min}(P)}} \|PT\|(\tilde{\sigma}^M + \|\Sigma_0\|) \\ &< -\lambda_{\max}\Big[(-C + T\Sigma_0)^T P \\ &\quad + P(-C + T\Sigma_0)\Big] \end{aligned} \qquad (7.14.15)$$

where $\tilde{\sigma}^M = \max\{(\sigma_i^M - \sigma_i^m)/2 : 1 \leq i \leq n\}$,

$$\Sigma_0 = \text{diag}\Big[(\sigma_1^m + \sigma_1^M)/2, \cdots, (\sigma_n^m + \sigma_n^M)/2\Big]$$

and $\overline{c} = \max\{c_i : 1 \leq i \leq n\}$.

A direct consequence of the above is the following result: Assume that $-C + T\Sigma_0$ is Hurwitz stable. Then the equilibrium $x_e = 0$ of system (7.14.11) is asymptotically stable if

$$\begin{aligned} 2\|P_1 T\|\tilde{\sigma}^M &+ 2\tau[\overline{c} + \|T\|(\tilde{\sigma}^M + \|\Sigma_0\|)] \\ &\times \sqrt{\frac{\lambda_{\max}(P_1)}{\lambda_{\min}(P_1)}} \|P_1 T\|(\tilde{\sigma}^M + \|\Sigma_0\|) < 1 \end{aligned} \qquad (7.14.16)$$

where $P_1 = P_1^T$ is positive definite and $(-C + T\Sigma_0)^T P_1 + P_1(-C + T\Sigma_0) = -E$, and where E is the identity matrix.

7.14. SUMMARY

When condition (7.14.13) [resp., (7.14.14)] or condition (7.14.15) [resp., (7.14.16)] are not satisfied, the equilibrium $x_e = 0$ of system (7.14.11) may still be asymptotically stable. This can be ascertained by the use of the linearization of system (7.14.11) given by

$$\dot{x}(t) = -C(x(t) + TD(0)x(t-\tau) \quad (7.14.17)$$

where

$$D(x) = \text{diag}[s'_1(x_1), \cdots, s'_n(x_n)].$$

Using the linearization (7.14.17), we then devised in the present chapter a method of obtaining an estimate of the domain of attraction of an asymptotically stable equilibrium $x_e = 0$ of system (7.14.11).

The chapter was concluded with a robust stability analysis of system (7.14.11). To this end, we employed a perturbation model for system (7.14.11) described by equations of the form

$$\dot{x}(t) = -(C + \Delta C)x(t) + (T + \Delta T)S(x(t-\tau)). \quad (7.14.18)$$

For *arbitrary bounded delays*, we established the following result in the present chapter: The equilibrium $x_e = 0$ of neural network (7.14.18) is asymptotically stable for any arbitrary bounded delay if

$$\begin{array}{c} 2\|P_0\| \cdot \|\Delta C\| + \|P_0 T\|^2 (\overline{\sigma}^M)^2 + \|P_0\|^2 \|\Delta T\|^2 (\overline{\sigma}^M)^2 \\ + 2\|P_0 T\| \cdot \|\Delta T\| \overline{\sigma}^M < 1 \end{array} \quad (7.14.19)$$

where $P_0 = \text{diag}[1/c_1, \cdots, 1/c_n]$ and $\overline{\sigma}^M = \max\{\sigma_i^M : 1 \leq i \leq n\}$.

For *fixed bounded delays*, we established the following results: The equilibrium $x_e = 0$ of neural network (7.14.18) is asymptotically stable if

$$\begin{array}{c} 2(\|P_1 T\| + \|P_1\| \cdot \|\Delta T\|)\tilde{\sigma}^M + 2\tau[(\|C\| + \|\Delta C\|) \\ + (\|T\| + \|\Delta T\|)(\tilde{\sigma}^M + \|\Sigma_0\|)]\sqrt{\dfrac{\lambda_{\max}(P)}{\lambda_{\min}(P)}} \\ \times (\|P_1 T\| + \|P_1\| \cdot \|\Delta T\|)(\tilde{\sigma}^M + \|\Sigma_0\|) \\ + 2(\|\Delta C\| + \|\Delta T\| \cdot \|\Sigma_0\|)\|P_1\| < 1 \end{array} \quad (7.14.20)$$

where P_1 is positive definite, $P_1(-C+T\Sigma_0)^T+(-C+T\Sigma_0)P_1 = -E$, E denotes the identity matrix,

$$\Sigma_0 = \text{diag}\left[(\sigma_1^m + \sigma_1^M)/2, \cdots, (\sigma_n^m + \sigma_n^M)/2\right],$$

$\tilde{\sigma}^M = \max\{(\sigma_i^M - \sigma_i^m)/2, \ i = 1, \cdots, n\}$, and where we assumed that $-C + T\Sigma_0$ is Hurwitz stable.

Finally, when the perturbation norms $\|\Delta C\|$ and $\|\Delta T\|$ are known a priori, the above results were used to obtain *estimates of the domain of attraction* of the equilibrium $x_e = 0$, similarly as in the case of unperturbed neural networks.

7.15 Notes and References

For discussions of electronic implementations of Hopfield neural networks by VLSI technology, refer to [7], [11], [24]. In such implementations, time delays are unavoidably introduced, and these in turn, may give rise to oscillations [1], [6], [17]. Hopfield neural networks with delays have received attention in several works (e.g., [2], [4], [8], [17] [19], [21] [22] [26]–[28]). Although most of these works address local stability issues, the global stability of Hopfield neural networks [17], [19], and [26] and Cohen-Grossberg neural networks [19], [27], have also been studied extensively. The results presented in Sections 7.1 through 7.5 of the present chapter are based on material developed in [19] and [26] while Sections 7.6 through 7.8 rely on material given in [19] and [27].

In [17], a special case of system (7.1.2) is considered, given by

$$\dot{x}(t) = -x(t) + T_1 S(x(t-\tau)). \tag{7.15.1}$$

This is clearly a special case of (7.3.1) [letting $C = E$, $T_0 = 0$, and $I = 0$ in (7.3.1)]. It is assumed in [17] that the components of $S(x)$ are identical sigmoidal functions. Linearizing (7.15.1) about the equilibrium $x_e = 0$, the authors of [17] obtained the bound

$$\tau\beta\lambda_{\min}(T_1) < \frac{\pi}{2} \tag{7.15.2}$$

for a sufficient condition of asymptotic stability. Relying on simulations and experimental evidence, it is *conjectured* in [17] that the bound (7.15.2) is also a sufficient condition for the global stability of (7.15.1). When applying Theorem 7.3.1 to system (7.15.1), one obtains the bound

$$\tau\beta\|T\| < 1 \qquad (7.15.3)$$

as a sufficient condition for global stability. Although condition (7.15.3) is more conservative than condition (7.15.2), it must be emphasized that the former is obtained by rigorous proof while the derivation of the latter involves experimentation and conjectures.

In addition to the above, we point to [4], where a global stability condition is established for a class of neural networks described by equations of the form (7.3.1), however, with $S(x)$ having saturation functions as components.

Finally, Sections 7.9 through 7.12 are based on material presented in [28].

Bibliography

[1] U an der Heiden. Analysis of Neural Networks. New York, NY: Springer-Verlag, 1980.

[2] TA Burton. Averaged neural networks. Neural Networks 6:677–680, 1993.

[3] E Cheres, ZL Palmor, S Gutman. Quantitative measures of robustness for systems including delayed perturbations. IEEE Transactions on Automatic Control 34:1203–1204, 1989.

[4] PP Civalleri, M Gilli, L Pandolfi. On stability of cellular neural networks with delay. IEEE Transactions on Circuits and Systems-I: Fundamental Theory and Applications 40:157–165, 1993.

[5] M Cohen, S Grossberg. Absolute stability of global pattern formation and parallel memory storage by competitive neural networks. IEEE Transactions on Systems, Man, and Cybernetics 13:815–826, 1983.

[6] BD Coleman, GH Renninger. Periodic solutions of certain nonlinear integral equations with a time lag. SIAM Journal on Applied Mathematics 31:111, 1976.

[7] JS Denker. Ed. Neural Networks for Computing. AIP Conference Proceedings, no 151, Snowbird, UT, 1986.

[8] M Gilli. Stability of cellular neural networks and delayed cellular neural networks with nonpositive templates and nonmonotonic output functions. IEEE Transactions on Circuits and Systems-I: Fundamental Theory and Applications 41:518–528, 1994.

[9] C Goffman. Calculus of Several Variables. New York, NY: Harper and Row, 1965.

[10] J Hale. Theory of Functional Differential Equations. Berlin, Germany: Springer-Verlag, 1977.

[11] JJ Hopfield, DW Tank. Computing with neural circuits: A model. Science 2:625–633, 1986.

[12] DG Kelly. Stability in contractive nonlinear neural networks. IEEE Transactions on Biomedical Engineering 37:231–242, 1990.

[13] DY Khusainov, EA Yun'kova. Estimation of magnitude of retardation in linear differential systems with deviated argument. Ukrainskii Matematicheskii Jhurnal 35:261–264, 1981.

[14] B Kosko. Neural Networks and Fuzzy Systems. Englewood Cliffs, NJ: Prentice-Hall, 1992.

[15] LM Li. Stability of linear neural delay-differential systems. Bulletin of Australian Mathematics Society 38:339–344, 1988.

[16] JH Li, AN Michel, W Porod. Qualitative analysis and synthesis of a class of neural networks. IEEE Transactions on Circuits and Systems 35:976–987, 1988.

[17] CM Marcus, RM Westervelt. Stability of analog neural networks with delay. Physical Review A 39:347–359, 1989.

[18] AN Michel, K Wang, B Hu. Qualitative Theory of Dynamical Systems–The Role of Stability Preserving Mappings. Second Edition. New York, NY: Marcel Dekker, 2001.

[19] AN Michel, K Wang, D Liu, H Ye. Qualitative limitations incurred in implementations of recurrent neural networks. IEEE Control Systems Magazine 15:52–65, 1995.

[20] RK Miller, AN Michel. Ordinary Differential Equations. New York, NY: Academic Press, 1982.

[21] T Roska, C Wu, M Balsi, LO Chua. Stability and dynamics of delay-type general and cellular neural networks. IEEE Transactions on Circuits and Systems-I: Fundamental Theory and Applications 39:487–490, 1992.

[22] T Roska, C Wu, LO Chua. Stability of cellular neural networks with dominant nonlinear and delay-type templates. IEEE Transactions on Circuits and Systems-I: Fundamental Theory and Applications 40:270–272, 1993.

[23] KK Shyu, JJ Yan. Robust stability of uncertain time-delay systems and its stabilization by variable structure control. International Journal of Control 57:237–246, 1993.

[24] DW Tank, JJ Hopfield. Collective computation in neuron-like circuits. Scientific American 257:104–114, 1984.

[25] K Wang, AN Michel. Qualitative analysis of dynamical systems determined by differential inequalities with applications to robust stability. IEEE Transactions on Circuits and Systems-I: Fundamental Theory and Applications 41:377–386, 1994.

[26] H Ye, AN Michel, K Wang. Global stability and local stability of Hopfield neural networks with delays. Physical Review E 50:4206–4213, 1994.

[27] H Ye, AN Michel, K Wang. Qualitative analysis of Cohen-Grossberg neural networks with multiple delays. Physical Review E 51:2611–2618, 1995.

[28] H Ye, AN Michel, K Wang. Robust stability of nonlinear time-delay systems with applications to neural networks. IEEE Transactions on Circuits and Systems-I: Fundamental Theory and Applications 43:532–543, 1996.

Chapter 8

Some Synthesis Methods for Associative Memories

8.1 Introduction: The Outer Product Method and the Projection Learning Rule

In this chapter we present several synthesis methods that are used in the realization of associative memories by means of artificial recurrent neural networks. In the present section we first give an overview of the *Outer Product Method* and the *Projection Learning Rule*, while in Section 8.2 we present some extensions to the latter. In the following two sections, we develop a third synthesis method to realize associative memories, called the *Eigenstructure Method*, using linear systems operating on a closed hypercube in Section 8.3, and a variety of other recurrent neural network models in Section 8.4. In the next two sections, we devise yet another synthesis method for realizing associative memories, which is based on the *Perceptron Training Algorithm*. A variety of recurrent neural network models are employed in Sections 8.5 and 8.6 in implementing this algorithm. Finally, in Section 8.7, a number of specific examples are considered to demonstrate the usefulness of the results presented.

Throughout the chapter we show how the various synthesis procedures are interrelated and we point to their strengths and weaknesses. Further, we provide guidelines that make possible the reduction of the number of undesired spurious memories, and in doing so, to enlarge the basins of attraction of the desired memories.

A. The Outer Product Method

Quite a few results for neural networks are motivated by Hebb's hypothesis [8], which may be summarized as follows [28]: "When units A and B are simultaneously excited, increase the strength between them." As pointed out in [28], this hypothesis is implemented by the Outer Product Method to a certain extent.

The Outer Product Method was introduced by Hopfield in [9] for neural networks described by [cf. (2.1.4)]

$$\begin{cases} du_i/dt = \sum_{j=1}^{n} T_{ij}v_j - b_i u_i + I_i \\ v_i = g(u_i), \quad i = 1, \cdots, n \end{cases} \quad (8.1.1)$$

and in [11] for asynchronous neural networks described by [cf. (2.1.1)]

$$\begin{cases} v_i(k+1) = \text{sgn}(u_i(k)), & 1 \leq i \leq n \\ u_i(k) = \sum_{j=1}^{n} T_{ij}v_j(k) + I_i, & 1 \leq i \leq n. \end{cases} \quad (8.1.2)$$

To store patterns α^i that are bipolar n-vectors, $i = 1, \cdots, m$, the parameter choices determined by the Outer Product Method are given by

$$\begin{cases} T = [T_{ij}] = \sum_{i=1}^{m} \alpha^i (\alpha^i)^T \\ I = (I_1, \cdots, I_n)^T = 0 \end{cases} \quad (8.1.3)$$

where the superscript T represents the transpose. The name *Outer Product Method* is motivated by the fact that the coefficient matrix T consists of the sum of outer products of the patterns to be stored. This method is also called correlation memory. In addition to Eq. (8.1.3), the Outer Product Method involves the differential form given below [10], by means of which new patterns can be learned by the network. We have,

$$\Delta T_{ij} = \eta \gamma_i \gamma_j$$

8.1. INTRODUCTION

where η is a small positive number that determines the learning rate of the network and $\gamma = (\gamma_1, \cdots, \gamma_n)^T \in \Re^n$ represents a new pattern for the network to learn.

In [9] and [11], Hopfield demonstrates that neural networks (8.1.1) and (8.1.2) have computational capabilities and are free of sustained oscillations, utilizing a Lyapunov-type argument. For example, in analyzing system (8.1.1), an energy function of the form

$$E(v) = -\frac{1}{2}v^T T v - v^T I + \sum_{j=1}^n b_j \int_0^{v_j} g^{-1}(\eta) d\eta \qquad (8.1.4)$$

is used. The time derivative of $E(v)$ along the solutions of system (8.1.1), denoted by $D_{(8.1.1)}E(v)$, is given by

$$\begin{aligned}
D_{(8.1.1)}E(v) &= \sum_{i=1}^n (\partial E/\partial v_i) \cdot (\partial v_i/\partial u_i) \cdot (du_i/dt) \\
&= \sum_{i=1}^n \left(-\sum_{j=1}^n T_{ij}v_j - I_i + b_i u_i\right) \cdot (\partial g(u_i)/\partial u_i) \cdot (du_i/dt) \\
&= -\sum_{i=1}^n (du_i/dt)^2 \cdot (\partial g(u_i)/\partial u_i) \\
&\leq 0.
\end{aligned}$$

The second equality above is true under the assumption that T is a symmetric matrix (i.e., $T_{ij} = T_{ji}$). The last inequality above is true since $(du_i/dt)^2 \geq 0$ and since $\partial g(u_i)/\partial u_i > 0$ because g is assumed to be monotonically increasing (recall that g is assumed to be a sigmoidal function). Moreover, $D_{(8.1.1)}E(v) = 0$ only when $du_i/dt = 0$ for $i = 1, \cdots, n$. But this will occur only at equilibrium points.

The function $E(v)$ is bounded from below and $E(v) \to \infty$ as $v_i \to \pm 1$ for any i [due to the integral terms in (8.1.4)]. Accordingly, we conclude that (8.1.1) cannot sustain oscillations, that all solutions of (8.1.1) seek local minima of $E(v)$, and that local minima of $E(v)$ correspond to the asymptotically stable equilibria of system (8.1.1). An oscillation of system (8.1.1) requires that $u(t) = u(t + \tau)$ for all t for some $\tau > 0$. In the present case, however, $E(v(t)) \neq E(v(t + \tau))$ since $E(v(t))$ is monotonically decreasing, unless $u(t)$ is at an equilibrium of (8.1.1).

A similar argument as above works for system (8.1.2), making use of an energy function of the form

$$E(v) = -\frac{1}{2}v^T T v - v^T I \qquad (8.1.5)$$

and replacing the derivative of $E(v)$ along the solutions of (8.1.1) with the first forward difference of $E(v)$ along the solutions of (8.1.2). The difference between expressions of the energy functions in (8.1.4) and (8.1.5) is in the integral terms given in Eq. (8.1.4). The implication of this difference is discussed in Hopfield's *high-gain argument* [11]. In this case, the input-output relationship of the neurons in the neural network (8.1.1) is expressed as $v_i = g(\lambda u_i)$, or equivalently, as

$$u_i = \frac{1}{\lambda} g^{-1}(v_i). \qquad (8.1.6)$$

In (8.1.6), $\lambda > 0$ denotes a parameter, called the *gain* of the function g. If λ is allowed to vary, then as $\lambda \to \infty$ each integral term

$$\frac{1}{\lambda} \int_0^{v_i} g^{-1}(\eta) d\eta$$

in (8.1.4) will become negligible for all $-1 < v_i < 1$, $i = 1, \cdots, n$. In this case, the extreme points of the energy function given in (8.1.5) will be arbitrarily close to corresponding extreme points of the energy function given in (8.1.4). Accordingly, if in a given design procedure we obtain an interconnection matrix T for system (8.1.2), then the same T may also be used for system (8.1.1), provided that the gain λ for the function g is sufficiently large.

Next, we outline the derivation of the Outer Product Method for neural network (8.1.2), originally given by Hopfield, making use of the function given in (8.1.5).

In [30], Tank and Hopfield consider the energy function

$$E(v) = -\frac{1}{2}\sum_{i=1}^{m}\left[(\alpha^i)^T v\right]^2 = -\frac{1}{2}v^T \left[\sum_{i=1}^{m}\alpha^i(\alpha^i)^T\right] v \qquad (8.1.7)$$

where α^i, $i = 1, \cdots, m$, are desired (asymptotically stable) equilibrium points for system (8.1.2). This function is of the same form as

8.1. INTRODUCTION

the one given in Eq. (8.1.5), provided that

$$I = 0 \text{ and } T = [T_{ij}] = \sum_{i=1}^{m} \alpha^i (\alpha^i)^T. \tag{8.1.8}$$

We note that the parameters given in (8.1.8) are identical to the ones specified earlier in the Outer Product Method given in (8.1.3).

The rationale for choosing the energy function (8.1.7) is as follows. If the vectors α^i, $i = 1, \cdots, m$, are mutually orthogonal [i.e., $(\alpha^i)^T \alpha^j = 0$ when $i \neq j$], then (8.1.7) yields

$$E(\alpha^i) = -\frac{n^2}{2}, \quad i = 1, \cdots, m$$

(since all entries of α^i are ± 1) and $E(v)$ assumes minima at the α^i, $i = 1, \cdots, m$. Since

$$T\alpha^i = \left[\sum_{j=1}^{m} \alpha^j (\alpha^j)^T\right] \alpha^i = n\alpha^i$$

it follows that each of the α^i is an equilibrium of the neural network (8.1.2) [or of the neural network (8.1.1) when the gain of the function g is sufficiently high].

For the more general case where the prototype patterns α^i, $i = 1, \cdots, m$, are not mutually orthogonal, the energy function $E(v)$ given in (8.1.7) does not necessarily assume a minimum at α^i, nor is the vector α^i necessarily an equilibrium for the network (8.1.2). More specifically, we have, e.g.,

$$T\alpha^i = \left[\sum_{j=1}^{m} \alpha^j (\alpha^j)^T\right] \alpha^i = n\alpha^i + \sum_{j=1, j \neq i}^{m} \alpha^j (\alpha^j)^T \alpha^i$$

which may be viewed as a "signal" $n\alpha^i$ plus a "noise term"

$$\sum_{j=1, j \neq i}^{m} \alpha^j (\alpha^j)^T \alpha^i.$$

If any component of the noise vector has magnitude larger than n and sign opposite to the corresponding component of α^i, then the vector α^i will not be an equilibrium of the network. We see that the noise term increases in magnitude as the number of prototype patterns (desired equilibria) increases.

Several simulation studies of the Outer Product Method suggest that this method is capable of storing reliably approximately $0.15n$ arbitrary prototype vectors [4] where n is the order of the network.

B. The Projection Learning Rule

An effective associative memory must at least guarantee that (i) each prototype pattern is an equilibrium of the network, and (ii) each prototype pattern is attractive. The Outer Product Method was shown to satisfy item (i) only for the special case where the prototype vectors are mutually orthogonal. Utilizing pseudo-inverse techniques, Personnaz et al. [25], [26] have developed a method that guarantees item (i), but not item (ii). Their result holds for arbitrary prototype vectors. However, to simplify the subsequent discussion, we will assume that the prototype vectors are linearly independent.

The neural network model considered in [25] and [26] is described by equations of the form [cf. (2.1.3)]

$$\begin{cases} v_i(k+1) = g(u_i(k)), & 1 \leq i \leq n \\ u_i(k) = \sum_{j=1}^{n} T_{ij} v_j(k) + I_i, & 1 \leq i \leq n \end{cases} \quad (8.1.9)$$

with $g(u) = \text{sgn}(u)$. System (8.1.9) is the synchronous counterpart to (8.1.2). Let $v = (v_1, \cdots, v_n)^T$, $T = [T_{ij}] = [T_{ji}]$, $I = (I_1, \cdots, I_n)^T$, and let $(Tv + I)_i$ denote the ith element of the vector $Tv + I$. It is straightforward to verify that a vector α^* is an equilibrium of the network if

$$(T\alpha^* + I)_i \alpha_i^* \geq 0, \quad i = 1, \cdots, n. \quad (8.1.10)$$

If it is desired to store m such patterns in the network, then a total of nm inequalities of the form (8.1.10) must be satisfied. One solution, established in [25] and [26], is presented in the following.

8.1. INTRODUCTION

For
$$-1 \leq I_i \leq 1, \quad i = 1, \cdots, n \qquad (8.1.11)$$
each of the prototype patterns will be an equilibrium of (8.1.9) if
$$T\alpha^k = \alpha^k, \quad k = 1, \cdots, m. \qquad (8.1.12)$$
Letting
$$\Sigma = \begin{bmatrix} \alpha^1 \vdots \cdots \vdots \alpha^m \end{bmatrix},$$
Eq. (8.1.12) yields the matrix equation
$$T\Sigma = \Sigma.$$
One solution to this set of nm linear equations is given by
$$T = \Sigma\Sigma^\dagger \qquad (8.1.13)$$
where $\Sigma^\dagger$ denotes the Moore-Penrose pseudo-inverse [1]. When the prototype vectors are linearly independent, we obtain
$$\Sigma^\dagger = (\Sigma^T \Sigma)^{-1} \Sigma^T$$
and
$$T = \Sigma(\Sigma^T \Sigma)^{-1} \Sigma^T. \qquad (8.1.14)$$

The computation of matrix T in Eq. (8.1.14) involves an $m \times m$ matrix inversion, which is much simpler than the inversion of an $n \times n$ matrix since usually m is much smaller than n. Furthermore, the pseudo-inverse can be calculated by an m-step iterative procedure [1], which eliminates the need for matrix inversions entirely.

In [26], the above method is referred to as the *Projection Learning Rule*, referring to the fact that the interconnection matrix T, when defined by Eq. (8.1.13), is the orthogonal projection matrix from $\Re^n$ onto the linear subspace spanned by the vectors α^k, $k = 1, \cdots, m$.

In the case where the prototype vectors are mutually orthogonal [i.e., $(\alpha^i)^T \alpha^j = 0$ if $i \neq j$ and $(\alpha^i)^T \alpha^j = n$ if $i = j$ for each $i, j = 1, \cdots, m$], we have
$$\Sigma^T \Sigma = nE \qquad (8.1.15)$$

where E is the $m \times m$ identity matrix. Equation (8.1.15) implies that

$$T = \frac{1}{n}\Sigma\Sigma^T.$$

Hence, in this special case, the Projection Learning Rule reduces to an equivalent of the Outer Product Method if we choose $I_i = 0$ in (8.1.11) [cf. (8.1.3)]. In all other cases, the Projection Learning Rule will guarantee that each prototype pattern is an equilibrium of the network, whereas the Outer Product Method does not provide such assurance.

In the case where $(\Sigma^T\Sigma)$ is an $n \times n$ invertible matrix, T will reduce to the $n \times n$ identity matrix. In fact, the identity matrix is always a solution to Eq. (8.1.12). However, this choice of an interconnection structure does not lead to interesting dynamics because if Eq. (8.1.11) is also satisfied, all of the 2^n possible binary (or bipolar) vectors will be stable. Thus, this design produces at least $(2^n - m)$ undesired stable equilibria. One case where $(\Sigma^T\Sigma)$ is $n \times n$ and invertible is when $m = n$ linearly independent patterns are to be stored.

Although the Projection Learning Rule is described here for system (8.1.2) operating in a synchronous mode [i.e., (8.1.9)], this method is equally applicable to the continuous-time model (8.1.1) when $g(u) = \text{sgn}(u)$. Let $B = \text{diag}(b_1, \cdots, b_n)$, $u = (u_1, \cdots, u_n)^T$, $T = [T_{ij}]$, $I = (I_1, \cdots, I_n)$, and $v_j = \text{sgn}(u_j)$, $j = 1, \cdots, n$, where $b_i \neq 0$, and u_i, T_{ij}, and I_i are all defined in (8.1.1). The condition for α^* to be an equilibrium of (8.1.1) is given by

$$0 = T\alpha^* - Bu + I.$$

A solution, equivalent to the Projection Learning Rule, is given by defining

$$u = B^{-1}(\alpha^* + I)$$

and choosing T and I to satisfy

$$T\alpha^* = \alpha^* \quad \text{and} \quad -1 \leq I_i \leq 1, \quad i = 1, \cdots, n.$$

8.2. PROJECTION LEARNING RULE

The Projection Learning Rule (8.1.13) results in the state $u^* = B^{-1}(\alpha^* + I)$ being an equilibrium and $\alpha_i^* = \text{sgn}(u_i^*)$, $i = 1, \cdots, n$.

It is verified in [26] by means of simulations of specific examples that for orthogonal prototype patterns each prototype will attract all initial states within a Hamming distance of $n/(2m)$.

The Projection Learning Rule constitutes an improvement over the Outer Product Method in the sense that the former guarantees that each prototype vector is stored as an equilibrium, whereas the latter does not provide this guarantee. An additional improvement, that of guaranteeing the attractivity of all prototype patterns, is provided in the methods developed in the subsequent sections of the present chapter.

8.2 Some Extensions to the Projection Learning Rule

In this section, we first present a synthesis method which incorporates stability results (developed in Section 5.6) into the Projection Learning Rule. Next, we develop an iterative learning algorithm based on the Projection Learning Rule.

A. Projection Learning Rule with Stability Constraints

Consider neural networks described by equations of the form,

$$\begin{cases} u_i(k+1) = \sum_{j=1}^{n} T_{ij} v_j(k) - a_i u_i(k) + I_i \\ v_i(k) = g(u_i(k)), \quad i = 1, \cdots, n, \end{cases} \quad (8.2.1)$$

where $T_{ij} \in \Re$, $a_i \in \Re$, $I_i \in \Re$, $g\colon \Re \to (-1,1)$ is monotonically increasing and continuously differentiable with $g(0) = 0$, $\lim_{\sigma \to \infty} g(\sigma) = +1$, and $\lim_{\sigma \to -\infty} g(\sigma) = -1$. We can rewrite equation (8.2.1) in vector form as

$$\begin{cases} u(k+1) = Tv(k) - Au(k) + I \\ v(k) = \bar{g}(u(k)) \end{cases} \quad (8.2.2)$$

where $T = [T_{ij}] \in \Re^{n \times n}$, $A = \text{diag}[a_1, \cdots, a_n]$, $I = (I_1, \cdots, I_n)^T \in \Re^n$, and $\bar{g} = [g, \cdots, g]^T : \Re^n \to (-1, 1)^n$.

Assume that we are given a set of vectors $v^i \in \Re^n$, $i = 1, \cdots, m$, to be stored as output vectors in neural network (8.2.2), corresponding to a set of asymptotically stable equilibria given by u^i, $i = 1, \cdots, m$. We will refer to $v^i \in \Re^n$, $i = 1, \cdots, m$, as *desired memory vectors* or *prototype vectors*. In order for u^i, $i = 1, \cdots, m$, to be equilibria of (8.2.2) we require that

$$u^i = Tv^i + I - Au^i \quad (8.2.3)$$

for $i = 1, \cdots, m$. If we write

$$L_m = \begin{bmatrix} v^1 & \vdots & \cdots & \vdots & v^m \end{bmatrix}$$

and

$$H_m = \begin{bmatrix} u^1 & \vdots & \cdots & \vdots & u^m \end{bmatrix},$$

(8.2.3) can be expressed as

$$H_m = TL_m + \tilde{I} - AH_m \quad (8.2.4)$$

where $\tilde{I} = \begin{bmatrix} I & \vdots & \cdots & \vdots & I \end{bmatrix} \in \Re^{n \times m}$. To solve A, T, and I from (8.2.4), we let

$$R_{m,j} = \begin{bmatrix} L_m^T & \vdots & Q_m & \vdots & H_{m,j}^T \end{bmatrix}, \quad j = 1, \cdots, n$$

and

$$W_{m,j} = [T_{j1}, \cdots, T_{jn}, I_j, -a_j], \quad j = 1, \cdots, n$$

where $H_{m,j} \in \Re^m$ is the jth row of H_m and $Q_m \in \Re^m$ is a column vector containing all ones. Equation (8.2.4) is equivalent to

$$H_{m,j}^T = R_{m,j} W_{m,j}^T, \quad j = 1, \cdots, n \quad (8.2.5)$$

where matrix $R_{m,j} \in R^{m \times (n+2)}$ and row vector $W_{m,j} \in R^{n+2}$. A well-known solution of (8.2.5) is given by

$$W_{m,j}^T = R_{m,j}^\dagger H_{m,j}^T, \quad j = 1, \cdots, n \quad (8.2.6)$$

8.2. PROJECTION LEARNING RULE

where $R_{m,j}^\dagger$ denotes a pseudo-inverse of $R_{m,j}$ which may not be unique (cf. [1]). When $R_{m,j}$ has full rank, its pseudo-inverse can be easily determined and in this case, (8.2.6) assumes the form

$$W_{m,j}^T = R_{m,j}^T (R_{m,j} R_{m,j}^T)^{-1} H_{m,j}^T, \quad j = 1, \cdots, n.$$

The A, T, and I obtained above will guarantee that the given set of vectors u^i, $i = 1, \cdots, m$, are equilibrium points of neural network (8.2.1) [or (8.2.2)]. To ensure that each of these vectors is asymptotically stable, i.e., to ensure that each of the prototype patterns, v^i, $i = 1, \cdots, m$, is attractive, we will require that

$$F_i = 1 - |a_i| - \sum_{j=1}^n |T_{ij}| > 0, \quad i = 1, \cdots, n. \quad (8.2.7)$$

The stability condition given in (8.2.7) is a consequence of the stability analysis results developed in Chapter 5 (see Section 5.6). In [19], an algorithm is presented which ensures that the constraints (8.2.7) are actually satisfied by the synthesized network.

B. An Iterative Projection Learning Algorithm

In this subsection, we assume that $a_i = 0$ for $i = 1, \cdots, n$.

Suppose that a neural network (8.2.2) has been designed in such a manner that the vectors $\{u^1, \cdots, u^m\}$ are stored as asymptotically stable equilibrium points and suppose that we desire to store an additional pattern (i.e., we wish to learn a new pattern)

$$v^{m+1} = \bar{g}(u^{m+1})$$

corresponding to an equilibrium point u^{m+1}. We define

$$L_{m+1} = \begin{bmatrix} v^1 & \vdots & \cdots & \vdots & v^m & \vdots & v^{m+1} \end{bmatrix} = \begin{bmatrix} L_m & \vdots & v^{m+1} \end{bmatrix}$$

$$H_{m+1} = \begin{bmatrix} u^1 & \vdots & \cdots & \vdots & u^m & \vdots & v^{m+1} \end{bmatrix} = \begin{bmatrix} H_m & \vdots & u^{m+1} \end{bmatrix}.$$

Let $H_{m+1,j} \in R^{m+1}$ denote the jth row of H_{m+1}. Then

$$H_{m+1,j} = \left[H_{m,j} \vdots u_j^{m+1}\right], \quad j = 1, \cdots, n$$

$$W_{m+1,j} = [T_{j1}, \cdots, T_{jn}, I_j, 0], \quad j = 1, \cdots, n$$

and

$$R_{m+1,j} = \left[L_{m+1}^T \vdots Q_{m+1} \vdots H_{m+1,j}^T\right]$$

$$= \left[L_{m+1}^T \vdots Q_{m+1} \vdots Z_{m+1}\right]$$

$$= \begin{bmatrix} L_m^T & \vdots & Q_m & \vdots & Z_m \\ \cdots & \vdots & \cdots & \vdots & \cdots \\ (v^{m+1})^T & \vdots & 1 & \vdots & 0 \end{bmatrix}$$

$$= \begin{bmatrix} R_{m,j} \\ \cdots \\ M_{m,j} \end{bmatrix}$$

$$= \begin{bmatrix} R_{m,j} \\ \cdots \\ M_m \end{bmatrix}$$

where u_j^{m+1} is the jth element of u^{m+1}, $M_{m,j} = \left[(v^{m+1})^T \vdots 1 \vdots 0\right] = M_m \in R^{n+2}$ (which is independent of j), and $Q_{m+1} \in R^{m+1}$ is a column vector containing all ones, and Z^{m+1} is a column vector containing all zeros. In order to express $W_{m+1,j}$ in terms of $W_{m,j}$ (and thus to obtain an iterative learning algorithm), we will require the following lemma from [32].

Lemma 8.2.1 Assume that $Z = [Y \vdots y] \in \Re^{n \times (k+1)}$ where Y consists of the first k columns of Z and $y \in \Re^n$ is the $k + 1$st column of Z. Then the pseudo-inverse of Z, $Z^\dagger$, can be expressed as

$$Z^\dagger = \begin{bmatrix} Y^\dagger - Y^\dagger y \eta \\ \cdots \\ \eta \end{bmatrix}$$

8.2. PROJECTION LEARNING RULE

where

$$\eta = \begin{cases} (y - YY^\dagger y)^\dagger, & \text{if } (E - YY^\dagger)y \neq 0 \\ (1 + y^T(YY^T)^\dagger y)^{-1} y^T (YY^T)^\dagger, & \text{if } (E - YY^\dagger)y = 0 \end{cases}$$

where E is the identity matrix. ∎

We will omit the proof of Lemma 8.2.1. For details concerning this proof, refer to Theorem 3.3 in [32].

Invoking Lemma 8.2.1, we now have

$$W_{m+1,j}^T = R_{m+1,j}^\dagger H_{m+1,j}^T$$

$$= \begin{bmatrix} R_{m,j} \\ \cdots \\ M_m \end{bmatrix}^\dagger \begin{bmatrix} H_{m,j}^T \\ \cdots \\ u_j^{m+1} \end{bmatrix}$$

$$= \begin{bmatrix} R_{m,j}^\dagger - b_m^T M_m R_{m,j}^\dagger \vdots b_m^T \end{bmatrix} \begin{bmatrix} H_{m,j}^T \\ \cdots \\ u_j^{m+1} \end{bmatrix}$$

$$= W_{m,j}^T - b_m^T M_m W_{m,j}^T + b_m^T u_j^{m+1}$$

(8.2.8)

where

$$b_m^T = \begin{cases} \left(M_m - M_m R_{m,j}^\dagger R_{m,j} \right)^\dagger, \\ \qquad \text{if } \left(E - R_{m,j}^T (R_{m,j}^T)^\dagger \right) M_m^T \neq 0 \\ \\ \left(R_{m,j}^T R_{m,j} \right)^\dagger M_m^T \left(1 + M_m (R_{m,j}^T R_{m,j})^\dagger M_m^T \right)^{-1}, \\ \qquad \text{if } \left(E - R_{m,j}^T (R_{m,j}^T)^\dagger \right) M_m^T = 0. \end{cases}$$

We can express (8.2.8) in vector form as

$$W_{m+1}^T = W_m^T + \Delta W_m^T \qquad (8.2.9)$$

where

$$\Delta W_m^T = b_m^T \left[(u^{m+1})^T - M_m W_m^T \right]. \qquad (8.2.10)$$

The preceding result enables us to store an additional pattern v^{m+1} (i.e., to add an additional equilibrium point u^{m+1} to the neural network corresponding to the pattern v^{m+1}), without affecting the patterns $v^1, \cdots, v^m$ already stored in the network. The asymptotic stability of the equilibrium points is guaranteed by choosing the matrix T using the above iterative algorithm, with the constraints given by (note that $a_i = 0$, $i = 1, \cdots, n$)

$$F_i = 1 - \sum_{i=1}^{n} |T_{ij}| > 0, \quad i = 1, \cdots, n \tag{8.2.11}$$

(refer to [19] for details on how to implement the constraints (8.2.11) algorithmically).

If we apply (8.2.9) and (8.2.10) starting from $m = 1$, we will have an iterative learning algorithm that enables us to store (learn) iteratively *all* of the desired equilibrium points $u^1, \cdots, u^m$.

8.3 The Eigenstructure Method

In the present section we develop a third synthesis method for the implementation of associative memories by artificial recurrent neural networks, called the *Eigenstructure Method*. In doing so, we first consider *linear systems operating on a closed hypercube*, introduced in Chapter 2. In the next section we will adapt this method to other types of neural networks [described by equations (2.2.4), (2.2.6), (2.3.4), (2.5.1), and (2.6.7)].

Recall that linear systems operating on a closed hypercube are described by equations of the form

$$\dot{x} = Tx + I, \quad x \in D^n \tag{8.3.1}$$

where $\dot{x}$ denotes the derivative of x with respect to time t, $T = [T_{ij}] \in \Re^{n \times n}$ is a constant matrix, $I = (I_1, \cdots, I_n)^T$ is a constant vector, and D^n denotes the closed unit hypercube in $\Re^n$, given by

$$D^n \triangleq \{x \in \Re^n : -1 \leq x_i \leq 1, \ i = 1, \cdots, n\}.$$

8.3. EIGENSTRUCTURE METHOD

In this section, we will concern ourselves with the design problem in which the desired memory vectors are located at the the corners of the hypercube D^n, i.e., we will consider the case where desired memory vectors are given by a set of *bipolar* vectors. We will use B^n to denote the corners of the hypercube D^n, i.e.,

$$B^n \triangleq \{x \in \Re^n : x_i = +1 \text{ or } x_i = -1\}.$$

In the following, we formulate the synthesis problem to be tackled in the present section.

Synthesis Problem Given m vectors in B^n, say $\alpha^1, \cdots, \alpha^m$, how can we properly choose a pair $\{T, I\}$ such that the resulting synthesized system (8.3.1) has the properties enumerated below?

1) $\alpha^1, \cdots, \alpha^m$ are asymptotically stable equilibrium points of system (8.3.1).

2) The system has no oscillatory solutions.

3) The total number of the spurious asymptotically stable equilibrium points [i.e., asymptotically stable equilibrium points of (8.3.1) contained in $B^n - \{\alpha^1, \cdots, \alpha^m\}$] is as small as possible.

4) The domain of attraction of each desired pattern α^i is as large as possible. ∎

In solving the above synthesis problem, we will employ the corollary given below which is a direct consequence of Case III of Theorem 4.4.1.

Corollary 8.3.1 If $\alpha \in B^n$ and if

$$T\alpha + I \in G(\alpha) \tag{8.3.2}$$

where

$$G(\alpha) \triangleq \{x \in \Re^n : x_i \alpha_i > 0, \ i = 1, \cdots, n\} \tag{8.3.3}$$

then α is an asymptotically stable equilibrium of (8.3.1). ∎

When in (8.3.1), $x = \alpha \in B^n$, we have

$$\min_{1 \leq i \leq n} \{(T\alpha + I)_i \cdot \alpha_i\} > 0$$

when (8.3.2) is satisfied, where $(T\alpha + I)_i$ denotes the ith component of $T\alpha + I$. This implies that $x = \alpha \in B^n$ is an asymptotically stable equilibrium of (8.3.1) according to Theorem 4.4.1.

In view of Corollary 8.3.1 and the results presented in Chapter 4, we can approach the preceding synthesis problem in the following manner.

Synthesis Strategy Given m vectors in B^n, say $\alpha^1, \cdots, \alpha^m$, find an $n \times n$ matrix $T = [T_{ij}]$ and a vector $I = (I_1, \cdots, I_n)^T$ such that:

1) T is symmetric.

2) For $i = 1, \cdots, m$,
$$\alpha^i = T\alpha^i + I. \tag{8.3.4}$$

3) All eigenvalues of T are negative with magnitude as large as possible. ∎

Remark 8.3.1 Following the above synthesis strategy, we have:

1) By Theorem 4.5.1, the synthesized system (8.3.1) will have no oscillatory solutions.

2) By Corollary 8.3.1, the α^i, $i = 1, \cdots, m$, are asymptotically stable equilibria of the synthesized system (8.3.1). ∎

Remark 8.3.2 We will show in a subsequent result (Theorem 8.3.2) that the smaller (i.e., the more negative) the eigenvalues of T are, the fewer spurious asymptotically stable equilibrium points for system (8.3.1) will exist. In general, this will result in larger domains of attraction for the remaining desired asymptotically stable equilibrium points. This will be accomplished by Part 3) of the preceding synthesis strategy. ∎

8.3. EIGENSTRUCTURE METHOD

Suppose now that we are given m vectors in B^n, say $\alpha^1, \cdots, \alpha^m$. Denote the linear subspace of $\Re^n$ generated by the $(m-1)$ vectors $(\alpha^1 - \alpha^m), \cdots, (\alpha^{m-1} - \alpha^m)$ by

$$L = \text{Span}(\alpha^1 - \alpha^m, \cdots, \alpha^{m-1} - \alpha^m)$$

and the affine subspace of $\Re^n$ generated by the vectors $\alpha^1, \cdots, \alpha^m$ by

$$L_a = \text{Aspan}(\alpha^1, \cdots, \alpha^m).$$

Then $L_a = L + \alpha^m$ (i.e., L_a is the affine subspace of $\Re^n$ generated by shifting L by α^m, i.e., $L + \alpha^m = \{y \in \Re^n : y = x + \alpha^m, x \in L\}$). Assume that $k = \text{rank}(L)$, that $\{u^1, \cdots, u^k\}$ is an orthonormal basis of L, and that $\{u^{k+1}, \cdots, u^n\}$ is an orthonormal basis of $L^\perp$. ($L^\perp$ denotes the orthogonal complement of L. Thus, if $x \in \Re^n$ and $Y \subset \Re^n$, then $x \perp Y$ means that $x^T \cdot y = 0$ for all $y \in Y$, and $Y^\perp = \{x \in \Re^n : x \perp Y\}$.) Let

$$U^+ = \begin{bmatrix} u^1 \vdots \cdots \vdots u^k \end{bmatrix},$$

$$U^- = \begin{bmatrix} u^{k+1} \vdots \cdots \vdots u^n \end{bmatrix},$$

$$T^+ = \begin{bmatrix} T^+_{ij} \end{bmatrix} = \sum_{i=1}^{k} u^i(u^i)^T = U^+(U^+)^T, \qquad (8.3.5)$$

$$T^- = \begin{bmatrix} T^-_{ij} \end{bmatrix} = \sum_{i=k+1}^{n} u^i(u^i)^T = U^-(U^-)^T, \qquad (8.3.6)$$

and let

$$T_\tau = T^+ - \tau T^- \quad \text{and} \quad I_\tau = \alpha^m - T_\tau \alpha^m$$

where $\tau \in \Re$ is a parameter. For this class of synthesized neural networks,

$$\frac{dx}{dt} = T_\tau x + I_\tau, \quad x \in D^n, \ \tau \in \Re, \qquad (8.3.7)$$

we have the following result.

Lemma 8.3.1

1) T^+ and T^- depend only on the given set $\{\alpha^1, \cdots, \alpha^m\}$ and they are independent of the choice of α^m and of the orthonormal basis $\{u^1, \cdots, u^n\}$ of $\Re^n$. This is also true for T_τ and I_τ, for any $\tau \in \Re$.

2) For any τ, T_τ is symmetric.

3) For any τ and for any $\alpha \in L_a$, $T_\tau \alpha + I_\tau = \alpha$. In particular, for each α^i, $i = 1, \cdots, m$, $T_\tau \alpha^i + I_\tau = \alpha^i$.

Proof: 1) The proof of Part 1 can be found in linear algebra texts (see, e.g., [20]).

2) Since

$$(T^+)^T = \left((U^+)(U^+)^T\right)^T = (U^+)(U^+)^T = T^+$$

it follows that T^+ is symmetric. Also T^- is symmetric, and thus $T_\tau = T^+ - \tau T^-$ is symmetric.

3) If $\alpha \in L_a$, there is a $\sigma = (\sigma_1, \cdots, \sigma_k) \in \Re^k$ such that

$$\alpha = \sigma_1 u^1 + \cdots + \sigma_k u^k + \alpha^m.$$

Then

$$\begin{aligned} T_\tau \alpha + I_\tau &= T_\tau(\sigma_1 u^1 + \cdots + \sigma_k u^k) + (T_\tau \alpha^m + I_\tau) \\ &= (\sigma_1 u^1 + \cdots + \sigma_k u^k) + \alpha^m \\ &= \alpha. \end{aligned}$$

■

From Remark 8.3.1 and Lemma 8.3.1, we obtain the following:

Theorem 8.3.1 With the parameter τ sufficiently large, the synthesized system (8.3.7) has the following properties:

1) Each $\alpha \in B^n \cap L_a$ is an asymptotically stable equilibrium point of (8.3.7). In particular, this is true for $\alpha^1, \cdots, \alpha^m$.

2) There are no oscillatory solutions.

■

8.3. EIGENSTRUCTURE METHOD

Remark 8.3.3 By Theorem 4.5.2, each $\alpha \in L_a \cap B^n$ is a local minimum of the energy function $E: D^n \to \Re$,

$$E(x) = -\frac{1}{2}x^T T_\tau x - x^T I_\tau.$$

In fact, it can be proved that each $\alpha \in L_a \cap B^n$ is a global minimum of the energy function E. ∎

In the following, we address spurious asymptotically stable equilibrium points of the synthesized system (8.3.7).

Theorem 8.3.2 For $-1 < \tau_1 < \tau_2$, if $\alpha \in B^n$ is an asymptotically stable equilibrium point of system (8.3.7) with $\tau = \tau_2$, then α is also an asymptotically stable equilibrium point of system (8.3.7) with $\tau = \tau_1$. The converse may not be true. This implies that when $\tau > -1$, the number of the spurious asymptotically stable equilibrium points of system (8.3.7) contained in B^n decreases as τ increases.

Proof: Take $\lambda_1 = (\tau_2 - \tau_1)/(1 + \tau_2)$ and $\lambda_2 = (1 + \tau_1)/(1 + \tau_2)$. Then $\lambda_1, \lambda_2 \geq 0$, $\lambda_1 + \lambda_2 = 1$, and

$$\begin{aligned}T_{\tau_1}\alpha + I_{\tau_1} &= T^+(\alpha - \alpha^m) - \tau_1 T^-(\alpha - \alpha^m) + \alpha^m \\ &= \lambda_1(T^+(\alpha - \alpha^m) + T^-(\alpha - \alpha^m) + \alpha^m) \\ &\quad + \lambda_2(T^+(\alpha - \alpha^m) - \tau_2 T^-(\alpha - \alpha^m) + \alpha^m) \\ &= \lambda_1 \alpha + \lambda_2(T_{\tau_2}\alpha + I_{\tau_2}),\end{aligned}$$

since $T^+(\alpha - \alpha^m) + T^-(\alpha - \alpha^m) = (T^+ + T^-)(\alpha - \alpha^m) = (\alpha - \alpha^m)$. If α is an asymptotically stable equilibrium point of system (8.3.7) with $\tau = \tau_2$, then by Corollary 8.3.1, we have

$$T_{\tau_2}\alpha + I_{\tau_2} \in G(\alpha).$$

In view of the definition of $G(\alpha)$ given by (8.3.3), it follows that

$$T_{\tau_1}\alpha + I_{\tau_1} = \lambda_1 \alpha + \lambda_2(T_{\tau_2}\alpha + I_{\tau_2}) \in G(\alpha)$$

since $\lambda_1 > 0$ and $\lambda_2 > 0$. By Corollary 8.3.1, α is an asymptotically stable equilibrium of system (8.3.7) with $\tau = \tau_1$. This implies that if α is an asymptotically stable equilibrium of system (8.3.7) with $\tau = \tau_2$, then α is also an asymptotically stable equilibrium of system (8.3.7) with $\tau = \tau_1$.

Clearly, the above also shows that the converse statement may not be true. ∎

In view of the preceding results, we are now in a position to give the following synthesis procedure.

Synthesis Procedure 8.3.1 Suppose that we are given m vectors $\alpha^1, \cdots, \alpha^m$ in B^n, which are to be stored as asymptotically stable equilibrium points for an n dimensional system (8.3.1). We proceed as follows:

1) Compute the $n \times (m-1)$ matrix:

$$Y = \left[\alpha^1 - \alpha^m \vdots \cdots \vdots \alpha^{m-1} - \alpha^m \right].$$

2) Perform a singular value decomposition of Y and obtain the matrices U, V and Σ such that $Y = U\Sigma V^T$, where U and V are unitary matrices and where Σ is a diagonal matrix with the singular values of Y on its diagonal. (This can be accomplished by standard computer routines.) Let

$$Y = \left[y^1 \vdots \cdots \vdots y^{m-1} \right]$$

$$U = \left[u^1 \vdots \cdots \vdots u^n \right]$$

and
$$k = \text{dimension of Span}(y^1, \cdots, y^{m-1}).$$

From the properties of singular value decomposition, we know that $k = \text{rank}(\Sigma)$, $\{u^1, \cdots, u^k\}$ is an orthonormal basis of $\text{Span}(y^1, \cdots, y^{m-1})$ and $\{u^1, \cdots, u^n\}$ is an orthonormal basis of $\Re^n$.

8.3. EIGENSTRUCTURE METHOD

3) Compute
$$T^+ = \left[T_{ij}^+\right] = \sum_{i=1}^{k} u^i (u^i)^T$$
$$T^- = \left[T_{ij}^-\right] = \sum_{i=k+1}^{n} u^i (u^i)^T.$$

4) Choose a large positive value for the parameter τ and compute
$$T_\tau = T^+ - \tau T^-$$
and
$$I_\tau = \alpha^m - T_\tau \alpha^m.$$

Then all vectors in $L_a \cap B^n$, where $L_a = \text{Aspan}(\alpha^1, \cdots, \alpha^m)$, including $\alpha^1, \cdots, \alpha^m$, will be stored as asymptotically stable equilibrium points in the system (8.3.7). ■

Remark 8.3.4 If we wish that in the synthesized system (8.3.7) the constant vector $I_\tau = 0$, we can modify Synthesis Procedure 8.3.1 as follows:

a) In step 1, take $Y = \begin{bmatrix} \alpha^1 \vdots \cdots \vdots \alpha^m \end{bmatrix}$.

b) In step 4, take $I_\tau = 0$.

Then all conclusions will remain unchanged. In particular, each $-\alpha^i$, $i = 1, \cdots, m$, will also be an asymptotically stable equilibrium point of the synthesized system (8.3.7) and the number of stored asymptotically stable equilibrium points of (8.3.7) will approximately be doubled. ■

We have shown earlier in Section 8.1 that the Projection Learning Rule is more general than the Outer Product Method. We have also shown that when the prototype patterns are mutually orthogonal, the Projection Learning Rule reduces to the Outer Product Method. It turns out that the method presented in this section, i.e., the Eigenstructure Method, is more general than the Projection Learning Rule and the Outer Product Method and constitutes a major improvement over these procedures. In particular, the Eigenstructure Method guarantees to store each prototype pattern as an asymptotically stable equilibrium of the network and each prototype pattern is attractive (i.e., an asymptotically stable equilibrium point or an output vector corresponding to an asymptotically stable equilibrium point). Consider

$$Y = \begin{bmatrix} \alpha^1 & \vdots & \cdots & \vdots & \alpha^m \end{bmatrix}.$$

If we denote the singular value decomposition of Y as

$$Y = \begin{bmatrix} U_1 & \vdots & U_2 \end{bmatrix} \begin{bmatrix} D & \vdots & 0 \\ \cdots & \cdots & \cdots \\ 0 & \vdots & 0 \end{bmatrix} \begin{bmatrix} V_1^T \\ \cdots \\ V_2^T \end{bmatrix} = U_1 D V_1^T,$$

then $Y^\dagger = V_1 D^{-1} U_1^T$ is the generalized (Moore-Penrose) pseudo-inverse of Y [2]. From the properties of singular value decomposition [1], [2], we have in (8.3.5)

$$T^+ = U^+(U^+)^T = U_1 U_1^T = YY^\dagger.$$

Therefore, when we choose $\tau = 0$, the Eigenstructure Method reduces in this special case to the Projection Learning Rule [cf. (8.1.13)]. When the prototype patterns are mutually orthogonal, we have in (8.3.5)

$$T^+ = U^+(U^+)^T = YY^\dagger = \frac{1}{n} YY^T. \tag{8.3.8}$$

Note that in (8.3.8) we have used the fact that

$$Y^\dagger = \left(Y^T Y\right)^{-1} Y^T = \frac{1}{n} Y^T$$

when the prototype patterns are mutually orthogonal. Clearly, in this case, the Eigenstructure Method reduces to the Outer Product Method if we choose $\tau = 0$ [cf. (8.1.3)].

8.4. EXTENSIONS TO EIGENSTRUCTURE METHOD

We conclude by noting that an *iterative procedure* for implementing the Eigenstructure Method (which is in the same spirit as the algorithm presented in Section 8.2B for the Projection Learning Rule) has been developed in [33]. We will, however, not pursue this topic further at this time.

8.4 Some Extensions to the Eigenstructure Method

In the present section we adapt the Eigenstructure Method to a number of different recurrent neural networks in the implementation of associative memories.

Neural Network (2.2.6) We restate Eq. (2.2.6) as

$$\begin{cases} \dot{x} = -Ax + Ty + I \\ y = \text{sat}(x) \end{cases} \quad (8.4.1)$$

where $A = \text{diag}[a_1, \cdots, a_n]$ with $a_i > 0$ and the function

$$\text{sat}(x) = (\text{sat}(x_1), \cdots, \text{sat}(x_n))^T$$

is defined by

$$\text{sat}(x_i) = \begin{cases} 1, & x_i > 1 \\ x_i, & -1 \leq x_i \leq 1 \\ -1, & x_i < -1. \end{cases}$$

We will refer to the output vector corresponding to an asymptotically stable equilibrium of (8.4.1) as a (stable) memory vector. In this case, the condition for a bipolar vector to be a memory vector is given by (cf. Lemma 6.6.1)

$$\beta = A^{-1}(T\alpha + I) \in F(\alpha) \quad (8.4.2)$$

where $\alpha \in B^n$ and

$$F(\alpha) \stackrel{\triangle}{=} \{x \in \Re^n : x_i \alpha_i > 1, \ i = 1, \cdots, n\}. \quad (8.4.3)$$

CHAPTER 8. SYNTHESIS METHODS

Given $\alpha^1, \cdots, \alpha^m$ to be stored as memory vectors for neural network (8.4.1), similarly to (8.3.2) or (8.3.4), we will now determine $\{A, T, I\}$, using

$$A^{-1}(T\alpha^i + I) \in F(\alpha^i), \quad i = 1, \cdots, m.$$

One of the solutions is presented in the following.

Synthesis Procedure 8.4.1

1) Choose A as the identify matrix (without loss of generality).

2) Choose

$$T = \mu T^+ - \tau T^- \quad \text{and} \quad I = \mu \alpha^m - T\alpha^m$$

where $\mu > 1$, $\tau > 0$, and T^+ and T^- are given as in (8.3.5) and (8.3.6), respectively.

Then, $\alpha^1, \cdots, \alpha^m$ will be stored as memory vectors in the synthesized system (8.4.1), each of which corresponds to an asymptotically stable equilibrium point of system (8.4.1) given by $\beta^i = \mu \alpha^i$, $i = 1, \cdots, m$. ∎

We emphasize that in order to apply the Eigenstructure Method developed earlier to a variety of neural network models, the key step is to derive conditions for a bipolar pattern to be a memory vector of the network, as in (8.3.2) and (8.4.2). The same procedure will be utilized in the following to adapt the Eigenstructure Method to other neural network models.

Neural Network (2.2.4) We restate Eq. (2.2.4) as

$$\begin{cases} \dot{x} = -Ax + Ty + I \\ y = S(x) = [s_1(x_1), \cdots, s_n(x_n)]^T \end{cases} \quad (8.4.4)$$

where $s_i(\cdot)$ represents a sigmoidal function. For (8.4.4), assume that there exist $\gamma_i > 0$ such that

$$s_i(x_i) \approx 1 \quad \text{when } x_i > \gamma_i$$

and

$$s_i(x_i) \approx -1 \quad \text{when } x_i < -\gamma_i$$

8.4. EXTENSIONS TO EIGENSTRUCTURE METHOD

for $i = 1, \cdots, n$. Without loss of generality, one can assume that $\gamma_i \geq 1$ for $i = 1, \cdots, n$. This is possible if one chooses, e.g.,

$$s_i(x_i) = \frac{2}{\pi} \arctan(x_i)$$

or

$$s_i(x_i) = \text{arctanh}(x_i) = \frac{e^{x_i} - e^{-x_i}}{e^{x_i} + e^{-x_i}}.$$

Due to the nature of the functions $s_i(\cdot)$, the design objective has to be modified to approximately store a set of desired bipolar patterns when using (8.4.4). Assume that $\alpha \in B^n$ is such a desired memory pattern to be stored in (8.4.4). Denote $\Gamma = \text{diag}[\gamma_1, \cdots, \gamma_n]$. For $x \in \Re^n$ such that $\Gamma^{-1}x \in F(\alpha)$, where $F(\alpha)$ is defined in (8.4.3), (8.4.4) can be written as

$$\dot{x} \approx -Ax + T\alpha + I \qquad (8.4.5)$$

since $S(x) \approx \alpha$ when $\Gamma^{-1}x \in F(\alpha)$. The unique equilibrium of (8.4.5),

$$\beta = A^{-1}(T\alpha + I)$$

is asymptotically stable and satisfies $S(\beta) \approx \alpha$ whenever $\Gamma^{-1}\beta \in F(\alpha)$. Thus, stable memories must satisfy the condition that

$$\Gamma^{-1}A^{-1}(T\alpha + I) \in F(\alpha). \qquad (8.4.6)$$

All the results established in the preceding can now be modified in accordance with (8.4.6). In particular, (8.4.6) and (8.4.2) are equivalent if we incorporate the matrix Γ into A. In this case, we obtain a solution for the synthesis of neural networks described by (8.4.4) using Synthesis Procedure 8.4.1 with matrix A chosen as Γ^{-1}.

Neural Network (2.5.1) We restate Eq. (2.5.1) as

$$\begin{cases} \dot{x} = -Ax + Ty + I \\ y = \text{sgn}(x) \end{cases} \qquad (8.4.7)$$

where $A = \text{diag}[a_1, \cdots, a_n]$ with $a_i > 0$. In this case, the condition for a bipolar vector to be a memory vector is captured in the following result.

Lemma 8.4.1 If $\alpha \in B^n$ and if

$$\beta = A^{-1}(T\alpha + I) \in G(\alpha) \tag{8.4.8}$$

where

$$G(\alpha) = \{x \in \Re^n : x_i \alpha_i > 0, \ i = 1, \cdots, n\}$$

then (α, β) is a pair of stable memory vector and asymptotically stable equilibrium point of (8.4.7). ∎

Clearly, if we choose A as the identity matrix, condition (8.4.8) becomes equivalent to (8.3.2) given in Corollary 8.3.1. We therefore can obtain a solution for the synthesis of neural networks described by (8.4.7) using Synthesis Procedure 8.3.1 by choosing the matrix A as the identity matrix. We note that in this case, matrix A can actually be chosen as any diagonal matrix with positive diagonal elements as is seen from (8.4.8). As a matter of fact, in this case, (8.4.8) is equivalent to

$$T\alpha + I \in G(\alpha) \tag{8.4.9}$$

as long as A is a diagonal matrix with positive diagonal elements.

Neural Network (2.3.4) We consider the case when $g(\cdot) = \text{sgn}(\cdot)$ and restate Eq. (2.3.4) as

$$\begin{cases} x(k+1) = -Ax(k) + Ty(k) + I \\ y(k) = \text{sgn}(x(k)). \end{cases} \tag{8.4.10}$$

Assume that $\alpha \in B^n$ is a desired memory pattern. We will require α to satisfy

$$\begin{cases} \beta = -A\beta + T\alpha + I \\ \alpha = \text{sgn}(\beta) \end{cases}$$

or equivalently,

$$\beta = (E + A)^{-1}(T\alpha + I) \in G(\alpha), \tag{8.4.11}$$

where E is the $n \times n$ identity matrix. Condition (8.4.11) is similar to (8.4.8), and thus, a similar procedure can be established for the synthesis of neural networks described by (8.4.10). In particular, we can use Synthesis Procedure 8.3.1 for the synthesis of (8.4.10) by choosing matrix A as $A = \text{diag}[a_1, \cdots, a_n]$ with $|a_i| < 1$, $i = 1, \cdots, n$. We note that the asymptotic stability of the equilibrium points of (8.4.10) require that $|a_i| < 1$, $i = 1, \cdots, n$, and that under these conditions, (8.4.11) becomes equivalent to (8.4.9).

Neural Network (2.6.7) We restate Eq. (2.6.7) as

$$x(k+1) = \text{sat}(Tx(k) + I). \tag{8.4.12}$$

In this case, the condition for a bipolar vector to be a memory vector becomes

$$\beta = T\alpha + I \in F(\alpha). \tag{8.4.13}$$

When (8.4.13) is satisfied, (α, β) is a pair of stable memory vector and asymptotically stable equilibrium point of (8.4.12). The synthesis of neural networks described by (8.4.12) using the Eigenstructure Method is therefore equivalent to the synthesis of neural networks described by (8.4.1) (with its matrix A chosen as the identity matrix). Therefore, Synthesis Procedure 8.4.1 is applicable to neural networks described by (8.4.12) if we simply skip the first step of the procedure.

8.5 Synthesis of Recurrent Neural Networks Based on the Perceptron Training Algorithm

We develop in the present section another synthesis procedure for recurrent neural networks which is based on a perceptron training algorithm.

We first introduce necessary preliminaries, including the perceptron training algorithm and its convergence theorem. A number of different types of perceptrons are described in [23] and [27]. The one which we will utilize is described by the relation

$$z = \text{sign}(Wu)$$

where $u = (u_1, \cdots, u_n, 1)^T$, $W = (w_1, \cdots, w_n, \theta)$, and

$$\text{sign}(\xi) = \begin{cases} 1, & \xi \geq 0 \\ -1, & \xi < 0. \end{cases}$$

This simple perceptron can perform pattern classification (between two classes C_1 and C_2). The weight vector W can be obtained by the following perceptron training algorithm (cf. [23] and [27]).

Perceptron Training Algorithm Given m training patterns α^k, $k = 1, \cdots, m$, which are known to belong to class C_1 (corresponding to $z = 1$) or C_2 (corresponding to $z = -1$). The weight vector W can be obtained by the following algorithm:

1) Initialize the weight vector $W(l)$ for $l = 0$.
2) For $l = 0, 1, \cdots$,

   - if $W(l)u(l) \geq 0$ and $u(l) \in C_2$, then update $W(l+1) = W(l) - \eta u(l)$,
   - if $W(l)u(l) < 0$ and $u(l) \in C_1$, then update $W(l+1) = W(l) + \eta u(l)$,
   - otherwise, $W(l+1) = W(l)$,

   where $u(l) = \alpha^k$ for some k, $1 \leq k \leq m$, and $\eta > 0$ is the perceptron learning rate.

3) Stop the training when no more updates for the weight vector W are needed, i.e., stop the training when all the training patterns can correctly be classified by W. ∎

The following result is well-known [23], [27] and will be stated without proof.

Perceptron Training Convergence Theorem The Perceptron Training Algorithm is convergent if and only if the two classes C_1 and C_2 are linearly separable. ∎

Recall that two classes of patterns are *linearly separable* if there exists a linear discriminant function which can classify the patterns as belonging to the correct class (without error) [34].

8.5. PERCEPTRON BASED TRAINING METHOD

Remark 8.5.1 It is noted that one can always continue the training of a perceptron until a weight vector W is obtained such that

$$\begin{cases} W\alpha^k > 0 & \text{if } \alpha^k \in C_1 \\ W\alpha^k < 0 & \text{if } \alpha^k \in C_2 \end{cases}$$

for $k = 1, \cdots, m$. ∎

In the sequel, the Perceptron Training Algorithm will be used to develop a synthesis procedure for associative memories realized by neural network (2.2.6), restated here as

$$\begin{cases} \dot{x} = -Ax + Ty + I \\ y = \text{sat}(x) \end{cases} \quad (8.5.1)$$

where $x \in \Re^n$, $\dot{x}$ denotes the derivative of x with respect to time t, $T = [T_{ij}] \in \Re^{n \times n}$ is the connections matrix, $I = (I_1, \cdots, I_n)^T$ is a bias vector, $A = \text{diag}[a_1, \cdots, a_n]$ with $a_i > 0$ and the function $\text{sat}(x) = (\text{sat}(x_1), \cdots, \text{sat}(x_n))^T$ is defined by

$$\text{sat}(x_i) = \begin{cases} 1, & x_i > 1 \\ x_i, & -1 \leq x_i \leq 1 \\ -1, & x_i < -1. \end{cases}$$

We will refer to the output vector corresponding to an asymptotically stable equilibrium of (8.5.1) as a (stable) memory vector. The output vector y in (8.5.1) is constrained to $y \in D^n$, where

$$D^n = \{x \in \Re^n : -1 \leq x_i \leq 1, \ i = 1, \cdots, n\}.$$

Generalizations of the perceptron based synthesis approach to other neural network models will be addressed in the next section.

From Lemma 6.6.1, we can see that for a vector $\alpha \in B^n$ to be a stable memory vector of neural network (8.5.1), we require that

$$A^{-1}(T\alpha + I) \in F(\alpha) \quad (8.5.2)$$

where

$$F(\alpha) \triangleq \{x \in \Re^n : x_i \alpha_i > 1, \ i = 1, \cdots, n\}.$$

Therefore, in order to solve the synthesis problem for neural networks described by (8.5.1), i.e., for a given set of vectors $\alpha^1, \cdots, \alpha^m$ in B^n to be stored as memory vectors of (8.5.1), one needs to determine A, T and I from

$$A^{-1}(T\alpha^k + I) \in F(\alpha^k) \text{ for } k = 1, \cdots, m. \quad (8.5.3)$$

Condition (8.5.3) can equivalently be written as

$$\begin{cases} T_i\alpha^k + I_i > a_i, & \text{if } \alpha_i^k = 1 \\ T_i\alpha^k + I_i < -a_i, & \text{if } \alpha_i^k = -1 \end{cases} \quad (8.5.4)$$

for $k = 1, \cdots, m$ and for $i = 1, \cdots, n$, where T_i represents the ith row of T, I_i denotes the ith element of I, and α_i^k is the ith entry of α^k. From (8.5.4) [or equivalently, from (8.5.3)], the following synthesis algorithm (design method) based on the Perceptron Training Algorithm is now established.

Synthesis Procedure 8.5.1 Suppose that we are given m vectors $\alpha^1, \cdots, \alpha^m$ in B^n which are to be stored as memory vectors in (8.5.1). We proceed as follows:

Using the Perceptron Training Algorithm, determine n perceptrons $W^i = (w_1^i, w_2^i, \cdots, w_{n+1}^i)$, $i = 1, \cdots, n$, such that

$$\begin{cases} W^i \overline{\alpha}^k \geq 0, & \text{if } \alpha_i^k = 1 \\ W^i \overline{\alpha}^k < 0, & \text{if } \alpha_i^k = -1 \end{cases} \quad (8.5.5)$$

for $k = 1, \cdots, m$, where $\overline{\alpha}^k = \begin{pmatrix} \alpha^k \\ \cdots \\ 1 \end{pmatrix}$.

Choose the matrix $A = \text{diag}[a_1, \cdots, a_n]$ with $a_i > 0$. For $i, j = 1, \cdots, n$, choose $T_{ij} = w_j^i$ if $i \neq j$, $T_{ii} = w_i^i + a_i\mu_i$ with $\mu_i > 1$, and $I_i = w_{n+1}^i$. ∎

The next result establishes the validity of the above synthesis algorithm.

8.5. PERCEPTRON BASED TRAINING METHOD

Theorem 8.5.1

1) The A, T and I obtained in Synthesis Procedure 8.5.1 satisfy condition (8.5.3); i.e., system (8.5.1) with A, T and I obtained in Synthesis Procedure 8.5.1 guarantees that the α^i, $i = 1, \cdots, m$, are output vectors corresponding to asymptotically stable equilibrium points of (8.5.1). Therefore, α^i, $i = 1, \cdots, m$, are (stable) memory vectors.

2) The perceptron training in Synthesis Procedure 8.5.1 will always converge.

Proof: 1) In view of the definition of $\overline{\alpha}^k$ and the choice of T_{ij} and I_i in Synthesis Procedure 8.5.1 with $a_i > 0$ and $\mu_i > 1$, one can see that for $i = 1, \cdots n$ and $k = 1, \cdots, m$, $W^i \overline{\alpha}^k \geq 0$ (when $\alpha_i^k = 1$) implies

$$T_{i1}\alpha_1^k + T_{i2}\alpha_2^k + \cdots + T_{ii}\alpha_i^k + \cdots + T_{in}\alpha_n^k + I_i \geq a_i \mu_i \alpha_i^k > a_i \quad (8.5.6)$$

and $W^i \alpha^k < 0$ (when $\alpha_i^k = -1$) implies

$$T_{i1}\alpha_1^k + T_{i2}\alpha_2^k + \cdots + T_{ii}\alpha_i^k + \cdots + T_{in}\alpha_n^k + I_i < a_i \mu_i \alpha_i^k < -a_i. \quad (8.5.7)$$

The above two expressions can be written in vector form as in (8.5.3). Therefore, according to Lemma 6.6.1, α^k, $k = 1, \cdots, m$, are indeed stable memory vectors of system (8.5.1).

2) Consider the ith perceptron's training in Synthesis Procedure 8.5.1. The training patterns $\overline{\alpha}^k$ in the algorithm are labeled according to the ith element α_i^k of α^k for $k = 1, \cdots, m$. Since every $\alpha^k \in B^n$, it is clear that the two classes in the present case are linearly separable and this is true for every i, $i = 1, \cdots, n$. ∎

Remark 8.5.2 From Lemma 6.6.1 and from the proof of Theorem 8.5.1 it is clear that in Synthesis Procedure 8.5.1 we are always required to choose $\mu_i > 1$. ∎

Remark 8.5.3 Condition (8.5.3) is also equivalent to

$$A^{-1}(T\alpha^k + I) = \Gamma_k \alpha^k \quad \text{for} \quad k = 1, \cdots, m \quad (8.5.8)$$

where $\Gamma_k = \text{diag}[e_1^k, \cdots, e_n^k]$ with $e_i^k > 1$ (to be determined) for $i = 1, \cdots, n$, $k = 1, \cdots, m$. From (8.5.6) and (8.5.7), it is clear that Synthesis Procedure 8.5.1 results in $e_i^k \geq \mu_i$. This implies that large μ_i in Synthesis Procedure 8.5.1 will result in large e_i^k for equation (8.5.8). If one chooses A as the identity matrix and

$$T\alpha^k + I = \mu \alpha^k \text{ for } k = 1, \cdots, m \qquad (8.5.9)$$

with every $e_i^k = \mu > 1$, then (8.5.3) is satisfied. We note that (8.5.9) is actually what Synthesis Procedure 8.4.1 solves. In a sense, Synthesis Procedure 8.5.1 solves a more general design problem [i.e., (8.5.8)] than Synthesis Procedure 8.4.1 [i.e., (8.5.9)]. ∎

Remark 8.5.4 It is clear from Synthesis Procedure 8.5.1 that one has the freedom to choose matrix $A = \text{diag}[a_1, \cdots, a_n]$ with $a_i > 0$ for system (8.5.1). Without loss of generality, one can usually choose $a_i = 1$, i.e., in Synthesis Procedure 8.5.1, A can be chosen as the identity matrix. ∎

Remark 8.5.5 The learning rate η in the Perceptron Training Algorithm can be any positive real number [23], [27]. If $\eta = 1$ or any other positive integer and if one chooses the initial W^i to be the zero vector or any vector with integer and zero components, then the matrix T and the vector I obtained from Synthesis Procedure 8.5.1 will have only integer components. It is noted that in VLSI implementations of neural networks, certain weights (e.g., integers) can be implemented *more* accurately than others (e.g., numbers with many decimal digits). The learning rate η specifies the step size of every update for the weight vector during the perceptron training. Large η results in large step size which implies a coarse searching in the solution space of W^i. In most cases, choosing η to be $0 < \eta < 1$ is desirable for perceptron training to converge quickly. ∎

Remark 8.5.6 From Synthesis Procedure 8.5.1 and Theorem 8.5.1, one can see that there are no restrictions on how many bipolar vectors can be stored as stable memories in system (8.5.1) designed by

8.5. PERCEPTRON BASED TRAINING METHOD

the present approach. This implies that the storage capacity (maximum allowable number m for the desired patterns) can be large. It will be seen (cf. Remarks 8.5.8 and 8.5.13 below), however, that there are certain constraints on the desired memory patterns if one wants to design a neural network (8.5.1) with some prespecified constraints on the diagonal elements of the connection matrix T. A more sophisticated definition of associative memory capacity has also been used in the literature [5], [6]. The capacity used in [5], [6] is defined as a measure of the ability of an associative memory to store a set of *unbiased random* binary patterns at a given error correction and recall accuracy level (e.g., 99%). We note that the definition used in [5], [6] may be more appropriate for the present synthesis approach. Using this definition, we will evaluate the capacity of the present synthesis approach by means of a specific example in Section 8.7 (Example 8.7.8). ∎

Remark 8.5.7 If one wishes that the above synthesis algorithm result in a system of form (8.5.1) with $I = 0$, one can modify (8.5.5) in Synthesis Procedure 8.5.1 as follows:

$$\begin{cases} W^i \alpha^k \geq 0 & \text{if } \alpha_i^k = 1 \\ W^i \alpha^k < 0 & \text{if } \alpha_i^k = -1 \end{cases}$$

where $W^i = [w_1^i, \cdots, w_n^i]$. Choose A and T as in Synthesis Procedure 8.5.1, and choose $I = 0$. Theorem 8.5.1 is still valid for this case. ∎

As pointed out in Remark 8.5.6, the storage capacity (maximum allowable number m for the desired patterns) in the present case can be very large. When the number of desired memory patterns becomes too large, the connection matrix T obtained from most known synthesis methods will be diagonally dominant or nearly diagonally dominant. A diagonally dominant connection matrix T will make almost every bipolar pattern (every corner of the hypercube) become a stable memory vector which results in many spurious memories (stable memories which are not desired) and which results in networks with no interesting dynamics. In practice, one has to consider a trade-off between the storage capacity and the number of spurious memories.

Generally speaking, large positive diagonal elements in the connection matrix T will result in a large number of spurious memories. The basins of attraction of desired memories will get smaller as the total number of spurious memories in a network gets larger. One of the goals of the synthesis approach in the present section is to design neural networks with constraints on the diagonal elements of the connection matrix (e.g., lower and/or upper bounded) so that the number of spurious memories may be reduced and the basins of attraction of desired memories may be increased.

If it is desired that neural network (8.5.1) has only bipolar stable memory vectors, Corollary 5.7.1 provides some guidelines on what *lower bounds* may be used for the diagonal elements of the connection matrix T. Note that in practice, it is usually desired to design neural networks with only bipolar stable memory vectors. Corollary 5.7.1 states that if we require that $T_{ii} \geq a_i$ for $i = 1, \cdots, n$, where $a_i > 0$ is the ith diagonal element of matrix A, then all the stable memory vectors of system (8.5.1) will be in B^n, i.e., the system will have no stable memories in $D^n - B^n$, where $D^n = \{x \in \Re^n : -1 \leq x_i \leq 1, i = 1, \cdots, n\}$.

For $\alpha, \gamma \in B^n$, define the Hamming distance between α and γ as

$$H(\alpha, \gamma) = \frac{1}{2} \sum_{i=1}^{n} |\alpha_i - \gamma_i|$$

i.e., $H(\alpha, \gamma)$ = the number of bits for which α and γ differ.

The next result summarizes some important properties of neural networks (8.5.1) with the connection matrix T having *upper bounds* on the diagonal elements.

Theorem 8.5.2 Suppose that $\alpha \in B^n$ is a stable memory vector of system (8.5.1) with $A = \text{diag}[a_1, \cdots, a_n]$, where $a_i > 0$ for $i = 1, \cdots, n$.

1) None of the vectors $\gamma \in B^n$ such that $H(\alpha, \gamma) = 1$ can

8.5. PERCEPTRON BASED TRAINING METHOD

become memory vectors of system (8.5.1) if $T_{ii} \leq a_i$ for $i = 1, \cdots, n$.

2) Assume that $T_{ii} \leq a_i$ for some i, $\gamma \in B^n$, $H(\alpha, \gamma) = 1$, and α and γ differ in the ith bit. Then, the ith component of the state of system (8.5.1) will move in the direction towards α if the system starts from $x(0) = \gamma$.

Proof: 1) From Lemma 6.6.1, $\alpha = [\alpha_1, \cdots, \alpha_n]^T \in B^n$ is a stable memory vector if (8.5.2) is satisfied. Assume that $\gamma = [\gamma_1, \cdots, \gamma_n]^T \in B^n$, $H(\alpha, \gamma) = 1$, and α and γ differ in the ith bit, $1 \leq i \leq n$, i.e., $\alpha_j = \gamma_j$ for $j \neq i$ and $\alpha_i = -\gamma_i$. According to (8.5.2), if $T_{ii} \leq a_i$, one has [cf. (8.5.4)]

$$\begin{cases} T_i\gamma + I_i = T_i\alpha + I_i + 2T_{ii}\gamma_i > a_i - 2T_{ii} \geq -a_i \\ \qquad \text{if } \gamma_i = -\alpha_i = -1 \\ T_i\gamma + I_i = T_i\alpha + I_i + 2T_{ii}\gamma_i < -a_i + 2T_{ii} \leq a_i \\ \qquad \text{if } \gamma_i = -\alpha_i = 1 \end{cases} \quad (8.5.10)$$

where T_i and I_i represent the ith row of T and the ith component of I, respectively. It is clear that there will be no equilibrium points of (8.5.1) in $F(\gamma)$ since (8.5.10) implies that $A^{-1}(T\gamma + I) \notin \overline{F(\gamma)}$, where $\overline{F(\gamma)}$ denotes the closure of $F(\gamma)$. Therefore, γ cannot be a stable memory vector of system (8.5.1). This conclusion is true for all $\gamma \in B^n$ such that $H(\alpha, \gamma) = 1$ if $T_{ii} \leq a_i$ for $i = 1, \cdots, n$.

2) Assume that $T_{ii} \leq a_i$, $\gamma \in B^n$, $H(\alpha, \gamma) = 1$, and α and γ differ in the ith bit. If system (8.5.1) starts from $x(0) = \gamma$, one can obtain for the ith component of the state of system (8.5.1)

$$\dot{x}_i(0) = -a_i x_i(0) + T_i \text{sat}(x(0)) + I_i = -a_i \gamma_i + T_i \gamma + I_i. \quad (8.5.11)$$

In view of (8.5.10), equation (8.5.11) implies that

$$\dot{x}_i(0) > -a_i \gamma_i - a_i = 0 \quad \text{when } \gamma_i = -1 \ (\alpha_i = 1)$$

and

$$\dot{x}_i(0) < -a_i \gamma_i + a_i = 0 \quad \text{when } \gamma_i = 1 \ (\alpha_i = -1).$$

Clearly, at $t = 0^+$, the ith component $x_i(t)$ of the state $x(t)$ will evolve in the direction towards α if $x(0) = \gamma$. ∎

Remark 8.5.8 The results in Theorem 8.5.2 indicate that it is very likely that every corner of the hypercube which is in the immediate neighborhood (with Hamming distance 1) of a stable memory vector is in the domain of attraction of that stable memory vector. Theorem 8.5.2 also implies that none of two desired patterns can have Hamming distance 1 if the diagonal elements of T are required to satisfy $T_{ii} \leq a_i$, $i = 1, \cdots, n$, where $a_i > 0$ is the ith diagonal element of matrix A. ∎

Remark 8.5.9 In view of the results in Corollary 5.7.1 and Theorem 8.5.2, in practice it is desired to design neural networks with $T_{ii} = a_i$ for $i = 1, \cdots, n$, where a_i is the ith diagonal element of matrix A. The constraints on the diagonal elements of matrix T given by $T_{ii} = a_i$ for $i = 1, \cdots, n$ will henceforth, in the present section, be referred to as the *optimal constraints*. Therefore, under such optimal constraints,

- a neural network will have only bipolar stable memory vectors; and

- every corner of the hypercube which is in the immediate neighborhood of a stable memory vector cannot become a memory vector and is very likely in the domain of attraction of that stable memory vector.

Our experimental results indicate that neural networks (8.5.1) which satisfy the optimal constraints have usually less spurious memories and larger basins of attraction for desired memories than networks which do not satisfy these constraints. ∎

Remark 8.5.10 When in system (8.5.1) $I = 0$, one can show that $\alpha \in B^n$ is a stable memory if and only if $-\alpha$ is a stable memory. This implies that Part 1 of Theorem 8.5.2 will be true for all $\gamma \in B^n$ such that $H(\alpha, \gamma) = 1$ or $H(\alpha, \gamma) = n - 1$ if $I = 0$ in (8.5.1). ∎

8.5. PERCEPTRON BASED TRAINING METHOD

Remark 8.5.11 From Synthesis Procedure 8.5.1, one knows that $T_{ii} = w_i^i + a_i \mu_i$ where μ_i is chosen such that $\mu_i > 1$. When the w_i^i obtained from Synthesis Procedure 8.5.1 satisfies the condition $w_i^i < 0$, one can choose $a_i > 0$, $T_{ii} = a_i$, and $\mu_i = 1 - w_i^i/a_i > 1$, or one can choose $a_i > 0$ and $T_{ii} < a_i$ such that $\mu_i = (T_{ii} - w_i^i)/a_i > 1$. It can easily be proved that a neural network design with the ith diagonal element of the connection matrix T satisfying $T_{ii} \leq a_i$, where $a_i > 0$ is the ith diagonal element of matrix A, can be obtained *if and only if* $w_i^i < 0$ from Synthesis Procedure 8.5.1. ∎

Remark 8.5.12 If the algorithm ends up with $w_i^i \geq 0$ for some i, then one can repeat the perceptron training with an initial weight W^i chosen to be

$$W^i = [w_1^i, \cdots, w_{i-1}^i, -\xi_i, w_{i+1}^i, \cdots, w_{n+1}^i]$$

with $\xi_i > 0$. Experiments show that this case will usually terminate with $w_i^i < 0$, if such a solution exists. ∎

Most of the existing synthesis methods in the literature cannot be applied if some or all of the diagonal elements of a connection matrix are constrained (e.g., $T_{ii} \leq a_i$) except for the methods developed in [24] and [29] where optimization techniques and linear programming methods are used. The next result provides necessary and sufficient conditions for the existence of a neural network design with diagonal elements of the connection matrix to be upper bounded.

Theorem 8.5.3 A neural network design with the ith diagonal element of T satisfying $T_{ii} \leq a_i$, where $a_i > 0$ is the ith diagonal element of matrix A, can be achieved if and only if the desired patterns $\alpha^1, \cdots, \alpha^m$ with the ith entry eliminated are linearly separable, where the two classes are determined according to the ith element of the desired patterns.

Proof: (Sufficiency) From Remark 8.5.1, it is always possible to generate perceptrons W^i by Synthesis Procedure 8.5.1 such that

$$\begin{cases} W^i \overline{\alpha}^k > 0 & \text{if } \alpha_i^k = 1 \\ W^i \overline{\alpha}^k < 0 & \text{if } \alpha_i^k = -1 \end{cases} \quad (8.5.12)$$

for $k = 1, \cdots, m$ and for $i = 1, \cdots, n$.

Assume that the desired patterns $\alpha^1, \cdots, \alpha^m$ with the ith entry eliminated are linearly separable for some i, $1 \leq i \leq n$, where the two classes are determined according to the ith element. One can now apply Synthesis Procedure 8.5.1 to train the perceptron W^i without using the ith element of the desired patterns (training patterns). In this case, equation (8.5.12) implies that when $\alpha_i^k = 1$,

$$w_1^i \alpha_1^k + \cdots + w_{i-1}^i \alpha_{i-1}^k + w_{i+1}^i \alpha_{i+1}^k + \cdots + w_{n+1}^i > 0 \qquad (8.5.13)$$

and when $\alpha_i^k = -1$,

$$w_1^i \alpha_1^k + \cdots + w_{i-1}^i \alpha_{i-1}^k + w_{i+1}^i \alpha_{i+1}^k + \cdots + w_{n+1}^i < 0 \qquad (8.5.14)$$

for $k = 1, \cdots, m$. Choose ε_i such that

$$0 < \varepsilon_i < \min_{1 \leq k \leq m} \left\{ \left| \sum_{j=1, j \neq i}^{n} w_j^i \alpha_j^k + w_{n+1}^i \right| \right\}. \qquad (8.5.15)$$

Let $w_i^i = -\varepsilon_i$. Then, it is clear from (8.5.13)–(8.5.15) that, when $\alpha_i^k = 1$

$$\sum_{j=1}^{n} w_j^i \alpha_j^k + w_{n+1}^i = \sum_{j=1, j \neq i}^{n} w_j^i \alpha_j^k + w_{n+1}^i + w_i^i \alpha_i^k$$

$$= \left| \sum_{j=1, j \neq i}^{n} w_j^i \alpha_j^k + w_{n+1}^i \right| - \varepsilon_i > 0$$

and when $\alpha_i^k = -1$

$$\sum_{j=1}^{n} w_j^i \alpha_j^k + w_{n+1}^i = -\left| \sum_{j=1, j \neq i}^{n} w_j^i \alpha_j^k + w_{n+1}^i \right| + \varepsilon_i < 0.$$

This implies that one can always obtain W^i with $w_i^i < 0$ and hence, to obtain the ith diagonal element of matrix T satisfying $T_{ii} \leq a_i$, where $a_i > 0$ is the ith diagonal element of matrix A (cf. Remark 8.5.11).

(*Necessity*) If the ith diagonal element of T can be chosen such that $T_{ii} \leq a_i$, where a_i is the ith diagonal element of A (i.e., if

8.5. PERCEPTRON BASED TRAINING METHOD

Synthesis Procedure 8.5.1 terminates with $w_i^i < 0$), then from (8.5.5) we obtain

$$w_1^i \alpha_1^k + \cdots + w_{i-1}^i \alpha_{i-1}^k + w_{i+1}^i \alpha_{i+1}^k + \cdots + w_{n+1}^i$$
$$\geq -w_i^i \alpha_i^k > 0 \quad \text{when} \quad \alpha_i^k = 1$$

and

$$w_1^i \alpha_1^k + \cdots + w_{i-1}^i \alpha_{i-1}^k + w_{i+1}^i \alpha_{i+1}^k + \cdots + w_{n+1}^i$$
$$< -w_i^i \alpha_i^k < 0 \quad \text{when} \quad \alpha_i^k = -1.$$

The above two expressions constitute a perceptron with the ith entry α_i^k of α^k deleted. Therefore, the desired patterns $\alpha^1, \cdots, \alpha^m$, with the ith entry eliminated, are linearly separable into two classes, determined according to the ith element. ∎

In order to apply Theorem 8.5.3, one has to train the perceptrons of Synthesis Procedure 8.5.1 to determine whether the training will converge, since in general there are no simple criteria for testing linear separability of two classes of patterns. It turns out, however, that a simple criterion is possible for this purpose in the present case in which all the training patterns are represented in a bipolar space. In our next result we provide a simple sufficient condition for the existence of a neural network design with the connection matrix T having upper bounds for the diagonal elements.

Theorem 8.5.4 Let

$$Y = [\alpha^1 \vdots \cdots \vdots \alpha^m] \tag{8.5.16}$$

and let $Y^i = [Y$ with the ith row deleted$]$. If

$$\text{rank}(Y) = \text{rank}(Y^i) \tag{8.5.17}$$

for some i, $1 \leq i \leq n$, then Synthesis Procedure 8.5.1 will lead to a neural network design with the ith diagonal element of T satisfying $T_{ii} \leq a_i$, where $a_i > 0$ is the ith diagonal element of matrix A.

Proof: If (8.5.17) is satisfied, the ith row of Y can be expressed as a linear combination of all the other rows of Y, i.e.,

$$y_i = \sum_{j=1, j \neq i}^{n} \lambda_j y_j$$

for some real numbers λ_j, where $y_j = [\alpha_j^1, \cdots, \alpha_j^m]$ represents the jth row of Y. The componentwise expression of the above equation yields

$$\alpha_i^k = \sum_{j=1, j \neq i}^{n} \lambda_j \alpha_j^k \quad \text{for } k = 1, \cdots, m. \tag{8.5.18}$$

According to Theorem 8.5.1, Synthesis Procedure 8.5.1 will always determine perceptrons with weights W^i, $i = 1, \cdots, n$. Consider the ith perceptron W^i for which (8.5.5) is true and for which $w_i^i \geq 0$. From (8.5.18), we obtain

$$W^i \overline{\alpha}^k = \sum_{j=1, j\neq i}^{n} w_j^i \alpha_j^k + (w_i^i + \varepsilon_i)\alpha_i^k - \varepsilon_i \alpha_i^k + w_{n+1}^i$$

$$= \sum_{j=1, j\neq i}^{n} w_j^i \alpha_j^k + (w_i^i + \varepsilon_i) \sum_{j=1, j\neq i}^{n} \lambda_j \alpha_j^k - \varepsilon_i \alpha_i^k + w_{n+1}^i$$

where $\varepsilon_i > 0$. We can now choose a new weight vector

$$\underline{W}^i = [\underline{w}_1^i, \underline{w}_2^i, \cdots, \underline{w}_{n+1}^i]$$

with $\underline{w}_j^i = w_j^i + \lambda_j(w_i^i + \varepsilon_i)$ for $i \neq j$ and $\underline{w}_i^i = -\varepsilon_i < 0$. Since $\underline{W}^i \overline{\alpha}^k = W^i \overline{\alpha}^k$, we see that (8.5.5) is also satisfied for $\underline{W}^i$, by assumption. From $\underline{W}^i$, it is now clear that the diagonal elements of the connection matrix T satisfying $T_{ii} \leq a_i$, where $a_i > 0$ is the ith diagonal element of matrix A, can be realized, since $\underline{w}_i^i < 0$ (cf. Remark 8.5.11). ∎

Remark 8.5.13 It is clear from Theorem 8.5.4 that if $\text{rank}(Y) = n$, then condition (8.5.17) can never be satisfied. Thus, if one wishes to design a neural network (8.5.1) with prespecified constraints on the diagonal elements of the connection matrix T so that fewer spurious memories and larger basins of attraction for the desired memories may be achieved, it is desirable for the prototype patterns to satisfy that $\text{rank}(Y) < n$, where Y is defined in (8.5.16). ∎

8.5. PERCEPTRON BASED TRAINING METHOD

The Synthesis Procedure 8.5.1 presented above will usually result in a nonsymmetric matrix T. In the following, we develop a procedure for the design of neural network (8.5.1) with symmetric matrix T.

For the T and I determined by Synthesis Procedure 8.5.1 with $\mu_i > 1$, choose $\Delta T = (T^T - T)/2$. Then, $T_s \triangleq T + \Delta T = (T+T^T)/2$ is a symmetric matrix. From Theorem 6.6.1, we note that if $\Delta A = 0$ and $\Delta I = 0$ and if

$$\|A^{-1}\Delta T\|_\infty = \|A^{-1}(T^T - T)\|_\infty/2 < \nu - 1$$

then the neural network (8.5.1), after perturbations, given by

$$\begin{cases} \dot{x} = -Ax + (T+\Delta T)y + I \\ y = \text{sat}(x) \end{cases}$$

will also store all the desired patterns α^i, $i = 1, \cdots, n$, as memory vectors, where ν is determined by

$$\nu = \min_{1 \leq k \leq m} \{\delta(\beta^k)\} > 1 \qquad (8.5.19)$$

with

$$\beta^k = A^{-1}(T\alpha^k + I) \text{ for } k = 1, \cdots, m \qquad (8.5.20)$$

and $\delta(x) \triangleq \min_{1 \leq i \leq n} \{|x_i|\}$ for $x \in \Re^n$.

The above observation gives rise to the possibility of designing a neural network (8.5.1) with a symmetric interconnection matrix, using the perceptron based training algorithm. Such a symmetric design procedure is summarized in the following.

Synthesis Procedure 8.5.2 Given m vectors $\alpha^1, \cdots, \alpha^m$ in B^n to be stored as stable memories of system (8.5.1) with *symmetric* interconnection matrix T, we proceed as follows:

1) According to Synthesis Procedure 8.5.1, determine A, T and I for system (8.5.1) with $\mu_i > 1$.

2) Compute $\beta^k = A^{-1}(T\alpha^k + I)$ for $k = 1, \cdots, m$ and let $\mu = \min_{1 \le k \le m} \{\delta(\beta^k)\}$.

3) If $T = T^T$ or $\mu \le 1 + \eta$, where η is a small positive number (e.g., $\eta = 0.01$), stop. Otherwise, go to step 4.

4) Compute $\Delta T = (T^T - T)/2$. If $\|A^{-1}\Delta T\|_\infty < \mu - 1$, choose $\lambda = 1$. Otherwise, choose

$$\lambda = \frac{\mu - 1}{\|A^{-1}\Delta T\|_\infty} - \varepsilon$$

where ε is a small positive number (e.g., $\varepsilon = 0.001$). Compute $\overline{T} = T + \lambda \Delta T$.

5) Compute $\overline{\beta}^k = A^{-1}(\overline{T}\alpha^k + I)$ for $k = 1, \cdots, m$, and compute

$$\nu = \min_{1 \le k \le m} \{\delta(\overline{\beta}^k)\} > 1.$$

6) Replacing μ by ν and replacing T by $\overline{T}$, go to step 3.

If one ends up with $T = T^T$, a solution has been determined for the symmetric design problem. If one ends up with $\mu < 1 + \eta$ and $T \ne T^T$, the symmetric design procedure is not successful in solving a symmetric T for the given problem. ∎

8.6 Some Extensions to the Perceptron Based Training Algorithm

In this section we present adaptations of the synthesis method based on the perceptron training algorithm (developed in the previous section) to several neural network models introduced in Chapter 2 [including networks described by (2.2.4), (2.3.4), (2.5.1), (2.6.1), and (2.6.7)]. We also provide appropriate modifications to the robustness analysis result given in Theorem 6.6.1, in order to be able to adapt Synthesis Procedure 8.5.2 to the above networks, resulting in symmetric network designs.

8.6. EXTENSIONS TO THE PERCEPTRON TRAINING 389

In the following, we will assume that $\alpha \in B^n$ is a desired memory pattern which is to be stored in a given neural network. We will use the conditions derived in Section 8.4 for a bipolar pattern to be a memory vector to make the applicability of the perceptron training algorithm evident.

Neural Network (2.2.4) We restate Eq. (2.2.4) as

$$\begin{cases} \dot{x} = -Ax + Ty + I \\ y = S(x) = [s_1(x_1), \cdots, s_n(x_n)]^T \end{cases} \quad (8.6.1)$$

where $s_i(\cdot)$ represents a sigmoidal function, and we assume that there exist $\gamma_i > 0$ such that

$$s_i(x_i) \approx 1 \quad \text{when } x_i > \gamma_i$$

and

$$s_i(x_i) \approx -1 \quad \text{when } x_i < -\gamma_i$$

for $i = 1, \cdots, n$. Without loss of generality, we can assume that $\gamma_i \geq 1$ for $i = 1, \cdots, n$. In this case, the design objective has to be modified to approximately store a set of desired bipolar patterns using (8.6.1) due to the nature of the functions $s_i(\cdot)$. Specifically, our objective will be to store a set of desired patterns, which are in the vicinity of the corners of the hypercube, as output vectors corresponding to a set of asymptotically stable equilibrium points of system (8.6.1). Similarly as in Section 8.4, we derive for $\alpha \in B^n$ to be a memory vector of (8.6.1) the condition

$$\Gamma^{-1} A^{-1}(T\alpha + I) \in F(\alpha). \quad (8.6.2)$$

We note that if we incorporate the matrix Γ into A, (8.6.2) will be equivalent to (8.5.2). Therefore, the synthesis of neural networks described by (8.6.1) can be accomplished by Synthesis Procedure 8.5.1 with matrix A replaced by $A\Gamma$, where $\Gamma = \text{diag}[\gamma_1, \cdots, \gamma_n]$.

Due to the nature of the functions $s_i(\cdot)$, optimal constraints can in general not easily be identified for the diagonal elements of matrix T in system (8.6.1). However, the constraints given by $T_{ii} = \gamma_i a_i$, $i = 1, \cdots, n$, may be considered to be nearly optimal in this case. As in Corollary 5.7.1, we can show for system (8.6.1) that as the values of T_{ii}, $i = 1, \cdots, n$, increase, the chance of having stable memory vectors in the unsaturated region of the sigmoidal functions $s_i(\cdot)$ will be reduced. On the other hand, following similar steps as in Theorem 8.5.2, we can also show that when $T_{ii} \leq \gamma_i a_i$ for $i = 1, \cdots, n$, there will be no stable memory vectors in the vicinity of the corners of the hypercube that are in the immediate neighborhood of a stable memory vector (i.e., within Hamming distance 1 from a stable memory vector).

The robustness analysis result given in Theorem 6.6.1 needs to be modified for the present case by replacing (6.6.5) with

$$\|A^{-1}\Delta A\|_\infty + \|A^{-1}\Delta T\|_\infty + \|A^{-1}\Delta I\|_\infty < \nu \tag{8.6.3}$$

where

$$\nu = \min_{1 \leq k \leq m} \left\{ \delta\left(\beta^k - (\gamma_1, \cdots, \gamma_n)^T\right) \right\} > 0$$

with

$$\beta^k = A^{-1}(T\alpha^k + I) \quad \text{for} \quad k = 1, \cdots, m \tag{8.6.4}$$

and $\delta(x) = \min_{1 \leq i \leq n} \{|x_i|\}$ for $x \in \Re^n$. When condition (8.6.3) is satisfied, the neural network

$$\begin{cases} \dot{x} = -(A + \Delta A)x + (T + \Delta T)y + (I + \Delta I) \\ y = S(x) \end{cases}$$

will also store $\alpha^i \in B^n$, $i = 1, \cdots, n$, as memory vectors if A, T, and I in (8.6.1) are designed using $\alpha^i \in B^n$, $i = 1, \cdots, n$, as prototype patterns. Again, we note that in this case we can only store a set of bipolar patterns approximately.

Neural Network (2.5.1) We restate Eq. (2.5.1) as

$$\begin{cases} \dot{x} = -Ax + Ty + I \\ y = \text{sgn}(x). \end{cases} \tag{8.6.5}$$

In this case, the condition for a bipolar vector to be a memory vector is given by

$$A^{-1}(T\alpha + I) \in G(\alpha)$$

8.6. EXTENSIONS TO THE PERCEPTRON TRAINING

where $G(\alpha) = \{x \in \Re^n : x_i \alpha_i > 0, \ i = 1, \cdots, n\}$, or equivalently,

$$T\alpha + I \in G(\alpha), \tag{8.6.6}$$

under the assumption that A is a diagonal matrix with positive diagonal elements. Therefore, synthesis algorithms similar to the ones developed in the present section, using perceptron training, can be formulated based on condition (8.6.6). For example, Synthesis Procedure 8.5.1 may now be adapted to neural network (8.6.5) in the following manner:

Synthesis Procedure 8.6.1 Suppose that $\alpha^1, \cdots, \alpha^m$ are given vectors in B^n which are to be stored as memory vectors for system (8.6.5). Using the Perceptron Training Algorithm, generate n perceptrons $W^i = [w_1^i, w_2^i, \cdots, w_{n+1}^i]$, $i = 1, \cdots, n$, such that

$$\begin{cases} W^i \overline{\alpha}^k \geq 0 & \text{if } \alpha_i^k = 1 \\ W^i \overline{\alpha}^k < 0 & \text{if } \alpha_i^k = -1 \end{cases}$$

for $k = 1, \cdots, m$, where $\overline{\alpha}^k = \begin{pmatrix} \alpha^k \\ \cdots \\ 1 \end{pmatrix}$.

Choose $A = \text{diag}[a_1, \cdots, a_n]$ with $a_i > 0$. For $i, j = 1, \cdots, n$, choose $T_{ij} = w_j^i$ if $i \neq j$, $T_{ii} = w_i^i + \mu_i$ with $\mu_i > 0$, and choose $I_i = w_{n+1}^i$. ∎

In the present case, all of the output vectors, including all of the memory vectors, are in B^n. Following similar steps as in Theorem 8.5.2, we can show that when $T_{ii} \leq 0$ for $i = 1, \cdots, n$ are satisfied, no two desired memory patterns can have Hamming distance 1. In addition, we can also show that every corner of the hypercube which is in the immediate neighborhood of a stable memory vector is very likely in the domain of attraction of that stable memory vector. Furthermore, the analysis results for system (8.6.5) developed in Section 3.8 show that when T is *symmetric* with $T_{ii} = 0$, $i = 1, \cdots, n$, stable output vectors of the system correspond to local minima of an energy function for (8.6.5) (refer to Theorem 3.8.1). We may thus view the present results as a complement to Theorem 3.8.1. Therefore, under the conditions of Theorem 3.8.1, in addition to the conclusions stated in that theorem, we have also shown that system (8.6.5) possesses the properties enumerated above.

When $a_i + \Delta a_i > 0$, $i = 1, \cdots, n$, the robustness analysis result of Theorem 6.6.1 assumes the form

$$\|\Delta T\|_\infty + |\Delta I|_\infty < \nu \qquad (8.6.7)$$

where

$$\nu = \min_{1 \leq k \leq m} \left\{ \delta\left(\beta^k\right) \right\} > 0 \qquad (8.6.8)$$

with

$$\beta^k = T\alpha^k + I \text{ for } k = 1, \cdots, m. \qquad (8.6.9)$$

Note that the bounds for allowable parameter perturbations provided in (8.6.7) are true as long as the perturbations of matrix A still guarantee that $A + \Delta A$ is a diagonal matrix with positive diagonal elements. The proof of this result follows similar steps as the proof of Theorem 6.6.1, taking into account the definition of $G(\alpha)$ in (8.3.3). When these conditions are satisfied, the neural network

$$\begin{cases} \dot{x} = -(A + \Delta A)x + (T + \Delta T)y + (I + \Delta I) \\ y = \text{sgn}(x) \end{cases}$$

will also store α^i, $i = 1 \cdots, n$, as memory vectors.

Neural Network (2.3.4) We restate Eq. (2.3.4) as

$$\begin{cases} x(k+1) = -Ax(k) + Ty(k) + I \\ y(k) = \text{sgn}(x(k)) \end{cases} \qquad (8.6.10)$$

where the activation function is chosen as $\text{sgn}(\cdot)$. In this case, the condition for a bipolar vector to be a memory vector is given by

$$(E + A)^{-1}(T\alpha + I) \in G(\alpha). \qquad (8.6.11)$$

Therefore, for the synthesis of neural networks described by (8.6.10), we can use Synthesis Procedure 8.6.1 by choosing matrix A as $A = \text{diag}[a_1, \cdots, a_n]$, with $|a_i| < 1$, $i = 1, \cdots, n$.

8.6. EXTENSIONS TO THE PERCEPTRON TRAINING 393

The optimal constraints, which can be determined similarly as in the case of neural network (8.6.5), are given by $T_{ii} \leq 0$, $i = 1, \cdots, n$. The robustness analysis result in Theorem 6.6.1 needs to be modified as follows: when $1 + a_i + \Delta a_i > 0$ and $|a_i + \Delta a_i| < 1$, $i = 1, \cdots, n$, then

$$\|\Delta T\|_\infty + |\Delta I|_\infty < \nu,$$

where ν and β^k are given as in (8.6.8) and (8.6.9). We note that under the conditions $1 + a_i + \Delta a_i > 0$, (8.6.11) will be equivalent to (8.6.6). Also, the conditions $|a_i + \Delta a_i| < 1$ are required for the asymptotic stability of the equilibrium points of (8.6.5).

Neural Network (2.6.1) We restate Eq. (2.6.1) as

$$\dot{x} = Tx + I, \quad x \in D^n \qquad (8.6.12)$$

where

$$D^n \triangleq \{x \in \Re^n : -1 \leq x_i \leq 1, \ i = 1, \cdots, n\}.$$

The condition for a bipolar vector to be a memory vector is given in this case by

$$T\alpha + I \in G(\alpha)$$

which is the same as (8.6.6) [for neural networks described by (8.6.5)]. Thus, in this case, Synthesis Procedure 8.6.1 applies.

Presently, the optimal constraints are given by $T_{ii} = 0$ for $i = 1, \cdots, n$. We note that the constraints $T_{ii} = 0$ for (8.6.12) may be viewed to be a consequence and complement of the results developed in Sections 4.4 and 8.3. In particular, Theorem 4.4.1 implies that when $T_{ii} \geq 0$, there will be no asymptotically stable equilibrium points of (8.6.12) in $D^n - B^n$, i.e., all of the asymptotically stable equilibrium points of (8.6.12) will be in B^n. Furthermore, Theorem 8.3.2 suggests that by choosing $\tau > -1$ sufficiently large in the calculation of $T = T^+ - \tau T^-$, we can reduce the number of asymptotically stable equilibrium points in B^n. We point out that when choosing large τ in $T = T^+ - \tau T^-$, we will also decrease the values of the diagonal elements of matrix T. By further extending the results of Theorem 8.3.2, and following similar arguments as in

Theorem 8.5.2, we can show that when $T_{ii} \leq 0$, every corner of the hypercube which is in the immediate neighborhood of an asymptotically stable equilibrium point of (8.6.12) cannot become an asymptotically stable equilibrium point and is very likely in the domain of attraction of that asymptotically stable equilibrium point.

The robustness analysis result in Theorem 6.6.1 assumes in the present case the form

$$\|\Delta T\|_\infty + |\Delta I|_\infty < \nu \qquad (8.6.13)$$

where ν and β^k are given as in (8.6.8) and (8.6.9). When condition (8.6.13) is satisfied, the neural network

$$\dot{x} = (T + \Delta T)x + (I + \Delta I), \quad x \in D^n$$

will also store the set of desired memory patterns, α^i, $i = 1, \cdots, m$, as asymptotically stable equilibrium points, provided that T and I in (8.6.12) are designed by storing α^i, $i = 1, \cdots, m$, as asymptotically stable equilibrium points.

Neural Network (2.6.7) We restate Eq. (2.6.7) as

$$x(k+1) = \text{sat}(Tx(k) + I). \qquad (8.6.14)$$

The condition for a bipolar vector to be a memory vector assumes in the present case the form

$$T\alpha + I \in F(\alpha)$$

which is identical to (8.5.2) [for neural networks described by (8.5.1) when A is the identity matrix]. In this case, Synthesis Procedure 8.5.1 applies, if we choose $a_i = 1$, $i = 1, \cdots, n$.

The optimal constraints for the present case are given by $T_{ii} = 1$ for $i = 1, \cdots, n$. These can partially be derived from the results developed earlier in Section 4.6. In particular, Theorem 4.6.1 implies that $T_{ii} \geq 1$ guarantees that (8.6.14) will have no asymptotically stable equilibrium points in $D^n - B^n$. On the other hand, we can prove

8.7. ILLUSTRATIVE EXAMPLES

that when $T_{ii} \leq 1$, every corner of the hypercube which is in the immediate neighborhood of an asymptotically stable equilibrium point of (8.6.14) cannot become an asymptotically stable equilibrium point and is very likely in the domain of attraction of that asymptotically stable equilibrium point.

The robustness analysis result of Theorem 6.6.1 needs to be modified in the present case as

$$\|\Delta T\|_\infty + |\Delta I|_\infty < \nu - 1 \qquad (8.6.15)$$

where

$$\nu = \min_{1 \leq k \leq m} \left\{ \delta\left(\beta^k\right) \right\} > 1$$

and the β^k are computed as in (8.6.9). When (8.6.15) is satisfied, the neural network

$$x(k+1) = \text{sat}\Big((T + \Delta T)x(k) + (I + \Delta I)\Big)$$

will also store α^i, $i = 1, \cdots, m$, as asymptotically stable equilibrium points.

8.7 Illustrative Examples

In this section, our primary objective is to demonstrate and evaluate the Synthesis Procedures 8.3.1 and 8.5.1. Additional examples will be provided in Chapter 9 for these synthesis procedures, coupled to neural network designs with constraints on the interconnection matrix T, including symmetry constraints and sparsity constraints.

Example 8.7.1 In this example, we illustrate the use of Synthesis Procedure 8.3.1. The dimension of the system is $n = 10$. Given are

$m = 5$ vectors specified by

$$\alpha^1 = \begin{bmatrix} -1 \\ 1 \\ -1 \\ 1 \\ 1 \\ 1 \\ -1 \\ 1 \\ 1 \\ 1 \end{bmatrix}, \quad \alpha^2 = \begin{bmatrix} 1 \\ 1 \\ -1 \\ -1 \\ 1 \\ -1 \\ 1 \\ -1 \\ 1 \\ 1 \end{bmatrix}, \quad \alpha^3 = \begin{bmatrix} -1 \\ 1 \\ 1 \\ 1 \\ -1 \\ -1 \\ 1 \\ -1 \\ 1 \\ -1 \end{bmatrix}, \quad \alpha^4 = \begin{bmatrix} 1 \\ 1 \\ -1 \\ 1 \\ -1 \\ 1 \\ -1 \\ 1 \\ 1 \\ 1 \end{bmatrix}, \quad \alpha^5 = \begin{bmatrix} 1 \\ -1 \\ -1 \\ -1 \\ 1 \\ 1 \\ 1 \\ -1 \\ -1 \\ -1 \end{bmatrix}.$$

It is desired that these vectors be asymptotically stable equilibrium points of system (8.3.1). From Synthesis Procedure 8.3.1, we obtain the following.

1) Compute the $n \times (m-1) = 10 \times 4$ matrix

$$Y = \begin{bmatrix} y^1 \vdots y^2 \vdots y^3 \vdots y^4 \end{bmatrix} = \begin{bmatrix} -2 & 0 & -2 & 0 \\ 2 & 2 & 2 & 2 \\ 0 & 0 & 2 & 0 \\ 2 & 0 & 2 & 2 \\ 0 & 0 & -2 & -2 \\ 0 & -2 & -2 & 0 \\ -2 & 0 & 0 & -2 \\ 2 & 0 & 0 & 2 \\ 2 & 2 & 2 & 2 \\ 2 & 2 & 0 & 2 \end{bmatrix}$$

where $y^i = \alpha^i - \alpha^5$ for $1 \leq i \leq 4$.

2) Perform a singular value decomposition of Y to obtain the matrices U, V, and Σ such that $Y = U\Sigma V^T$. We have $k = $ rank of $\Sigma = 4$. (In MATLAB, singular value decomposition [1], [2] is performed using a function called svd.)

3) Compute

$$T^+ = \begin{bmatrix} T_{ij}^+ \end{bmatrix} = u^1 \left(u^1\right)^T + \cdots + u^4 \left(u^4\right)^T$$

8.7. ILLUSTRATIVE EXAMPLES

and
$$T^- = \left[T_{ij}^-\right] = u^5 \left(u^5\right)^T + \cdots + u^{10} \left(u^{10}\right)^T.$$

4) Choose the parameter $\tau = 10$ and compute
$T_\tau = T^+ - \tau T^-$

$$= \begin{bmatrix}
-2.1314 & -0.6423 & -2.1679 & -2.5693 & -3.1314 & 0.2409 \\
-0.6423 & -7.0292 & 0.4015 & 0.8832 & -0.6423 & -2.4891 \\
-2.1679 & 0.4015 & -7.2701 & 1.6058 & -2.1679 & -1.5255 \\
-2.5693 & 0.8832 & 1.6058 & -6.4672 & -2.5693 & 1.0438 \\
-3.1314 & -0.6423 & -2.1679 & -2.5693 & -2.1314 & 0.2409 \\
0.2409 & -2.4891 & -1.5255 & 1.0438 & 0.2409 & -4.9416 \\
0.4015 & -0.4818 & 1.1241 & -1.9270 & 0.4015 & -2.5693 \\
-0.4015 & 0.4818 & -1.1241 & 1.9270 & -0.4015 & 2.5693 \\
-0.6423 & 2.9708 & 0.4015 & 0.8832 & -0.6423 & -2.4891 \\
1.5255 & 2.5693 & -2.3285 & -0.7226 & 1.5255 & -0.9635
\end{bmatrix}$$

$$\begin{bmatrix}
0.4015 & -0.4015 & -0.6423 & 1.5255 \\
-0.4818 & 0.4818 & 2.9708 & 2.5693 \\
1.1241 & -1.1241 & 0.4015 & -2.3285 \\
-1.9270 & 1.9270 & 0.8832 & -0.7226 \\
0.4015 & -0.4015 & -0.6423 & 1.5255 \\
-2.5693 & 2.5693 & -2.4891 & -0.9635 \\
-6.9489 & -3.0511 & -0.4818 & -1.6058 \\
-3.0511 & -6.9489 & 0.4818 & 1.6058 \\
-0.4818 & 0.4818 & -7.0292 & 2.5693 \\
-1.6058 & 1.6058 & 2.5693 & -5.1022
\end{bmatrix}.$$

and
$$I_\tau = \alpha^m - T_\tau \alpha^m = \begin{bmatrix}
0.7226 \\
3.5328 \\
-4.5766 \\
3.1314 \\
0.7226 \\
4.1752 \\
3.2920 \\
-3.2920 \\
3.5328 \\
-2.8905
\end{bmatrix}.$$

By Corollary 8.3.1 (or Theorem 4.4.1), we determine that $\alpha^1, \cdots, \alpha^5$ are asymptotically stable equilibrium points of the synthesized system

$$\dot{x} = T_\tau x + I_\tau, \quad \tau = 10 \qquad (8.7.1)$$

with the constraints

$$-1 \leq x_i \leq 1, \quad 1 \leq i \leq n.$$

By Theorem 4.4.1, we determine that system (8.7.1) has 8 additional asymptotically stable equilibrium points which are not in B^n, and are given by

$$\alpha_1' = \begin{bmatrix} -1 \\ 1 \\ 0 \\ 0 \\ 1 \\ -1 \\ 1 \\ -1 \\ 1 \\ 0 \end{bmatrix}, \alpha_2' = \begin{bmatrix} 1 \\ 1 \\ 0 \\ 0 \\ -1 \\ -1 \\ 1 \\ -1 \\ 1 \\ 0 \end{bmatrix}, \alpha_3' = \begin{bmatrix} -1 \\ 0 \\ 0 \\ 0 \\ 1 \\ 0 \\ 1 \\ -1 \\ 0 \\ -1 \end{bmatrix}, \alpha_4' = \begin{bmatrix} 1 \\ 0 \\ 0 \\ 0 \\ -1 \\ 0 \\ 1 \\ -1 \\ 0 \\ -1 \end{bmatrix}, \alpha_5' = \begin{bmatrix} -1 \\ 0 \\ 0 \\ 1 \\ 0 \\ 1 \\ 0 \\ 0 \\ 0 \\ -1 \end{bmatrix},$$

$$\alpha_6' = \begin{bmatrix} -1 \\ -0.4741 \\ -0.3664 \\ 0.2470 \\ 1 \\ 1 \\ 0.4870 \\ -0.4870 \\ -0.4741 \\ -1 \end{bmatrix}, \alpha_7' = \begin{bmatrix} 1 \\ -0.4741 \\ -0.3664 \\ 0.2467 \\ -1 \\ 1 \\ 0.4870 \\ -0.4870 \\ -0.4741 \\ -1 \end{bmatrix}, \alpha_8' = \begin{bmatrix} 0 \\ 0 \\ 0 \\ 1 \\ -1 \\ 1 \\ 0 \\ 0 \\ 0 \\ -1 \end{bmatrix}.$$

Also by Theorem 4.4.1, we determine that system (8.7.1) has 70 unstable equilibrium points. ■

8.7. ILLUSTRATIVE EXAMPLES

Example 8.7.2 In order to ascertain how typical the results of Example 8.7.1 are, we repeat it 30 times, using different sets of given vectors to be stored as asymptotically stable equilibrium points of system (8.3.1). Each set contains $m = 5$ vectors. For each set of vectors, we synthesize system (8.3.1) as in Example 8.7.1. Table 8.4.1 summarizes these results.

Table 8.4.1: Results of Example 8.7.2

average total number of asymptotically stable equilibrium points of the synthesized system	9.90
average total number of asymptotically stable equilibrium points of the synthesized system in $B^n \cap L_a$	7.07
average total number of asymptotically stable equilibrium points of the synthesized system in $B^n - L_a$	0
average total number of asymptotically stable equilibrium points of the synthesized system in $D^n - B^n$	2.83
average total number of unstable equilibrium points of the synthesized system	52.45
average total number of vectors in the given data unsuccessfully synthesized as asymptotically stable equilibrium points of the synthesized system	0

Example 8.7.3 In this example, we show that Synthesis Procedure 8.3.1 with the parameter τ positive can be used to synthesize the analog Hopfield model (cf. Section 2.4). Consider the (generalized) Hopfield model with ten neurons, described by

$$dx/dt = H(x)(-S(x) + Tx + I) \qquad (L)$$

where $x \in (-1, 1)^{10}$, $S(x) = (s(x_1), \cdots, s(x_{10}))^T$,

$$s(\rho) = \frac{2}{\lambda \pi} \tan\left(\frac{\pi}{2}\rho\right),$$

$H(x) = \text{diag}[1/s'(x_1), \cdots, 1/s'(x_{10})]$, and $\lambda = 100$. Suppose we want to store $m = 5$ vectors, say, $\gamma^1, \cdots, \gamma^5$, in the system (L) as stable memories and suppose the exact locations of these five vectors are not important but should be located in particular regions such that the sign of their components are the same as the given data in Example 8.7.1, i.e., $\alpha_j^i = \text{sgn}(\gamma_j^i)$, $1 \leq i \leq 5$, $1 \leq j \leq 10$, where α_j^i and γ_j^i are the jth components of vectors α^i and γ^i, respectively. Using the same T_τ and I_τ with $\tau = 10$ obtained in Example 8.7.1, we obtain

$$dx/dt = H(x)(-S(x) + T_\tau x + I_\tau). \qquad (8.7.2)$$

It seems that *efficient* methods of determining *all* of the asymptotically stable equilibrium points of *high dimensional* analog Hopfield models have not appeared in the literature. In the case of unstable equilibrium points, the situation is even worse. The close relationship between system (8.3.1) and the analog Hopfield model (8.7.2) suggests, as pointed out in Remark 4.5.2, that the set of asymptotically stable equilibrium points of (8.3.1) and the set of asymptotically stable equilibrium points of (8.7.2) are approximately the same. To verify this observation, using the present example, we simulate system (8.7.2) by Runge-Kutta method with step length 0.01. In doing so, we use *initial vectors* $\alpha^1, \cdots, \alpha^5$, respectively, to determine the five asymptotically stable equilibrium points of (8.7.2) given by

$$\gamma^1 \approx \begin{bmatrix} -.99592 \\ .99599 \\ -.99600 \\ .99598 \\ .99594 \\ .99600 \\ -.99588 \\ .99588 \\ .99599 \\ .99588 \end{bmatrix}, \gamma^2 \approx \begin{bmatrix} -.99594 \\ .99599 \\ -.99600 \\ -.99588 \\ .99594 \\ -.99586 \\ .99598 \\ -.99598 \\ .99599 \\ .99588 \end{bmatrix}, \gamma^3 \approx \begin{bmatrix} .99592 \\ .99599 \\ .99586 \\ .99598 \\ -.99592 \\ -.99586 \\ .99598 \\ -.99598 \\ .99599 \\ -.99598 \end{bmatrix},$$

8.7. ILLUSTRATIVE EXAMPLES

$$\gamma^4 \approx \begin{bmatrix} .99594 \\ .99599 \\ -.99600 \\ .99598 \\ -.99592 \\ .99600 \\ -.99588 \\ .99588 \\ .99599 \\ .99588 \end{bmatrix}, \quad \gamma^5 \approx \begin{bmatrix} .99594 \\ -.99587 \\ -.99600 \\ -.99588 \\ .99594 \\ .99600 \\ .99598 \\ -.99598 \\ -.99587 \\ -.99598 \end{bmatrix}.$$

Furthermore, with the initial vectors $\alpha'_1, \cdots, \alpha'_8$ (determined in Example 8.7.1), we obtain, respectively, the eight asymptotically stable equilibrium points of (8.7.2) given by

$$\bar{\gamma}^1 \approx \begin{bmatrix} -9.9593e-1 \\ 9.9597e-1 \\ -1.5740e-3 \\ 1.7863e-3 \\ 9.9593e-1 \\ -9.9584e-1 \\ 9.9597e-1 \\ -9.9597e-1 \\ 9.9597e-1 \\ -1.8422e-3 \end{bmatrix}, \quad \bar{\gamma}^2 \approx \begin{bmatrix} 9.9593e-1 \\ 9.9597e-1 \\ -1.5740e-3 \\ 1.7863e-3 \\ -9.9593e-1 \\ -9.9584e-1 \\ 9.9597e-1 \\ -9.9597e-1 \\ 9.9597e-1 \\ -1.8422e-3 \end{bmatrix}, \quad \bar{\gamma}^3 \approx \begin{bmatrix} -9.9594e-1 \\ 2.7891e-3 \\ -2.0755e-3 \\ 2.5102e-3 \\ 9.9592e-1 \\ 1.8154e-3 \\ 9.9593e-1 \\ -9.9593e-1 \\ 2.7891e-3 \\ -9.9592e-1 \end{bmatrix},$$

$$\bar{\gamma}^4 \approx \begin{bmatrix} 9.9592e-1 \\ 2.7809e-3 \\ -2.0777e-3 \\ 2.5124e-3 \\ -9.9594e-1 \\ 1.7904e-3 \\ 9.9593e-1 \\ -9.9593e-1 \\ 2.7809e-3 \\ -9.9592e-1 \end{bmatrix}, \quad \bar{\gamma}^5 \approx \begin{bmatrix} -9.9595e-1 \\ 2.0514e-3 \\ -2.7120e-3 \\ 9.9590e-1 \\ 3.9224e-3 \\ 9.9593e-1 \\ 2.5567e-3 \\ -2.5567e-3 \\ 2.0514e-3 \\ -9.9592e-1 \end{bmatrix}, \quad \bar{\gamma}^6 \approx \begin{bmatrix} -9.8968e-1 \\ -4.7226e-1 \\ -3.6780e-1 \\ 2.4001e-1 \\ 9.9746e-1 \\ 9.9529e-1 \\ 4.9090e-1 \\ -4.9090e-1 \\ -4.7226e-1 \\ -9.9804e-1 \end{bmatrix},$$

$$\bar{\gamma}^7 \approx \begin{bmatrix} -9.9746e-1 \\ -4.7226e-1 \\ -3.6780e-1 \\ 2.4002e-1 \\ -9.8968e-1 \\ 9.9529e-1 \\ 4.9090e-1 \\ -4.9090e-1 \\ -4.7226e-1 \\ -9.9804e-1 \end{bmatrix}, \quad \bar{\gamma}^8 \approx \begin{bmatrix} 3.9078e-3 \\ 2.0472e-3 \\ -2.7143e-3 \\ 9.9590e-1 \\ -9.9595e-1 \\ 9.9593e-1 \\ 2.5570e-3 \\ -2.5570e-3 \\ -2.0472e-3 \\ -9.9592e-1 \end{bmatrix},$$

where "$e-1$" denotes 10^{-1}. Thus, in the present example, the set of asymptotically stable equilibrium points for system (8.3.1) and the set of asymptotically stable equilibrium points for the corresponding (generalized) Hopfield model (8.7.2) (using the same matrix T and vector I) are indeed approximately identical, as discussed in Remark 4.5.2, and the former can be directly used to estimate the latter. ∎

Example 8.7.4 To illustrate how to estimate the domain of attraction of each asymptotically stable equilibrium point of system (8.3.1), we consider an example given by

$$\dot{x} = Tx + I, \quad -1 \leq x_i \leq 1, \quad i = 1, 2, 3 \tag{8.7.3}$$

where $x \in D^3$,

$$T = \begin{bmatrix} -2.6667 & -3.6667 & -3.6667 \\ -3.6667 & -2.6667 & -3.6667 \\ -3.6667 & -3.6667 & -2.6667 \end{bmatrix}$$

and

$$I = \begin{bmatrix} 3.6667 \\ 3.6667 \\ 3.6667 \end{bmatrix}.$$

This system is synthesized by Synthesis Procedure 8.3.1 with the given prototype patterns

$$\alpha^1 = \begin{bmatrix} -1 \\ 1 \\ 1 \end{bmatrix}, \quad \alpha^2 = \begin{bmatrix} 1 \\ -1 \\ 1 \end{bmatrix}, \quad \alpha^3 = \begin{bmatrix} 1 \\ 1 \\ -1 \end{bmatrix}.$$

8.7. ILLUSTRATIVE EXAMPLES

This system has three asymptotically stable equilibrium points α^1, α^2, and α^3, and four unstable equilibrium points given by

$$\beta^1 = \begin{bmatrix} 1 \\ 0 \\ 0 \end{bmatrix}, \quad \beta^2 = \begin{bmatrix} 0 \\ 1 \\ 0 \end{bmatrix}, \quad \beta^3 = \begin{bmatrix} 0 \\ 0 \\ 1 \end{bmatrix}, \quad \beta^4 = \begin{bmatrix} 0.3667 \\ 0.3667 \\ 0.3667 \end{bmatrix}.$$

For this particular example, the domain of attraction of each α^i can be determined by inspection of the symmetry of the set $\{\alpha^1, \alpha^2, \alpha^3\}$ and Span$(\alpha^1, \alpha^2, \alpha^3)$ relative to the axis passing through the point $x_0 = [1,1,1]^T$, as illustrated in Fig. 8.7.1. For example, the domain of attraction of α^1 is the polygon with vertices given by α^1, γ^1, γ^2, γ^3, γ^4, where

$$\gamma^1 = \begin{bmatrix} -1 \\ -1 \\ 1 \end{bmatrix}, \quad \gamma^2 = \begin{bmatrix} 1 \\ 1 \\ 1 \end{bmatrix}, \quad \gamma^3 = \begin{bmatrix} -1 \\ 1 \\ -1 \end{bmatrix}, \quad \gamma^4 = \begin{bmatrix} -1 \\ -1 \\ -1 \end{bmatrix}.$$

In Fig. 8.7.1, we see that all unstable equilibrium points are located on the boundaries of the domains of attraction of $\alpha^1, \alpha^2, \alpha^3$. In general, the domain of attraction of an asymptotically stable equilibrium point of system (8.3.1) may approximately be determined by the set of unstable equilibrium points of (8.3.1) in its vicinity. ∎

Example 8.7.5 We consider in this example patterns made up of 9×9 small boxes. Each pattern corresponds to a vector in $\Re^{81}$ with each component value varying from -1 to 1 determined by the grey level (cf. Fig. 8.7.2) in the corresponding box. If the grey level in a box is black (white) the value of the corresponding component is 1 (-1). Suppose that we wish to synthesize a system (8.3.1), with dimension $n = 81$, which will "remember" certain Chinese characters. Since many Chinese characters can be separated into two basic components, using the present synthesis procedure, we only need to synthesize a system (8.3.1) by employing these basic components. The resulting system will automatically "remember" all possible combinations of the above components. For instance, let us consider a data set $\{\alpha^1, \cdots, \alpha^{31}\}$, where each α^i, $1 \leq i \leq 30$, corresponds to a

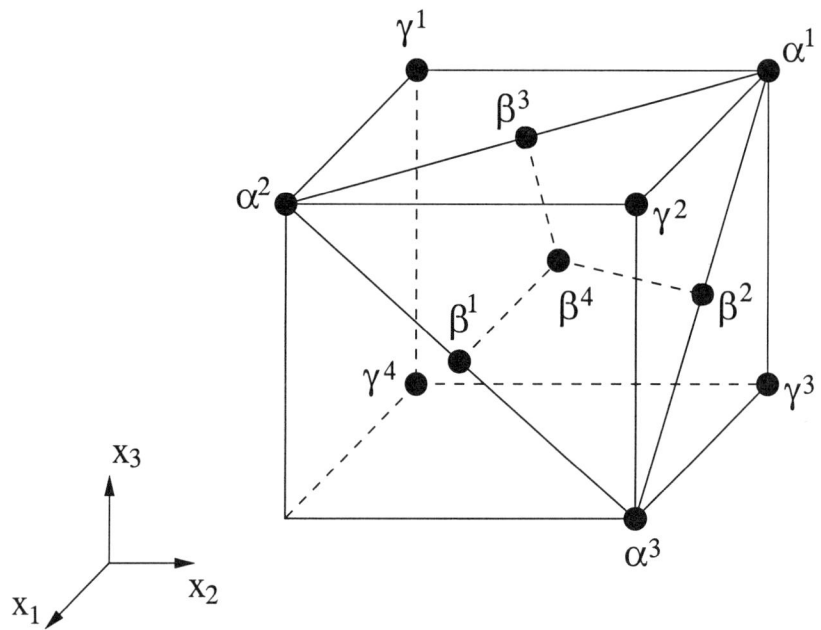

Figure 8.7.1: Location of Aspan($\alpha^1, \alpha^2, \alpha^3$).

8.7. ILLUSTRATIVE EXAMPLES

Chinese character in Fig. 8.7.3, respectively. In particular,

$$\alpha^7 = \begin{bmatrix} -1 & -1 & -1 & -1 & -1 & -1 & -1 & -1 & -1 \\ -1 & -1 & -1 & -1 & -1 & -1 & -1 & -1 & -1 \\ 1 & 1 & 1 & 1 & -1 & -1 & -1 & -1 & -1 \\ 1 & -1 & -1 & 1 & -1 & -1 & -1 & -1 & -1 \\ 1 & 1 & 1 & 1 & -1 & -1 & -1 & -1 & -1 \\ 1 & -1 & -1 & 1 & -1 & -1 & -1 & -1 & -1 \\ 1 & 1 & 1 & 1 & -1 & -1 & -1 & -1 & -1 \\ -1 & -1 & -1 & -1 & -1 & -1 & -1 & -1 & -1 \\ -1 & -1 & -1 & -1 & -1 & -1 & -1 & -1 & -1 \end{bmatrix}$$

and

$$\alpha^{18} = \begin{bmatrix} -1 & -1 & -1 & -1 & -1 & 1 & 1 & 1 & 1 \\ -1 & -1 & -1 & -1 & -1 & 1 & -1 & -1 & 1 \\ -1 & -1 & -1 & -1 & -1 & 1 & 1 & 1 & 1 \\ -1 & -1 & -1 & -1 & -1 & 1 & -1 & -1 & 1 \\ -1 & -1 & -1 & -1 & -1 & 1 & 1 & 1 & 1 \\ -1 & -1 & -1 & -1 & -1 & 1 & -1 & -1 & 1 \\ -1 & -1 & -1 & -1 & -1 & 1 & -1 & -1 & 1 \\ -1 & -1 & -1 & -1 & -1 & 1 & -1 & -1 & 1 \\ -1 & -1 & -1 & -1 & 1 & -1 & -1 & 1 & 1 \end{bmatrix}.$$

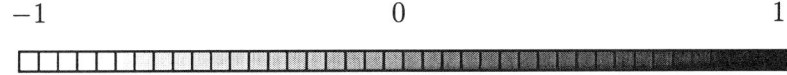

Figure 8.7.2: Grey levels.

The Chinese character corresponding to α^7 means "sun" and the Chinese character corresponding to α^{18} means "moon." Also, in the

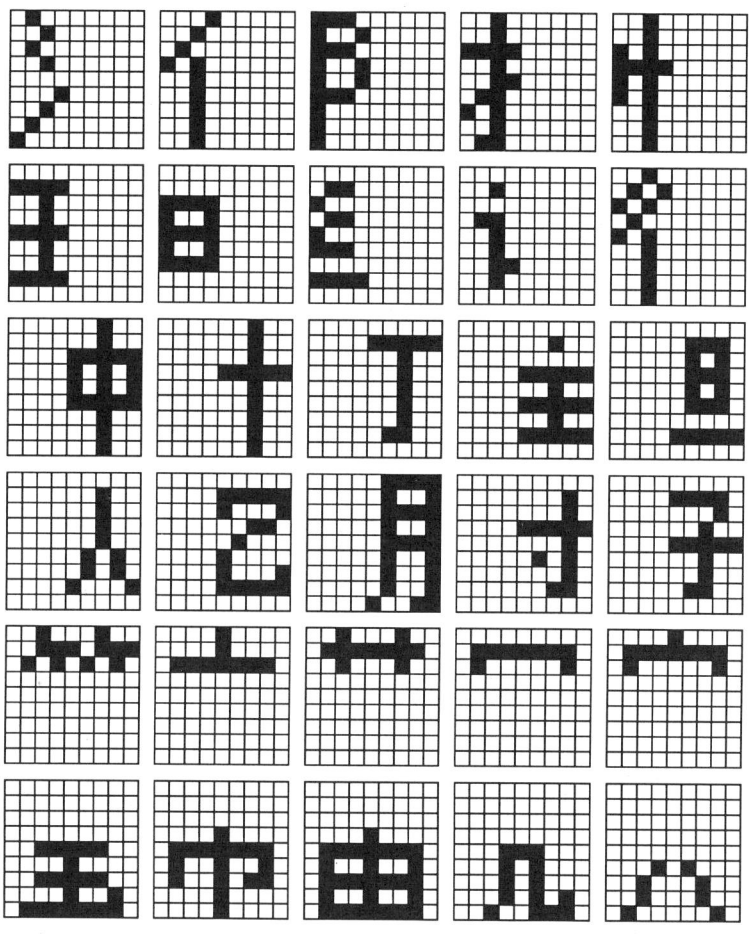

Figure 8.7.3: 30 Chinese characters.

8.7. ILLUSTRATIVE EXAMPLES

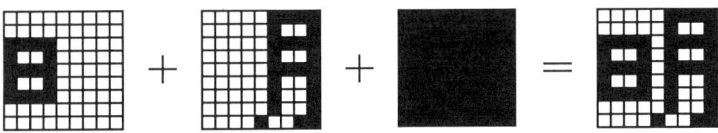

Figure 8.7.4: Two basic Chinese characters, "sun" and "moon", together form the Chinese character "bright".

given data set, α^{31} corresponds to "nothing," i.e.,

$$\alpha^{31} = \begin{bmatrix} 1 & 1 & 1 & 1 & 1 & 1 & 1 & 1 & 1 \\ 1 & 1 & 1 & 1 & 1 & 1 & 1 & 1 & 1 \\ 1 & 1 & 1 & 1 & 1 & 1 & 1 & 1 & 1 \\ 1 & 1 & 1 & 1 & 1 & 1 & 1 & 1 & 1 \\ 1 & 1 & 1 & 1 & 1 & 1 & 1 & 1 & 1 \\ 1 & 1 & 1 & 1 & 1 & 1 & 1 & 1 & 1 \\ 1 & 1 & 1 & 1 & 1 & 1 & 1 & 1 & 1 \\ 1 & 1 & 1 & 1 & 1 & 1 & 1 & 1 & 1 \\ 1 & 1 & 1 & 1 & 1 & 1 & 1 & 1 & 1 \end{bmatrix}.$$

With these desired patterns, we can generate combinations of Chinese characters which are made up of some of the basic modules in Fig. 8.7.3. For instance, a new Chinese character can be generated as

$$\alpha^* = \alpha^7 + \alpha^{18} + \alpha^{31} \in \text{Span}(\alpha^1, \cdots, \alpha^{31}) \cap B^{81}$$

which means "bright" (cf. Fig. 8.7.4).

To simplify our calculation, we will synthesize system (8.3.1) as discussed in Remark 8.3.4, resulting in $I_\tau = 0$. In this case, we have $L_a = \text{Aspan}(\alpha^1, \cdots, \alpha^{31}) = \text{Span}(\alpha^1, \cdots, \alpha^{31})$, and by Theorem 8.3.1, α^* will be an asymptotically stable equilibrium point of the synthesized system. To illustrate this, we generate an initial pattern γ by adding zero-mean Gaussian noise with standard deviation SD= 1 to α^*. A simulation run of the synthesized system (performed on a Sun SPARC Station, using MATLAB) with γ as the initial state is depicted in Fig. 8.7.5. The desired pattern α^* is recovered in 24

408   CHAPTER 8. SYNTHESIS METHODS

steps. The initial pattern γ is shown in the upper left corner of Fig. 8.7.5. We note that γ has more than 30 bits which differ from α^*. The iteration of the simulation evolves from left to right in each row and from the top row to the bottom row.

Simulation results show that all the other vectors corresponding to the combinations of patterns given in Fig. 8.7.3 are asymptotically stable equilibrium points of the synthesized system. ∎

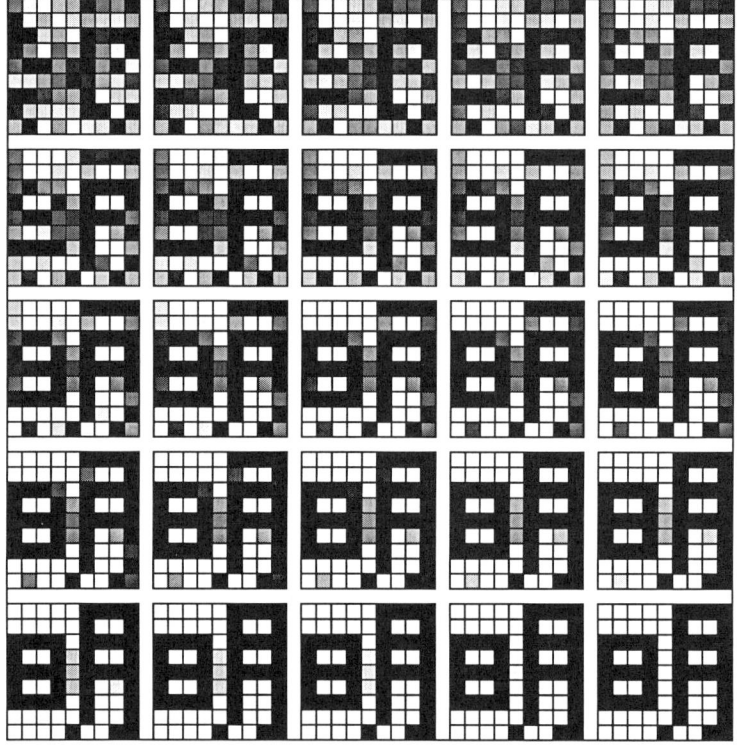

Figure 8.7.5: The Chinese character composed of pattern number 7 and number 18.

Example 8.7.6 A neural network with 12 neurons ($n = 12$) is considered with the objective of storing the 12 ($m = 12$) patterns

8.7. ILLUSTRATIVE EXAMPLES

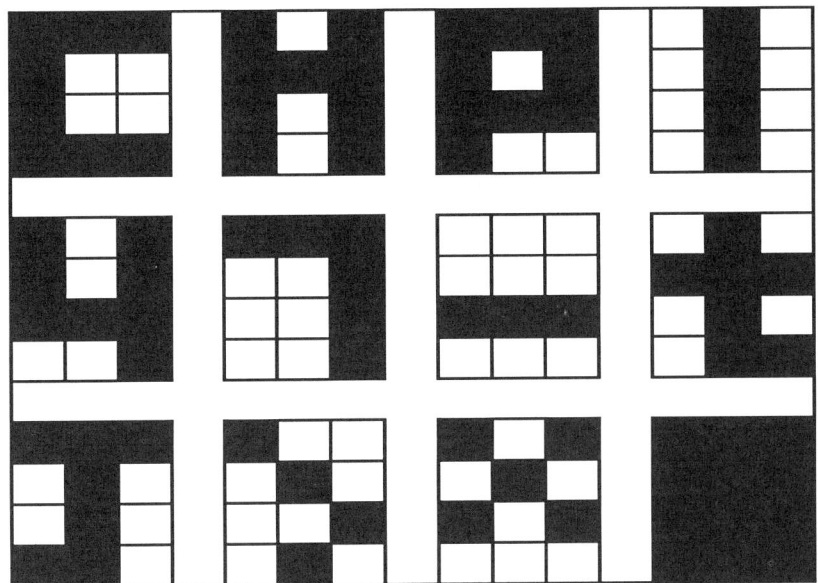

Figure 8.7.6: The twelve desired memory patterns.

$\alpha^1, \cdots, \alpha^{12}$ shown in Fig. 8.7.6 as memories. As indicated in this figure, twelve boxes are used to represent each pattern (in $\Re^{12}$), with each box corresponding to a vector component which is allowed to assume values between -1 and 1 according to the grey levels shown in Fig 8.7.2. In this example, a neural network (8.5.1) with A equal to the identity matrix and satisfying the optimal constraints, i.e., with every diagonal element of T equal to 1 ($T_{ii} = a_i = 1$), will be designed.

The objective is to utilize Synthesis Procedure 8.5.1 to design a non-symmetric neural network with all the diagonal elements equal to 1. In Synthesis Procedure 8.5.1, the initial weight W^i is chosen to be the zero vector and the perceptron learning rate is chosen to be $\eta = 0.1$. (Symmetric design procedures will be evaluated and illustrated in Section 9.5.) It turns out that the desired patterns do not satisfy the rank condition of Theorem 8.5.4 when $i = 2, 5, 8, 10, 11, 12$. Still, all the w_i^i obtained by using Synthesis Procedure 8.5.1, along with Remark 8.5.12, are less than 0. Therefore, a connection matrix T with every diagonal element equal to 1 can be obtained. A is determined to be the identity matrix, T is determined as

$$T = \begin{bmatrix} 1 & -1.2 & 9.2 & 0.4 & 2.2 & 0 & -1 & -4.4 & 4.6 & 2.4 & 2.2 & 0.2 \\ -0.3 & 1 & 5.9 & -3.3 & -4.9 & 5.5 & -9.3 & 3.9 & -6.7 & 7.7 & 6.3 & -0.9 \\ 8.9 & 3.9 & 1 & -0.1 & 0.3 & 0.9 & 4.5 & -0.5 & -0.9 & 5.7 & -5.1 & 1.3 \\ -1.5 & 0.5 & -0.9 & 1 & -0.3 & 6.7 & 7.1 & 3.3 & -2.3 & 4.7 & 2.1 & 5.3 \\ 1.8 & -19 & 0.4 & -2.6 & 1 & 11 & -10.2 & -6.2 & 4.8 & 4.6 & 24 & -10.6 \\ 0 & 2.8 & 1 & 6 & 2 & 1 & -4.6 & 3.6 & 5.2 & -0.6 & -5.2 & 5 \\ -0.3 & -5.7 & 3.5 & 7.3 & -2.3 & -3.9 & 1 & 2.1 & 4.1 & 4.1 & -3.7 & -0.1 \\ -15.4 & 7.8 & 4.6 & 8.6 & -1.6 & 20 & 6 & 1 & -2.6 & -5 & 7.8 & -23.4 \\ 6.2 & -5.8 & 0.6 & -1.4 & 2.4 & 6 & 4.6 & 0 & 1 & -2.8 & -4.2 & -1 \\ 5.3 & 5.5 & 7.3 & 7.7 & 3.1 & 0.9 & 4.3 & -3.5 & -4.5 & 1 & 4.3 & -2.3 \\ 2.9 & 6.1 & -4.3 & 1.7 & 6.3 & -5.1 & -4.1 & 1.9 & -3.7 & 2.3 & 1 & 1.7 \\ -1.5 & -0.7 & 5.1 & 7.3 & 0.7 & 10.5 & -1.3 & -6.5 & -4.7 & -6.9 & 6.7 & 1 \end{bmatrix}$$

and I is determined to be

$$I = [6,\ 5.5,\ 2.5,\ -0.7,\ 12.8,\ -2.8,\ 2.3,\ 17.6,\ 4,\ -9.3,\ 2.7,\ -1.5]^T.$$

Using Lemma 6.6.1, one can determine that neural network (8.5.1) with the $\{A, T, I\}$ determined as above has 8 spurious memory points in B^n. From Corollary 5.7.1, one can see that these 8 vectors are the only spurious memory vectors in D^n in this case since $T_{ii} \geq a_i$ for $i = 1, \cdots, n$ are satisfied. To see whether the neural network has in this case other stable memories in D^n, 5000 simulation runs

8.7. ILLUSTRATIVE EXAMPLES

with randomly chosen initial states in D^n are performed. From these runs, no more spurious memory vectors in D^n are discovered. In the present case, the synthesized neural network may not be globally stable, since the matrix T is not symmetric, and thus, periodic solutions may exist. (However, all 5000 simulation runs terminated at stable equilibria.) Simulation results also show that every $\gamma \in B^n$ such that $H(\alpha^k, \gamma) = 1$ for each k, $1 \leq k \leq 12$, is indeed in the domain of attraction of α^k. Using Theorem 6.6.1, one can determine as in (6.6.4) [cf. (8.5.19)] $\nu = 7$, which implies that the allowable upper bound for parameter perturbations in neural network (8.5.1) is given by

$$\|A^{-1}\Delta A\|_\infty + \|A^{-1}\Delta T\|_\infty + |A^{-1}\Delta I|_\infty$$
$$= \|\Delta A\|_\infty + \|\Delta T\|_\infty + |\Delta I|_\infty < \nu - 1 = 6. \qquad \blacksquare$$

Example 8.7.7 The objective of this example is to study the effects of the diagonal elements of the connection matrix T on the spurious memories in neural networks described by (8.5.1), and to compare the Eigenstructure Method (Synthesis Procedure 8.4.1), the method based on the perceptron training algorithm (Synthesis Procedure 8.5.1), and the method of [29]. The same network as in Example 8.7.6 will be used. As seen in that example, under the optimal constraints ($T_{ii} = a_i = 1$ for $i = 1, \cdots, n$) with $\nu = 7$, the network has a total of 8 spurious memories in D^n. Table 8.5.2 shows the results for the neural network designed using Synthesis Procedure 8.5.1 which stores the $m = 12$ patterns in Fig. 8.7.6 as stable memories. Different constraints for the diagonal elements of matrix T given by $T_{ii} = 4, 3, 2, 1, 0, -1, -2, -3$ are considered in the design examples (cf. Remark 8.5.11 for how to achieve $T_{ii} \leq a_i$).

The value of ν is also computed in accordance with (8.5.19) for each case considered. From Table 8.5.2, one can see that the total number of spurious memories in a network which satisfies the optimal constraints are generally smaller than the total number of spurious memories in a network which does not satisfy the optimal constraints. Also, the total number of spurious memories in a network change little with respect to the value of ν when the optimal constraints are

Table 8.5.2: Comparison results of Example 8.7.7.

	Number of spurious memories in B^n	Number of spurious memories in D^n-B^n
$T_{ii}=4$	4084 ($\nu=3.6$), 357 ($\nu=4$) 64 ($\nu=7$), 20 ($\nu=14$) 16 ($\nu=28$), 12 ($\nu=56$)	0
$T_{ii}=3$	4084 ($\nu=2.6$), 95 ($\nu=4$) 32 ($\nu=7$), 16 ($\nu=14$) 12 ($\nu=28$), 10 ($\nu=56$)	0
$T_{ii}=2$	3876 ($\nu=1.6$), 30 ($\nu=4$) 18 ($\nu=7$), 12 ($\nu=14$) 11 ($\nu=28$), 9 ($\nu=56$)	0
$T_{ii}=1$ (optimal constraints)	6 ($\nu=1.2$), 9 ($\nu=4$) 8 ($\nu=7$), 8 ($\nu=14$) 9 ($\nu=28$), 9 ($\nu=56$)	0
$T_{ii}=0$	3 ($\nu=4$), 5 ($\nu=14$)	≥ 6 ($\nu=4$) ≥ 4 ($\nu=14$)
$T_{ii}=-1$	0 ($\nu=4$), 3 ($\nu=14$)	≥ 10 ($\nu=4$) ≥ 8 ($\nu=14$)
$T_{ii}=-2$	0 ($\nu=4$), 2 ($\nu=14$)	≥ 10 ($\nu=4$) ≥ 8 ($\nu=14$)
$T_{ii}=-3$	0 ($\nu=4$), 1 ($\nu=14$)	≥ 10 ($\nu=4$) ≥ 11 ($\nu=14$)
Synthesis Procedure 8.4.1	1382 ($\nu=1.6$), 874 ($\nu=4$) 874 ($\nu=7$), 874 ($\nu=14$) 874 ($\nu=28$), 874 ($\nu=56$)	0
method of [29] with $T_{ii}=1$	15 ($\nu=1.7$), 17 ($\nu=4$) 14 ($\nu=7$), 13 ($\nu=14$) 12 ($\nu=28$), 13 ($\nu=56$)	0
method of [29] with $T_{ii}=3$	644 ($\nu=4$), 183 ($\nu=5$) 69 ($\nu=7$), 24 ($\nu=14$) 18 ($\nu=28$), 17 ($\nu=56$)	0

8.7. ILLUSTRATIVE EXAMPLES

satisfied. However, when the optimal constraints are not satisfied, the total number of spurious memories depends heavily on the value of ν (especially when $T_{ii} = 2, 3, 4$).

For the same problem as above, results for neural networks designed using Synthesis Procedure 8.4.1 and the method of [29] are also compared in the table. Since Synthesis Procedure 8.4.1 does not have any control over the diagonal elements of the connection matrix T, the network designed by this procedure will usually have more spurious memories than the network designed using Synthesis Procedure 8.5.1 and using the method of [29]. The latter two design methods are comparable to each other in terms of the total number of spurious memories. However, in general, neural networks designed using Synthesis Procedure 8.5.1 and the method of [29] will not be globally stable, while neural networks designed using Synthesis Procedure 8.4.1 will *always* be globally stable. It is noted that when the number of desired patterns is small (e.g., when $m \leq 5$), all three methods yield comparable results. It is also noted that approaches using Synthesis Procedures 8.4.1 and 8.5.1 are simpler to implement and usually take less computational time than the design method of [29]. ∎

Example 8.7.8 The objective of this example is to study the capacity of associative memories designed using Synthesis Procedure 8.5.1 and to compare this with the study in [5], [6]. In the present example, capacity is defined as a measure of the ability of an associative memory to store a set of unbiased random binary patterns at a given error correction and recall accuracy level (cf. [5], [6]). For each test, 10 sets of m random bipolar patterns $(2 < m \leq n)$ are generated with memory size $n = 16, 32$, and 64. The results shown are based on ensemble averages over 10 tests. The empirical data show that the capacity of system (8.5.1) with high recall accuracy $(RA > 99\%)$ is approximately linear to the pattern dimension (i.e., $m \approx n$). When the number of stored patterns exceeds n, system (8.5.1) looses its error correction ability (for the given $RA > 99\%$). The results shown in Figs. 8.7.7 and 8.7.8 are comparable to the Ho-Kashyap recording [6] with certain improvement. For example, it is concluded in [6] that

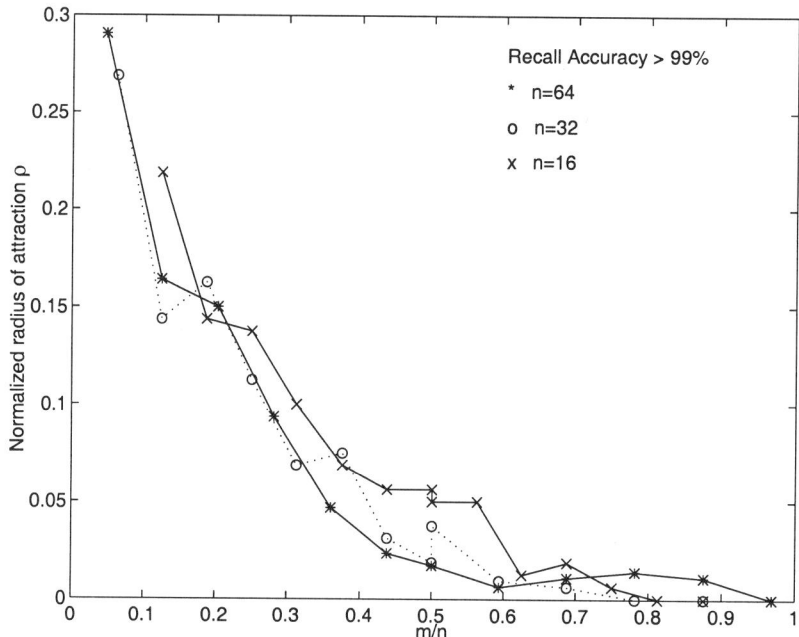

Figure 8.7.7: Capacity performance of Synthesis Procedure 8.5.1

the Ho-Kashyap recording requires $m/n < 0.5$, while in the present case, m/n can be very close to 1. ∎

8.8 Summary

In the present chapter, we concerned ourselves with associative memory synthesis problems using different types of neural networks. We first reviewed the Outer Product Method for the design of (asynchronous) neural networks described by equations of the form

$$\begin{cases} v_i(k+1) = \text{sgn}(u_i(k)), & 1 \leq i \leq n \\ u_i(k) = \sum_{j=1}^{n} T_{ij} v_j(k) + I_i, & 1 \leq i \leq n. \end{cases} \quad (8.8.1)$$

8.8. SUMMARY

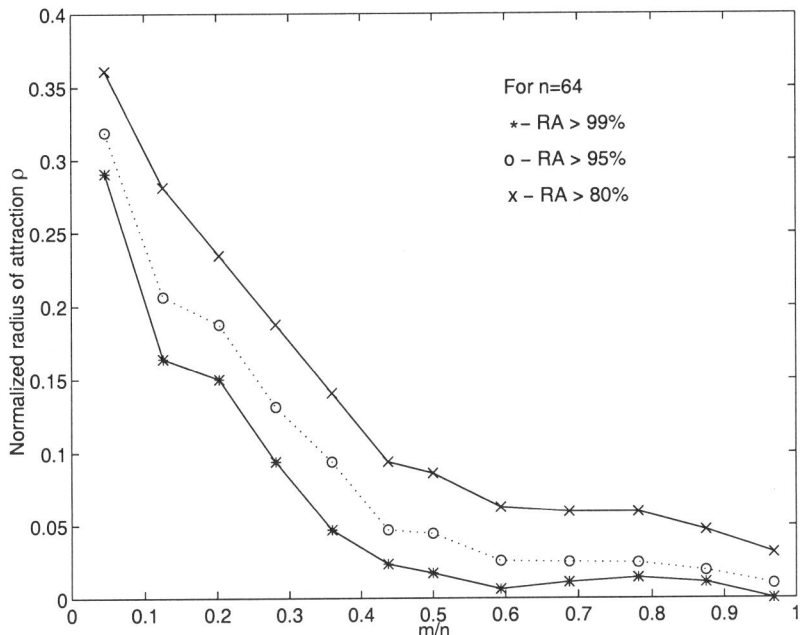

Figure 8.7.8: Capacity performance of Synthesis Procedure 8.5.1 for various RA ranges ($n = 64$)

Using the Outer Product Method, T and I are chosen as

$$\begin{cases} T = [T_{ij}] = \sum_{i=1}^{m} \alpha^i (\alpha^i)^T \\ I = (I_1 \cdots, I_n)^T = 0 \end{cases} \quad (8.8.2)$$

where $\alpha^i \in B^n$, $i = 1, \cdots, m$, are prototype patterns to be stored as memory vectors in network (8.8.1). It was argued that the Outer Product Method presented in (8.8.2) can also be applied to neural networks described by equations of the form

$$\begin{cases} du_i/dt = \sum_{j=1}^{n} T_{ij} v_j - b_i u_i + I_i \\ v_i = g(u_i), \quad i = 1, \cdots, n, \end{cases} \quad (8.8.3)$$

when the gain of the function g is sufficiently large. It was shown that when the prototype patterns are not mutually orthogonal, the Outer

Product Method cannot guarantee to store all the desired patterns as equilibrium points of the designed neural network.

Next, we reviewed the Projection Learning Rule for the design of neural networks described by equations of the form

$$\begin{cases} v_i(k+1) = g(u_i(k)), & 1 \leq i \leq n \\ u_i(k) = \sum_{j=1}^{n} T_{ij}v_j(k) + I_i, & 1 \leq i \leq n \end{cases} \quad (8.8.4)$$

with $g(u) = \text{sgn}(u)$. This is the synchronous counterpart to (8.8.1). Using the Projection Learning Rule, T and I in (8.8.4) were determined as

$$\begin{cases} T = \Sigma\Sigma^\dagger \\ -1 \leq I_i \leq 1, & i = 1, \cdots, n \end{cases} \quad (8.8.5)$$

where $\Sigma = [\alpha^1 \vdots \cdots \vdots \alpha^m]$ and $\Sigma^\dagger$ denotes the Moore-Penrose pseudo-inverse. It was shown that the Projection Learning Rule guarantees to store all the desired patterns as equilibrium points in a network, but in general does not guarantee to store them as asymptotically stable equilibrium points. It was also shown that when all the prototype patterns are mutually orthogonal, the Projection Learning Rule reduces to the Outer Product Method.

The Projection Learning Rule can be combined with the stability analysis results developed in Chapter 5 (see Section 5.6) to obtain a design method with constraints so that all the prototype patterns become asymptotically stable equilibria of the neural network. We accomplished this by the use of neural networks described by equations of the form

$$\begin{cases} u_i(k+1) = \sum_{j=1}^{n} T_{ij}v_j(k) - a_i u_i(k) + I_i \\ v_i(k) = g(u_i(k)), & i = 1, \cdots, n. \end{cases} \quad (8.8.6)$$

Combining the Projection Learning Rule with the stability results of Section 5.6, we obtained neural network parameters using the Projection Learning Rule (or, pseudo-inverse method) with constraints given by

$$F_i = 1 - |a_i| - \sum_{j=1}^{n} T_{ij} > 0, \quad i = 1, \cdots, n.$$

8.8. SUMMARY

Finally, for neural networks described by (8.8.6), we developed an *iterative* learning algorithm in the spirit of the Projection Learning Rule, assuming (for convenience) that $a_i = 0$, $i = 1, \cdots, n$.

Next, we developed a third synthesis approach, called the Eigenstructure Method. This method was first introduced in the design of neural networks described by equations of the form

$$\dot{x} = Tx + I, \quad x \in D^n. \tag{8.8.7}$$

In the Eigenstructure Method, we first construct the matrix

$$Y = \begin{bmatrix} \alpha^1 - \alpha^m \vdots \cdots \vdots \alpha^{m-1} - \alpha^m \end{bmatrix},$$

where the $\alpha^1, \cdots, \alpha^m$ denote the memory patterns to be stored in (8.8.7). We then perform a singular value decomposition of Y to obtain

$$Y = \begin{bmatrix} U_1 \vdots U_2 \end{bmatrix} \begin{bmatrix} D & \vdots & 0 \\ \cdots & \cdots & \cdots \\ 0 & \vdots & 0 \end{bmatrix} \begin{bmatrix} V_1^T \\ \cdots \\ V_2^T \end{bmatrix}.$$

The parameters which make up T and I are determined by

$$\begin{cases} T = T^+ - \tau T^- \\ I = \alpha^m - T\alpha^m \end{cases}$$

where $T^+ = U_1 U_1^T$, $T^- = U_2 U_2^T$, and τ is a parameter chosen as $\tau > -1$. We then showed that the Eigenstructure Method guarantees that the designed network will store all the desired patterns as asymptotically stable equilibrium points of (8.8.7). We also showed that when choosing $\tau > -1$, the number of spurious memories contained in B^n will decrease as τ increases. Similar synthesis procedures were also devised for various other neural network models discussed in Chapter 2.

Next, we developed another synthesis approach which is based on the perceptron training algorithm. In doing so, we considered neural networks described by equations of the form

$$\begin{cases} \dot{x} = -Ax + Ty + I \\ y = \text{sat}(x). \end{cases} \tag{8.8.8}$$

We formulated the design problem as a set of linear inequalities for which the use of the perceptron training algorithm becomes evident. In this approach, we obtained n perceptrons given by $W^i = (w_1^i, w_2^i, \cdots, w_{n+1}^i)$, $i = 1, \cdots, n$, such that

$$\begin{cases} W^i \overline{\alpha}^k \geq 0 & \text{if } \alpha_i^k = 1 \\ W^i \overline{\alpha}^k < 0 & \text{if } \alpha_i^k = -1 \end{cases}$$

for $k = 1, \cdots, m$, where $\overline{\alpha}^k = \begin{pmatrix} \alpha^k \\ \cdots \\ 1 \end{pmatrix}$. Choose $A = \text{diag}[a_1, \cdots, a_n]$ with $a_i > 0$. For $i, j = 1, \cdots, n$, choose $T_{ij} = w_j^i$ if $i \neq j$, $T_{ii} = w_i^i + a_i \mu_i$ with $\mu_i > 1$, and $I_i = w_{n+1}^i$. We showed that the perceptron training in the above synthesis procedure will always converge.

In comparing the Eigenstructure Method with the perceptron based training approach, we utilized the identical neural network model, given in (8.8.8). In both approaches, we solved the parameters $\{A, T, I\}$, using the requirement that

$$A^{-1}(T\alpha^k + I) \in F(\alpha^k), \quad k = 1, \cdots, m, \qquad (8.8.9)$$

where $F(\alpha) = \{x \in \Re^n : x_i \alpha^i > 1, \ i = 1, \cdots, n\}$. However, in the case of the Eigenstructure Method, we had to choose a special case of (8.8.9) given by

$$T\alpha^k + I = \mu \alpha^k, \quad k = 1, \cdots, m$$

with $\mu > 1$. The Eigenstructure Method presented in this chapter will always yield a globally stable neural network design with symmetric matrix T, while the perceptron based training approach will usually lead to a network design with nonsymmetric matrix T (which need not necessarily be globally stable). To obtain a neural network design with symmetric matrix T, using the perceptron training algorithm, we utilized the robustness analysis results of Section 6.6. For this method, a solution does not always exist.

For neural networks described by (8.8.8), we established results which show that when we impose certain constraints on the diagonal elements of matrix T, the network will possess certain desirable properties. In particular, when requiring that $T_{ii} \geq a_i$, $i = 1, \cdots, n$, all of the memory vectors [output vectors corresponding to the asymptotically stable equilibrium points of (8.8.8)] will be in B^n; and when $T_{ii} \leq a_i$, $i = 1, \cdots, n$, every corner of the hypercube which is in the immediate neighborhood of a stable memory vector may itself not become a stable memory and is very likely in the domain of attraction of that stable memory vector. Combining the above, we referred to the constraints given by $T_{ii} = a_i$, $i = 1, \cdots, n$, as "optimal constraints."

Next, we showed that the necessary and sufficient conditions under which a designed neural network (8.8.8) satisfies the preceding constraints is that $T_{ii} \leq a_i$, $i = 1, \cdots, n$. We also extended the synthesis approach based on the perceptron training algorithm to several neural network models originally discussed in Chapter 2. Similar optimal constraints were established for each of the neural network models considered. To facilitate the design of other neural networks with symmetric connection matrix, using the perceptron training algorithm, we established results similar to Theorem 6.6.1 for each of the models considered. These results provided allowable bounds on parameter perturbations under which a desired set of bipolar patterns will still be memory vectors after parameter perturbations.

Finally, the Eigenstructure Method and the Perceptron Training Based Method were applied to several specific examples to demonstrate the strengths and weaknesses of these synthesis procedures.

8.9 Notes and References

Suitable sources for the Outer Product Method include [9]–[11] and [30]. The development of the Projection Learning Rule is presented in [25] and [26]. Our summary and comparison of these methods, given in Section 8.1, was influenced by a discussion of these methods in [18].

Section 8.2 is based on [19] and [32].

Section 8.3 is based on [14]. For more complete disclosures on the development of the Eigenstructure Method, refer to [12]–[14], [16], [17], [21], and [22].

In MATLAB, an implementation of the Eigenstructure Method is included as part of its Neural Network Toolbox. The function for the Eigenstructure Method in MATLAB's Neural Network Toolbox is called **newhop** [3].

Section 8.4 which contains adaptations of the Eigenstructure Method to a variety of neural networks, is based in part on [13] and [17]. Additional extensions of the Eigenstructure Method are addressed, e.g., in [31] and [33].

Sections 8.5 and 8.6 are based on material developed in [15]. The perceptron algorithm and related materials (including the convergence theorem for this algorithm), were made public several decades ago [23], [27]. This topic has become standard fare in contemporary texts on artificial neural networks (cf., e.g., [7] and [34]).

The examples presented in Section 8.7 are based on material presented in [14], [15], and [17].

Bibliography

[1] A Albert. Regression and the Moore-Penrose Pseudo-Inverse. New York, NY: Academic Press, 1972.

[2] R Bronson. Matrix Operation. New York, NY: McGraw-Hill, 1989.

[3] H Demuth, M Beale. Neural Network Toolbox for Use with MATLAB. Natick, MA: MathWorks, 1998.

[4] JS Denker. Neural Networks for Computing. AIP Conference Proceedings, no 151, Snowbird, UT, 1986.

[5] MH Hassoun. Associative Neural Memories: Theory and Implementation. New York, NY: Oxford University Press, 1993.

[6] MH Hassoun, AM Youssef. Associative neural memory capacity and dynamics. Proceedings of the International Joint Conference on Neural Networks, San Diego, CA, 1990, vol 1, pp 763–769.

[7] S Haykin. Neural Networks: A Comprehensive Foundation. Upper Saddle River, NJ: Prentice-Hall, 1999.

[8] DO Hebb. The Organization of Behavior. New York, NY: Wiley, 1949.

[9] JJ Hopfield. Neural networks and physical systems with emergent collective computational abilities. Proceedings of the National Academy of Sciences USA 79:2554–2558, 1982.

[10] JJ Hopfield, DI Feinstein, RE Palmer. 'Unlearning' has a stabilizing effect in collective memories. Nature 304:158–159, 1983.

[11] JJ Hopfield. Neurons with graded response have collective computational properties like those of two-state neurons. Proceedings of the National Academy of Sciences USA 81:3088–3092, 1984.

[12] JH Li, AN Michel, W Porod. Qualitative analysis and synthesis of a class of neural networks. IEEE Transactions on Circuits and Systems 35:976–987, 1988

[13] JH Li, AN Michel, W Porod. Analysis and synthesis of a class of neural networks: Variable structure systems with infinite gains. IEEE Transactions on Circuits and Systems 36:713–731, 1989.

[14] JH Li, AN Michel, W Porod. Analysis and synthesis of a class of neural networks: Linear systems operating on a closed hypercube. IEEE Transactions on Circuits and Systems 36:1405–1422, 1989.

[15] D Liu, Z Lu. A new synthesis approach for feedback neural networks based on the perceptron training algorithm. IEEE Transactions on Neural Networks 8:1468–1482, 1997.

[16] D Liu, AN Michel. Dynamical Systems with Saturation Nonlinearities: Analysis and Design. Lecture Notes in Control and Information Sciences, vol 195. Berlin, Germany: Springer-Verlag, 1994.

[17] D Liu, AN Michel. Sparsely interconnected neural networks for associative memories with applications to cellular neural networks. IEEE Transactions on Circuits and Systems-II: Analog and Digital Signal Processing 41:295–307, 1994.

[18] AN Michel, JA Farrell. Associative memories via neural networks. IEEE Control Systems Magazine 10:6–17, 1990.

[19] AN Michel, JA Farrell, HF Sun. Analysis and synthesis techniques for Hopfield type synchronous discrete time neural networks with applications to content addressable memory. IEEE Transactions on Circuits and Systems 37:1356–1366, 1990.

[20] AN Michel, CJ Herget. Applied Algebra and Functional Analysis. New York, NY: Dover Publications, 1993.

[21] AN Michel, D Liu. Theory and applications of sparsely interconnected neural networks. Neural, Parallel and Scientific Computations 4:305–324, 1996.

[22] AN Michel, J Si, G Yen. Analysis and synthesis of a class of discrete-time neural networks described on hypercubes. IEEE Transactions on Neural Networks 2:32–46, 1991.

[23] ML Minsky, SA Papert. Perceptrons: An Introduction to Computational Geometry. Cambridge, MA: M.I.T. Press, 1969 and 1988 (expanded version).

[24] R Perfetti. A synthesis procedure for brain-state-in-a-box neural networks. IEEE Transactions on Neural Networks 6:1071–1080, 1995.

[25] L Personnaz, I Guyon, G Dreyfus. Information storage and retrieval in spin-glass like neural networks. Journal de Physique Lettres 46:L359–L365, 1985.

[26] L Personnaz, I Guyon, G Dreyfus. Collective properties of neural networks: New learning mechanism. Physical Review A 34:4217–4228, 1986.

[27] F Rosenblatt. Principles of Neurodynamics. New York, NY: Spartan, 1962.

[28] DE Rumelhart, KL McClelland. Eds. Parallel Distributed Processing, vol 1. Cambridge, MA: MIT Press, 1986.

[29] G Seiler, AJ Schuler, JA Nossek. Design of robust cellular neural networks. IEEE Transactions on Circuits and Systems-I: Fundamental Theory and Applications 40:358–364, 1993.

[30] DW Tank, JJ Hopfield. Simple 'neural' optimization networks: An A/D converter, signal decision circuit, and a linear programming circuit. IEEE Transactions on Circuits and Systems 33:533–541, 1986.

[31] ZB Xu, GQ Hu, CP Kwong. Some efficient strategies for improving the eigenstructure method in synthesis of feedback neural networks. IEEE Transactions on Neural Networks 7:233–245, 1996.

[32] G Yen, AN Michel. A learning and forgetting algorithm in associative memories: Results involving pseudo inverse. IEEE Transactions on Circuits and Systems 38:1193–1205, 1991.

[33] G Yen, AN Michel. A learning and forgetting algorithm in associative memories: The Eigenstructure Method. IEEE Transactions on Circuits and Systems-II: Analog and Digital Signal Processing 39:212–225, 1992.

[34] JM Zurada. Introduction to Artificial Neural Systems. St. Paul, MN: West Publishing Company, 1992.

Chapter 9

Effects of Interconnection Constraints

9.1 Introduction

In the present chapter, we continue to concern ourselves with the implementation of associative memories by means of artificial neural networks. One of the major difficulties encountered in VLSI implementations of artificial neural networks is the realization of extremely large numbers of interconnections in the network. To reduce the number of connections is therefore of great interest from a practical point of view. Many of the existing synthesis procedures for associative memories were developed for fully interconnected neural networks and they do not result in neural networks with *prespecified partial* or *sparse interconnection structure*. Synthesis procedures for neural networks with arbitrarily (prespecified) sparse interconnection structure, or equivalently, with sparse coefficient matrix, constitute a major addition to the development of neural network theory, and such procedures have potentially many practical applications, especially in the areas of associative memories and pattern recognition. (We will define the precise meaning of sparse coefficient matrix later.)

In one of the few existing works dealing with *sparsity constraints* (using the discrete-time Hopfield model), it is proposed to transform a given neural network into a partially connected or cellular network [6]. However, as pointed out in [6], "the application of the suggested transformation algorithm is severely limited by its quickly growing complexity."

Using the results of Section 8.3, we will develop in Section 9.2 a synthesis procedure based on the Eigenstructure Method for neural networks with sparse coefficient matrices in which the interconnection structure is prespecified. We will develop this synthesis procedure for neural networks described by equations of the form [cf. (2.2.6)]

$$\begin{cases} \dot{x} = -Ax + Ty + I \\ y = \text{sat}(x) \end{cases} \quad (9.1.1)$$

where $x \in \Re^n$, $\dot{x}$ denotes the derivative of x with respect to time t, $A = \text{diag}[a_1, \cdots, a_n]$ with $a_i > 0$, $T = [T_{ij}] \in \Re^{n \times n}$ is a constant matrix, $I = [I_1, \cdots, I_n]^T$ is a constant vector, and the activation function sat($\cdot$) is defined by

$$\text{sat}(x_i) = \begin{cases} 1, & x_i > 1 \\ x_i, & -1 \leq x_i \leq 1 \\ -1, & x_i < -1. \end{cases}$$

Our method is equally applicable to other neural network models introduced in Chapter 2. In Section 9.3, we will introduce a sparse synthesis method based on the perceptron training algorithm presented in Section 8.5. In Section 9.4, we will apply the sparse synthesis techniques developed in Sections 9.2 and 9.3 and the robustness analysis results established in Section 6.6 in the design of a class of cellular neural networks for associative memories. We will show that under certain restrictions on the interconnection structure, system (9.1.1) is equivalent to a class of zero-input, nonsymmetric cellular neural networks. Finally, in Section 9.5, we consider several specific examples to demonstrate the applicability of the synthesis procedures advocated herein. Special emphasis will be placed on cellular neural networks and networks with different sparse interconnection structures.

9.2 The Eigenstructure Method in the Synthesis of Sparsely Interconnected Neural Networks

The synthesis technique developed in Section 8.3 results in general in neural networks with *symmetric* and *non-sparse* coefficient matrix T. However, fully interconnected artificial neural networks with even a moderate number of neurons give rise to large numbers of *line-crossings* resulting from the network interconnections, and thus pose formidable obstacles in VLSI implementations. For these reasons, it is desirable to establish synthesis procedures which result in interconnecting structures which do not involve large numbers of connections.

Using the results of Section 8.3, we develop in the following a design procedure for artificial neural networks which results in few line-crossings or no line-crossings at all in the interconnections, and which does not require the interconnection matrix to be symmetric. *Cellular neural networks*, which we will address later in this chapter (with applications to associative memories), are special cases of such *sparsely interconnected artificial neural networks*.

We begin by introducing some necessary terminology.

A matrix $S = [S_{ij}] \in \Re^{n \times n}$ is said to be an *index matrix*, if it satisfies $S_{ij} = 1$ or 0. The restriction of matrix $W = [W_{ij}] \in \Re^{n \times n}$ to an index matrix S, denoted by $W|S$, is defined by $W|S = [h_{ij}]$, where

$$h_{ij} = \begin{cases} W_{ij}, & \text{if } S_{ij} = 1 \\ 0, & \text{otherwise.} \end{cases}$$

We will say that (9.1.1) is a *neural network with a sparse coefficient matrix* if $T = T|S$ for some given index matrix S, where for at least one pair (i, j), $S_{ij} = 0$.

Sparse Design Problem Given an $n \times n$ index matrix $S = [S_{ij}]$ with $S_{ii} \neq 0$ for $i = 1, \cdots, n$, and m vectors $\alpha^1, \cdots, \alpha^m$ in B^n, choose $\{A, T, I\}$ with $T = T|S$ in such a manner that $\alpha^1, \cdots, \alpha^m$ are (stable) memory vectors of system (9.1.1). ∎

Remark 9.2.1 In the literature, an $n \times n$ matrix is said to be *sparse*, if its number of nonzero elements $\ll n^2$. The definition of *sparse coefficient matrix* given in the present book is more general and includes the usual definition of sparse matrix as a special case. The sparse design problem considered herein, is in fact, more appropriately called an *indexed design problem*. We will use the term *sparse design* in the present book since we wish to be able to make comparisons with the fully connected case. ∎

We recall that according to Lemma 6.6.1, for the synthesis of neural networks described by (9.1.1), we need to solve $\{A, T, I\}$ from

$$A^{-1}(T\alpha^i + I) \in F(\alpha^i), \quad i = 1, \cdots, m, \qquad (9.2.1)$$

where
$$F(\alpha) \triangleq \{x \in \Re^n : x_i \alpha_i > 1, \; i = 1, \cdots, n\}.$$

One special case of (9.2.1) is given by

$$T\alpha^i + I = \mu \alpha^i, \quad i = 1, \cdots, m. \qquad (9.2.2)$$

A solution for our sparse design problem is now obtained in accordance with (9.2.2) as follows.

Synthesis Procedure 9.2.1 Suppose that we are given an $n \times n$ index matrix $S = [S_{ij}]$ with $S_{ii} \neq 0$ for $i = 1, \cdots, n$, and m vectors $\alpha^1, \cdots, \alpha^m$ in B^n which are to be stored as memory vectors in (9.1.1). We proceed as follows:

1) Choose matrix A as the identity matrix.
2) Choose a real number $\mu > 1$ and m vectors $\beta^1, \cdots, \beta^m$, such that $\beta^i = \mu \alpha^i$.
3) Compute the $n \times (m-1)$ matrices

$$Y = \left[y^1 \vdots \cdots \vdots y^{m-1} \right] = \left[\alpha^1 - \alpha^m \vdots \cdots \vdots \alpha^{m-1} - \alpha^m \right],$$

9.2. EIGENSTRUCTURE SPARSE DESIGN

and

$$Z = \begin{bmatrix} z^1 & \vdots & \cdots & \vdots & z^{m-1} \end{bmatrix} = \begin{bmatrix} \beta^1 - \beta^m & \vdots & \cdots & \vdots & \beta^{m-1} - \beta^m \end{bmatrix}.$$

We denote $y^i = (y_1^i, \cdots, y_n^i)^T$ and $z^i = (z_1^i, \cdots, z_n^i)^T$ for $i = 1, \cdots, m-1$.

4) Denote the ith row of the index matrix S by

$$S_i = (S_{i1}, \cdots, S_{in}).$$

For each $i = 1, \cdots, n$, construct two sets M_i and N_i, such that $M_i \cup N_i = \{1, \cdots, n\}$, $M_i \cap N_i = \{\emptyset\}$, and $S_{ij} = 1$ if $j \in M_i$, $S_{ij} = 0$ if $j \in N_i$. Let $M_i = \{\sigma_i(1), \cdots, \sigma_i(m_i)\}$, where $m_i = \sum_{j=1}^{n} S_{ij}$ and $\sigma_i(k) < \sigma_i(l)$ if $1 \leq k < l \leq m_i$.

(Note that m_i is the number of nonzero elements in the ith row of matrix S.)

5) For $i = 1, \cdots, n$ and $l = 1, \cdots, m-1$, let

$$y_{Ii}^l = \left(y_{\sigma(1)}^l, \cdots, y_{\sigma(m_i)}^l\right)^T.$$

6) For $i = 1, \cdots, n$, compute the $m_i \times (m-1)$ matrices

$$Y_i = (y_{Ii}^1, \cdots, y_{Ii}^{m-1}),$$

and the $1 \times (m-1)$ vectors

$$Z_i = (z_i^1, \cdots, z_i^{m-1}).$$

7) For $i = 1, \cdots, n$, perform singular value decompositions of Y_i, and obtain

$$Y_i = [U_{i1} \vdots U_{i2}] \begin{bmatrix} D_i & \vdots & 0 \\ \cdots & \cdots & \cdots \\ 0 & \vdots & 0 \end{bmatrix} \begin{bmatrix} V_{i1}^T \\ \cdots \\ V_{i2}^T \end{bmatrix},$$

where $D_i \in \Re^{p_i \times p_i}$ is a diagonal matrix with the nonzero singular values of Y_i on its diagonal and $p_i = \text{rank}(Y_i)$.

8) Compute for $i = 1, \cdots, n$,
$$G_i = (G_{i1}, \cdots, G_{im_i}) = Z_i V_{i1} D_i^{-1} U_{i1}^T + W_i U_{i2}^T$$
where W_i is an arbitrary $1 \times (m_i - p_i)$ real vector.

9) The matrix $T = [T_{ij}]$ is determined as follows:
$$T_{ij} = \begin{cases} 0, & \text{if } S_{ij} = 0 \\ G_{ik}, & \text{if } S_{ij} \neq 0 \text{ and if } j = \sigma_i(k). \end{cases} \qquad (9.2.3)$$

10) The bias vector $I = (I_1, \cdots, I_n)^T$ is computed by
$$I_i = \beta_i^m - T_i \alpha^m$$
for $i = 1, \cdots, n$, where T_i is the ith row of T.

Then, $\alpha^1, \cdots, \alpha^m$ will be stored as memory vectors for system (9.1.1) with A, T, and I determined as above. The states β^i corresponding to α^i, $i = 1, \cdots, m$, will be asymptotically stable equilibrium points of the synthesized system. ∎

Remark 9.2.2 If in the above synthesis procedure, we choose
$$A = \text{diag}[a_1, \cdots, a_n]$$
with $a_i > 0$, we need to change Z_i in step 6 to $Z_i = (a_i z_i^1, \cdots, a_i z_i^{m-1})$ and I_i in step 10 to $I_i = a_i \beta_i^m - T_i \alpha^m$. ∎

Remark 9.2.3 If in the index matrix S there are $q > 1$ identical rows, we can design the corresponding q rows of matrix T simultaneously. For such cases, we need to alter slightly steps 5–9 above. We will demonstrate this idea by means of an example in Section 9.5. We will also demonstrate in Section 9.5 that by special choices of the index matrix S, Synthesis Procedure 9.2.1 can result in a network with few line-crossings, or with no line-crossings at all. ∎

Our next result addresses the existence of solutions for the sparse design problem and the validity of the above design procedure.

9.2. EIGENSTRUCTURE SPARSE DESIGN

Theorem 9.2.1

1) Solutions for the sparse design problem always exist if $S_{ii} = 1$ for $i = 1, \cdots, n$.
2) Synthesis Procedure 9.2.1 guarantees that $T = T|S$.
3) Synthesis Procedure 9.2.1 guarantees that all vectors in $L_a \cap B^n$, including $\alpha^1, \cdots, \alpha^m$, are stored as memory vectors of system (9.1.1), where $L_a = \text{Aspan}(\alpha^1, \cdots, \alpha^m)$.
4) Synthesis Procedure 9.2.1 can be applied to any set of desired memory patterns $\alpha^1, \cdots, \alpha^m \in B^n$.

Proof: The present synthesis procedure solves matrix T from $TY = Z$ [cf. (9.2.2)] with $T = T|S$. According to the choice of T in step 9, we see that $G_i Y_i = Z_i$ is required in steps 7 and 8 of Synthesis Procedure 9.2.1. Thus, G_i in step 8 is a solution for the sparse design procedure *if and only if*

$$\text{rank}[Y_i] = \text{rank} \begin{bmatrix} Y_i \\ \cdots \\ Z_i \end{bmatrix}.$$

This condition is satisfied if $S_{ii} = 1$, $i = 1, \cdots, n$, since under the present conditions, Z_i becomes a row vector which is one of the rows in Y_i multiplied by μ. (This argument is also true if we choose $A = \text{diag}[a_1, \cdots, a_n]$ with $a_i > 0$.) This proves Part 1 of the theorem.

Part 2 is clear from (9.2.3).

To prove Part 3 of the theorem, we first check the equilibrium conditions (cf. Lemma 6.6.1) for $\alpha^1, \cdots, \alpha^m$, in which case we require that $T\alpha^l + I = A\beta^l = \beta^l$, for $l = 1, \cdots, m$, where $\beta^l = \mu \alpha^l$ and $\mu > 1$ [and hence, $\beta^l \in F(\alpha)$]. Using the notation given in the design procedure, we write for $l = 1, \cdots, m-1$, $y_{Ii}^l = Y_i e_l$, where $e_l \in \Re^{m-1}$ is a column vector with all elements zero except the lth element, which is 1 (cf. step 6 of Synthesis Procedure 9.2.1). Also, we have for $i = 1, \cdots, n$,

$$U_{i2}^T y_{Ii}^l = 0 \text{ for } l = 1, \cdots, m-1,$$

and
$$Z_i V_{i1} D_i^{-1} U_{i1}^T Y_i = Z_i.$$

The first equation is clear from the properties of the singular value decomposition. To verify the second equation, we recall that $Y_i = U_{i1} D_i V_{i1}^T$ and we assume that Z_i is the jth row of Y_i multiplied by μ (without loss of generality). Then, $Z_i = \mu \cdot R_j V_{i1}^T$, where R_j is the jth row of $U_{i1} D_i$, and from the properties of the singular value decomposition, we have

$$\begin{aligned} Z_i V_{i1} D_i^{-1} U_{i1}^T Y_i &= \mu \cdot R_j V_{i1}^T \cdot V_{i1} D_i^{-1} U_{i1}^T \cdot U_{i1} D_i V_{i1}^T \\ &= \mu \cdot R_j V_{i1}^T \\ &= Z_i, \end{aligned}$$

since $U_{i1}^T U_{i1} = V_{i1}^T V_{i1} = D_i^{-1} D_i =$ the $p_i \times p_i$ identity matrix (where p_i is defined in step 7 of the design procedure). According to steps 8, 9, and 10 of the design procedure, we compute for $i = 1, \cdots, n$,

$$T_i y^l = G_i y_{Ii}^l,$$

and
$$\begin{aligned} T_i \alpha^l + I_i &= T_i y^l + T_i \alpha^m + I_i \\ &= G_i y_{Ii}^l + T_i \alpha^m + \beta_i^m - T_i \alpha^m \\ &= Z_i V_{i1} D_i^{-1} U_{i1}^T Y_i e_l + W_i U_{i2}^T y_{Ii}^l + \beta_i^m \\ &= Z_i e_l + \beta_i^m \\ &= z_i^l + \beta_i^m \\ &= \beta_i^l - \beta_i^m + \beta_i^m \\ &= \beta_i^l. \end{aligned}$$

Hence, $T\alpha^l + I = \beta^l$ for $l = 1, \cdots, m-1$. For $l = m$, $T\alpha^m + I = \beta^m$ is clear from step 10. Next, we note that the above results imply that
$$T(\alpha^l - \alpha^m) = \beta^l - \beta^m \quad \text{for} \quad l = 1, \cdots, m-1,$$

and that for every vector $\alpha \in L_\alpha \cap B^n$, there is a $\sigma = (\sigma_1, \cdots, \sigma_{m-1}) \in \Re^{m-1}$ such that

$$\alpha = \sigma_1(\alpha^1 - \alpha^m) + \cdots + \sigma_{m-1}(\alpha^{m-1} - \alpha^m) + \alpha^m.$$

9.2. EIGENSTRUCTURE SPARSE DESIGN

Thus, for every vector $\alpha \in L_\alpha \cap B^n$, we have

$$\begin{aligned}
T\alpha + I &= T(\sigma_1(\alpha^1 - \alpha^m) + \cdots + \sigma_{m-1}(\alpha^{m-1} - \alpha^m)) + T\alpha^m + I \\
&= \sigma_1(\beta^1 - \beta^m) + \cdots + \sigma_{m-1}(\beta^{m-1} - \beta^m) + \beta^m \\
&= \mu(\sigma_1(\alpha^1 - \alpha^m) + \cdots + \sigma_{m-1}(\alpha^{m-1} - \alpha^m) + \alpha^m) \\
&= \mu\alpha \\
&\triangleq \beta.
\end{aligned}$$

Clearly, $\beta \in F(\alpha)$ since $\mu > 1$. By Lemma 6.6.1, we see that the states β^i corresponding to α^i, $i = 1, \cdots, m$, as well as the states which correspond to the output vectors in $L_\alpha \cap B^n$ other than α^i, will be asymptotically stable equilibrium points of system (9.1.1). Therefore, all vectors in $L_\alpha \cap B^n$, including $\alpha^1, \cdots, \alpha^m$, will be stored as memory vectors for system (9.1.1).

Part 4 follows from the fact that the present synthesis approach for neural networks is an extension of the Eigenstructure Method introduced in Section 8.3 and the Eigenstructure Method does not pose any constraints on the desired memory patterns. ∎

Remark 9.2.4 It is emphasized that Part 1 of Theorem 9.2.1 does not imply or require that S_{ij}, $i \neq j$, be zero. ∎

Remark 9.2.5 If we wish that the above procedure results in a system of form (9.1.1) with $I = 0$, we can modify Synthesis Procedure 9.2.1 as follows:

a) In step 3, let $Y = \begin{bmatrix} \alpha^1 & \vdots & \cdots & \vdots & \alpha^m \end{bmatrix}$ and $Z = \begin{bmatrix} \beta^1 & \vdots & \cdots & \vdots & \beta^m \end{bmatrix}$.

b) In step 10, let $I = 0$.

Then all conclusions will remain unchanged. In particular, all vectors in $\mathrm{Span}(\alpha^1, \cdots, \alpha^m) \cap B^n$, including $\pm\alpha^1, \cdots, \pm\alpha^m$, are stored as memory vectors of system (9.1.1). ∎

Synthesis Procedure 9.2.1 results usually in neural networks with nonsymmetric interconnection matrix T. To obtain a sparse design with symmetric matrix T for neural networks described by (9.1.1), we follow the same arguments as in Section 8.5 and develop a synthesis procedure similar to Synthesis Procedure 8.5.2, summarized as follows. Note that in this case, we require that $S = S^T$.

Synthesis Procedure 9.2.2 Suppose that we are given m vectors $\alpha^1, \cdots, \alpha^m$ in B^n which are to be stored as stable memory vectors for system (9.1.1), and an index matrix $S = S^T$ with $S_{ii} = 1$ for $i = 1, \cdots, n$. One can now proceed as follows to generate a symmetric design:

1) Determine A, $T = T|S$ and I for system (9.1.1) with $\mu > 1$ according to the Synthesis Procedure 9.2.1.

2) Compute $\beta^k = A^{-1}(T\alpha^k + I)$ for $k = 1, \cdots, m$ and let $\mu = \min_{1 \leq k \leq m} \{\delta(\beta^k)\}$.

3) If $T = T^T$ or $\mu \leq 1 + \eta$, where η is a small positive number (e.g., $\eta = 0.01$), stop. Otherwise, go to step 4.

4) Compute $\Delta T = (T^T - T)/2$. If $\|A^{-1}\Delta T\|_\infty < \mu - 1$, choose $\lambda = 1$. Otherwise, choose

$$\lambda = \frac{\mu - 1}{\|A^{-1}\Delta T\|_\infty} - \varepsilon$$

where ε is a small positive number (e.g., $\varepsilon = 0.001$). Compute $\overline{T} = T + \lambda \Delta T$.

5) Compute $\overline{\beta}^k = A^{-1}(\overline{T}\alpha^k + I)$ for $k = 1, \cdots, m$, and compute

$$\nu = \min_{1 \leq k \leq m} \{\delta(\overline{\beta}^k)\} > 1.$$

6) Replacing μ by ν and replacing T by $\overline{T}$, go to step 3.

If one ends up with $T = T^T$, a solution has been found for the symmetric design problem. If one ends up with $\mu < 1 + \eta$ and $T \neq T^T$, the present design procedure is not successful in solving for a symmetric T in the given problem. ∎

With the results of Section 8.3, we can also extend the Eigenstructure Method to other neural network models introduced in Chapter 2 with *sparse interconnecting structure*. We omit the details.

9.3 The Perceptron Based Training Algorithm in the Synthesis of Sparsely Interconnected Neural Networks

The Synthesis Procedure 8.5.1 developed in Section 8.5 can also be modified to solve the Sparse Design Problem introduced in the preceding section. We summarize this procedure in the following.

Synthesis Procedure 9.3.1 Suppose that we are given an $n \times n$ index matrix $S = [S_{ij}]$ with $S_{ii} \neq 0$ for $i = 1, \cdots, n$, and m vectors $\alpha^1, \cdots, \alpha^m$ in B^n which are to be stored as memory vectors for (9.1.1). We proceed as follows:

Using the Perceptron Training Algorithm, obtain n perceptrons

$$W^i = (w_1^i, w_2^i, \cdots, w_{n+1}^i), \quad i = 1, 2, \cdots, n$$

where w_j^i is preset to zero if $S_{ij} = 0$, such that

$$\begin{aligned} W^i \overline{\alpha}^k \geq 0 & \quad \text{if } \alpha_i^k = 1 \\ W^i \overline{\alpha}^k < 0 & \quad \text{if } \alpha_i^k = -1. \end{aligned}$$

Choose the matrix $A = \text{diag}[a_1, \cdots, a_n]$ with $a_i > 0$. For $i, j = 1, \cdots, n$, choose $T_{ij} = w_j^i$ if $i \neq j$, $T_{ii} = w_i^i + a_i \mu_i$ with $\mu_i > 1$, and $I_i = w_{n+1}^i$. ∎

The Synthesis Procedure 9.3.1 is a modification of the Synthesis Procedure 8.5.1 in which one needs to preset $w_j^i = 0$ if $S_{ij} = 0$. The convergence of the perceptron training in the sparse design algorithm can also be proved, following similar lines as in the proof of Theorem 8.5.1 (letting $S_{ii} = 1$ for $i = 1, \cdots, n$).

As was shown in Section 8.5, when we place certain constraints on the diagonal elements of the connection matrix T, neural network (9.1.1) will possess certain desirable properties. In particular, we have shown that when we require that $T_{ii} \geq a_i$, $i = 1, \cdots, n$, neural network (9.1.1) will have only bipolar stable memory vectors; and when we require that $T_{ii} \leq a_i$, every corner of the hypercube which is in the immediate neighborhood of a stable memory vector can itself not become a stable memory and is very likely in the domain of attraction of that stable memory vector. If one wishes to achieve a sparse neural network design with constraints on the diagonal components of the connection matrix T, the following results provide necessary and sufficient conditions and a simple criterion for the existence of such a design. The proofs of these results follow similar lines as the proofs of Theorems 8.5.3 and 8.5.4.

Theorem 9.3.1 Suppose that in the index matrix S, $S_{ii} = 1$ for $i = 1, \cdots, n$. A sparse neural network design with the ith diagonal element of T satisfying $T_{ii} \leq a_i$, where $a_i > 0$ is the ith diagonal element of matrix A, can be achieved if and only if the patterns

$$\alpha^1|S_i^T, \ \cdots, \ \alpha^m|S_i^T$$

with the ith entry eliminated are linearly separable. Here, S_i denotes the ith row of the index matrix S and the two classes of patterns are determined according to the ith element of the desired patterns. ∎

Theorem 9.3.2 Suppose that in the index matrix S, $S_{ii} = 1$ for $i = 1, \cdots, n$. Let S_i be the ith row of the index matrix S, let

$$Q = \left[\alpha^1|S_i^T \vdots \cdots \vdots \alpha^m|S_i^T \right]$$

and let

$$Q^i = \left[Q \text{ with the } i^{th} \text{ row deleted} \right].$$

If

$$\text{rank}(Q) = \text{rank}(Q^i)$$

for some i, $1 \leq i \leq n$, then Synthesis Procedure 9.3.1 can lead to a sparse design with the ith diagonal element of T satisfying $T_{ii} \leq a_i$, where $a_i > 0$ is the ith diagonal element of matrix A. ∎

9.3. PERCEPTRON TRAINING SPARSE SYNTHESIS

Remark 9.3.1 All results of Section 8.5 concerning constraints on the diagonal elements of T apply in the present case as well. In particular, we will demonstrate the applicability of the results of Section 8.5 to the present sparsity design, using several examples given in Section 9.5. ∎

The Synthesis Procedure 9.3.1 results usually in neural networks with nonsymmetric interconnection matrix T. To obtain a sparse design with symmetric matrix T for neural networks described by (9.1.1), we modify Synthesis Procedure 8.5.2 as follows.

Synthesis Procedure 9.3.2 Given m vectors $\alpha^1, \cdots, \alpha^m$ in B^n to be stored as stable memory vectors for system (9.1.1) and given an index matrix $S = S^T$ with $S_{ii} = 1$ for $i = 1, \cdots, n$, one can proceed in the following manner to generate a symmetric design:

1) Determine A, $T = T|S$ and I for system (9.1.1) with $\mu_i > 1$ according to Synthesis Procedure 9.3.1.

2) Compute $\beta^k = A^{-1}(T\alpha^k + I)$ for $k = 1, \cdots, m$ and let $\mu = \min_{1 \leq k \leq m} \{\delta(\beta^k)\}$.

3) If $T = T^T$ or $\mu \leq 1 + \eta$, where η is a small positive number (e.g., $\eta = 0.01$), stop. Otherwise, go to step 4.

4) Compute $\Delta T = (T^T - T)/2$. If $\|A^{-1}\Delta T\|_\infty < \mu - 1$, choose $\lambda = 1$. Otherwise, choose

$$\lambda = \frac{\mu - 1}{\|A^{-1}\Delta T\|_\infty} - \varepsilon$$

where ε is a small positive number (e.g., $\varepsilon = 0.001$). Compute $\overline{T} = T + \lambda \Delta T$.

5) Compute $\overline{\beta}^k = A^{-1}(\overline{T}\alpha^k + I)$ for $k = 1, \cdots, m$, and compute

$$\nu = \min_{1 \leq k \leq m} \{\delta(\overline{\beta}^k)\} > 1.$$

6) Replace μ by ν and replace T by $\overline{T}$. Go to step 3.

If one ends up with $T = T^T$, a solution has been found for the present design problem. If one ends up with $\mu < 1 + \eta$ and $T \neq T^T$, the present design procedure is not successful in solving a symmetric T for the given problem. ∎

9.4 Synthesis of Cellular Neural Networks for Associative Memories

Cellular neural networks, introduced in [4], have found several successful applications in image processing and pattern recognition (see, for example, [5], [13]–[16]). On the other hand, applications of cellular neural networks to associative memories, utilizing the Outer Product Method (the Hebbian rule), seem to have been somewhat less successful [18]. As is shown in Section 8.1, the Outer Product Method does not guarantee that every desired memory pattern is stored as an equilibrium point (memory point) of the synthesized system when the desired patterns are not mutually orthogonal. Moreover, the storage capacity of networks designed by the Outer Product Method is known to be low.

In the present section, we employ the sparse synthesis techniques developed in the previous sections in the design of cellular neural networks with applications to associative memories.

A special class of *two-dimensional cellular neural networks* is described by ordinary differential equations of the form (see [4])

$$\begin{cases} \dot{x}_{ij} = -a_{ij}x_{ij} + \sum_{C(k,l) \in N_r(i,j)} T_{ij,kl}\,\text{sat}(x_{kl}) + I_{ij} \\ y_{ij} = \text{sat}(x_{ij}) \end{cases} \quad (9.4.1)$$

where $1 \leq i \leq M$, $1 \leq j \leq N$, $a_{ij} > 0$, and x_{ij} and y_{ij} are the states and the outputs of the network, respectively. The basic unit in a cellular neural network is called a *cell*. In (9.4.1), there are $M \times N$ such cells arranged in an $M \times N$ array. The cell in the ith row and the jth column is denoted by $C(i,j)$, and an *r-neighborhood* $N_r(i,j)$

9.4. CELLULAR NEURAL NETWORK SYNTHESIS

of the cell $C(i,j)$ for a positive integer r is defined by

$$N_r(i,j) \triangleq \{C(k,l): \max\{|k-i|, |l-j|\} \leq r, \ 1 \leq k \leq M, \ 1 \leq l \leq N\}.$$

Remark 9.4.1 Note that system (9.4.1) characterizes a special class of continuous-time cellular neural networks with square grids, piecewise linear processors, and memoryless interactions. (For details concerning the classification of cellular neural networks, see [3].) ∎

Remark 9.4.2 In the original cellular neural network model introduced by Chua and Yang [4],

$$a_{ij} = \frac{1}{R_x C}$$

(R_x and C are constants), $I_{ij} = I_c$ (I_c is a constant), and $T_{ij,kl} = T_{kl,ij}$. We will not make these assumptions in (9.4.1). In the applications of cellular neural networks to image processing and pattern recognition, in addition to the bias terms $I_{ij} = I_c$, one frequently requires nonzero input terms

$$\sum_{C(k,l) \in N_r(i,j)} B_{ij,kl} \, u_{kl}$$

in the first equation of (9.4.1), where u_{ij} represents the inputs of the network. In the present application, we consider zero inputs ($u_{ij} \equiv 0$ for all i and j) and a constant *bias vector* $I = (I_{11}, I_{12}, \cdots, I_{MN})^T$. This renders (9.4.1) equivalent to a *nonsymmetric* cellular neural network model by setting the inputs in the original model equal to constants (cf. [2] and [4]). Under these circumstances, we will refer to (9.4.1) as a (zero-input) *nonsymmetric cellular neural network*. ∎

A. Design of Nonsymmetric Cellular Neural Networks

Using the above nomenclature, we choose a matrix $Q = [Q_{ij,kl}] \in \Re^{MN \times MN}$ as

$$Q_{ij,kl} = \begin{cases} 1, & \text{if } C(k,l) \in N_r(i,j) \\ 0, & \text{otherwise} \end{cases} \tag{9.4.2}$$

and we let $S = Q = [S_{ij}] \in \Re^{n \times n}$, where $n = M \times N$. With this notation, we see that in order for (9.1.1) [or (2.2.6)] to be equivalent to the nonsymmetric cellular neural network model (9.4.1), we require in (9.1.1) that $T = T|S$, where $S = Q$ and Q is defined in (9.4.2). Thus, the cellular neural network model (9.4.1) is a special case of the neural network model (9.1.1) where the n neurons are arranged in an $M \times N$ array (if $n = M \times N$) and the interconnection structure is confined to local neighborhoods of radius r. Hence, Synthesis Procedure 9.2.1 and its modified version (cf. Remark 9.2.5) can be applied directly to the design of the cellular neural network (9.4.1) based on the index matrix $S = Q$, where Q is determined in (9.4.2). By Theorem 9.2.1, for any given integer $r > 0$ and any set of m vectors $\alpha^1, \cdots, \alpha^m$ in B^{MN}, we can always design a cellular neural network (9.4.1) which will store $\alpha^1, \cdots, \alpha^m$ as (stable) memory vectors.

B. Space-Invariant Cloning Template Design

Cellular neural networks are characterized by local connections constrained to a neighborhood defined as a cell. When the connection weights maintain the same values from cell to cell, a cellular neural network is said to have a *space-invariant cloning template*. Otherwise, the cellular neural network has *space-varying cloning templates*.

The synthesis method in the preceding subsection will lead to space-varying cloning templates for (9.4.1). Many applications of cellular neural networks to image processing and pattern recognition have made use of space-invariant cloning templates (see, e.g., [5], [13]–[16]). We will develop in this subsection a design method for cellular neural networks with space-invariant cloning templates.

For a cellular neural network described by (9.4.1) with $n = M \times N$ cells and with neighborhood radius r, we can use a $(2r+1) \times (2r+1)$ (space-invariant) cloning template to describe the connection matrix T. We use p_k, $k = 1, \cdots, (2r+1)^2$, to denote these elements and we

9.4. CELLULAR NEURAL NETWORK SYNTHESIS

write

$$P_T = \begin{bmatrix} p_1 & p_2 & \cdots & p_{(2r+1)} \\ p_{(2r+1)+1} & p_{(2r+1)+2} & \cdots & p_{2\times(2r+1)} \\ \vdots & \vdots & \ddots & \vdots \\ \cdots & \cdots & \cdots & p_{(2r+1)^2} \end{bmatrix} \in \Re^{(2r+1)\times(2r+1)}. \tag{9.4.3}$$

If a cellular neural network (9.4.1) has a cloning template P_T, the connection matrix T will consist of only zeros and p_k's. The index matrix S can in this case be expressed as

$$S = \sum_{k=1}^{(2r+1)^2} S^k, \tag{9.4.4}$$

where $S^k = [S_{ij}^k] \in \Re^{n\times n}$, and for $k = 1, \cdots, (2r+1)^2$,

$$S_{ij}^k = \begin{cases} 1, & \text{if } T_{ij} = p_k, \text{ i.e., if the } ij\text{th} \\ & \text{element of } T \text{ corresponds to the} \\ & k\text{th element of the template} \\ 0, & \text{otherwise.} \end{cases} \tag{9.4.5}$$

S^k describes how the $(2r+1)^2$ elements of the cloning template are distributed in the connection matrix T. For the A, T, and I determined by the Synthesis Procedure 9.2.1 with $\mu > 1$, let us compute

$$f_k = \left(\sum_{i,j} S_{ij}^k\right)^{-1} \sum_{S_{ij}^k=1} T_{ij} \quad \text{for } k = 1, \cdots, (2r+1)^2. \tag{9.4.6}$$

Let $G = [G_{ij}] \in \Re^{n\times n}$, where

$$G_{ij} = \begin{cases} f_k, & \text{if } S_{ij}^k = 1 \text{ for } k = 1, \cdots, (2r+1)^2 \\ 0, & \text{otherwise.} \end{cases} \tag{9.4.7}$$

Let $\Delta T = G - T$. Then, $T + \Delta T = G$ is a matrix with cloning template specified by f_k, $k = 1, \cdots, (2r+1)^2$. From Theorem 6.6.1, we note that if $\Delta A = 0$, $\Delta I = 0$, and if

$$\|A^{-1}\Delta T\|_\infty = \|G - T\|_\infty < \nu - 1 \tag{9.4.8}$$

where ν is obtained as

$$\nu = \min_{1\leq k\leq m}\{\delta(\beta^k)\} > 1 \quad (9.4.9)$$

with

$$\beta^k = A^{-1}(T\alpha^k + I) \text{ for } k = 1, \cdots, m$$

and $\delta(x) \triangleq \min_{1\leq i\leq n}\{|x_i|\}$ for $x \in \Re^n$, the perturbed neural network will also store all the desired patterns as stable memories, with connection matrix $T + \Delta T$ which has a cloning template specified by f_k, $k = 1,\cdots,(2r+1)^2$.

The above observation gives rise to the possibility of designing a cellular neural network (9.4.1) with connection matrix T specified by a cloning template. In the following, we develop an *iterative algorithm* (design procedure) which in most cases will result in a cellular neural network (9.4.1) with connection matrix specified by a cloning template. In doing so, we apply Lemma 6.6.1 [i.e., condition (9.2.1)] and Theorem 6.6.1 [i.e., condition (9.4.8)] *iteratively*. Let G be defined as in (9.4.7) and let $\Delta T = G - T$, where $T = T|S$ is obtained by Synthesis Procedure 9.2.1 with $\mu > 1$. For the given μ, suppose that $\|\Delta T\|_\infty \geq \mu - 1$. We can find a λ, $0 < \lambda < 1$, such that $\lambda\|\Delta T\|_\infty < \mu - 1$, and we let $T_1 = T + \lambda\Delta T$. We use this T_1 as the *new* connection matrix for our cellular neural network (9.4.1). According to Theorem 6.6.1, we see that $\alpha^1,\cdots,\alpha^m$ are still stable memory vectors of system (9.4.1) with coefficient matrix T_1. Using Lemma 6.6.1, we can determine the corresponding asymptotically stable equilibrium points as $\overline{\beta}^k = A^{-1}(T_1\alpha^k + I)$ for $k = 1,\cdots,m$. Clearly, we have $\overline{\beta}^k \in F(\alpha^k)$. Using Theorem 6.6.1, we can determine the upper bound $\nu - 1$ for the permissible perturbation ΔT from equation (9.4.9), where we use $\overline{\beta}^k$ in place of β^k. We *repeat* the above procedure, until we determine a coefficient matrix T which is specified by a cloning template (i.e., $T = G$) or arrive at $\nu \leq 1 + \eta$ (where η is a small positive number).

We are now in a position to summarize a cloning template design procedure for cellular neural networks.

9.4. CELLULAR NEURAL NETWORK SYNTHESIS

Synthesis Procedure 9.4.1 Given are positive integers r, n, M, and N with $n = M \times N$, and m vectors $\alpha^1, \cdots, \alpha^m$ in B^n which are to be stored as stable memory vectors for cellular neural network (9.4.1). We proceed as follows.

1) Compute the matrix Q as in (9.4.2) and denote $S = Q = [S_{ij}] \in \Re^{n \times n}$. Compute S^k for $k = 1, \cdots, (2r+1)^2$, as in (9.4.5).

2) According to Synthesis Procedure 9.2.1, we choose A as the identity matrix and we determine $T = T|S$ and I for cellular neural network (9.4.1) with a $\mu > 1 + \eta$ (e.g., $\mu = 30$, $\eta = 0.001$).

3) Compute G as in (9.4.6) and (9.4.7).

4) If $T = G$ or $\mu \leq 1 + \eta$, stop. Otherwise go to step 5.

5) Compute $\Delta T = G - T$. If $\|\Delta T\|_\infty < \mu - 1$, choose $\lambda = 1$. Otherwise, choose

$$\lambda = \frac{\mu - 1}{\|\Delta T\|_\infty} - \varepsilon$$

where ε is a small positive number (e.g., $\varepsilon = 0.01$). Compute $T_1 = T + \lambda \Delta T$.

6) Compute

$$\overline{\beta}^k = A^{-1}(T_1 \alpha^k + I) \text{ for } k = 1, \cdots, m,$$

and compute

$$\nu = \min_{1 \leq k \leq m} \{\delta(\overline{\beta}^k)\} > 1.$$

7) Replacing μ by ν and T by T_1, go to step 3.

If we end up with $T = G$, we have found a solution for the present cloning template design problem, and $\alpha^1, \cdots, \alpha^m$ will be stored as stable memory vectors for system (9.4.1) with A, T, and I determined as above. If we end up with $\nu \leq 1 + \eta$ and $T \neq G$, our design procedure is not successful in solving the given cloning template design problem. ∎

Experimental results indicate that the above procedure will frequently succeed in determining a matrix T which is indeed specified by a cloning template.

Remark 9.4.3 The above design procedure will usually result in a space-invariant cloning template and in *space-varying* bias terms. Space-invariant bias can be achieved by either designing a cellular neural network with $I = 0$, or by modifying Synthesis Procedure 9.4.1 so that a similar iterative procedure (steps 3 to 7 above) is used for vector I by initially choosing $\Delta I = [\Delta I_1, \cdots, \Delta I_n]^T$ with

$$\Delta I_i = \left(\frac{1}{n}\sum_{i=1}^{n} I_i\right) - I_i.$$
■

Remark 9.4.4 The Synthesis Procedure 9.4.1 presented above will normally result in a nonsymmetric coefficient matrix T since the resulting cloning template is usually not endowed with the special structure required to render a symmetric matrix T [refer, e.g., to equation (9.5.4)]. We can apply the symmetric design procedure developed in the previous section (e.g., Synthesis Procedures 9.2.2 and 9.3.2) to determine a *symmetric* connection matrix T_s which also satisfies the condition $T_s|S = T_s$, and then, starting with T_s, and using Synthesis Procedure 9.4.1 of the present section, we can determine a connection matrix T which is *symmetric* and which is also *specified by a cloning template*. Such capability is of great interest since cellular neural network (9.4.1) will be *globally stable* when T is symmetric. ■

Remark 9.4.5 The f_k, $k = 1, \cdots, (2r+1)^2$, computed in (9.4.6), denote the target values for the cloning template with each element representing the average of all the elements appearing at the locations corresponding to the same template element in the matrix T. We note that there may be other ways of computing the f_k's. Simulation results show that the choice in (9.4.6) works very well (cf. Example 9.5.5). ■

C. A Design Method Based on Perceptron Training

In this subsection, we apply the perceptron training technique in the synthesis of cellular neural networks with space-invariant cloning template.

From the given α^k, $k = 1, \cdots, m$, define

$$\gamma^{ki} = \left(\gamma_1^{ki}, \cdots, \gamma_{(2r+1)^2}^{ki}\right)^T \qquad (9.4.10)$$

for $k = 1, \cdots, m$ and for $i = 1, \cdots, n$. Here

$$\gamma_l^{ki} = \begin{cases} \alpha_j^k, & \text{if the } l\text{th connection weight of the } i\text{th cell corresponds to the } j\text{th element on the } i\text{th row of } T \\ 0, & \text{otherwise.} \end{cases} \qquad (9.4.11)$$

Solutions for the synthesis problem of cellular neural network (9.4.1) [or (9.1.1)] are determined from

$$\begin{cases} T_i \alpha^k + I_i > a_i & \text{if } \alpha_i^k = 1 \\ T_i \alpha^k + I_i < -a_i & \text{if } \alpha_i^k = -1 \end{cases} \qquad (9.4.12)$$

for $k = 1, \cdots, m$ and for $i = 1, \cdots, n$, where T_i represents the ith row of T, I_i denotes the ith element of I, and α_i^k is the ith entry of α^k. If the connection matrix T has a space-invariant cloning template P_T as in (9.4.3) and a space-invariant bias term b, (9.4.12) can be written as

$$\begin{cases} [p_1, \cdots, p_{(2r+1)^2}] \gamma^{ki} + b > 1, & \text{if } \gamma_c^{ki} = 1 \\ [p_1, \cdots, p_{(2r+1)^2}] \gamma^{ki} + b < -1, & \text{if } \gamma_c^{ki} = -1 \end{cases} \qquad (9.4.13)$$

for $k = 1, \cdots, m$ and for $i = 1, \cdots, n$, where γ_c^{ki} denotes the center element of γ^{ki} and the subscript

$$c = \frac{(2r+1)^2 + 1}{2}. \qquad (9.4.14)$$

We note that (9.4.13) is simply a rearrangement of (9.4.12) where T and I are determined from P_T and b.

The following procedure constitutes a synthesis algorithm for the design of cellular neural networks with space-invariant cloning template based on the perceptron training algorithm.

Synthesis Procedure 9.4.2 Using the Perceptron Training Algorithm, obtain one perceptron $W = \left(w_1, w_2, \cdots, w_{(2r+1)^2+1}\right)$, such that
$$\begin{cases} W\overline{\gamma}^{ki} > 0, & \text{if } \gamma_c^{ki} = 1 \\ W\overline{\gamma}^{ki} < 0, & \text{if } \gamma_c^{ki} = -1 \end{cases}$$
for $k = 1, \cdots, m$ and for $i = 1, \cdots, n$, where $\overline{\gamma}^{ki} = \begin{pmatrix} \gamma^{ki} \\ \cdots \\ 1 \end{pmatrix}$ and γ^{ki} are determined by (9.4.10) and (9.4.11).

Choose A as the identity matrix. For $l = 1, \cdots, (2r+1)^2$, choose $p_l = w_l$ if $l \neq c$, $p_c = w_c + \mu$ with $\mu > 1$, and set $I = [I_1, \cdots, I_n]^T$ with $I_i = w_{(2r+1)^2+1}$ for $i = 1, \cdots, n$, where c is given in (9.4.14). Then construct T from P_T according to the interconnecting structure specified by the neighborhood radius r. ∎

We note that when designing cellular neural networks with space-invariant cloning template and space-invariant bias term, we will also require a_i to be space-invariant, i.e., we will require that matrix A be a diagonal matrix with the identical positive diagonal element.

In the remainder of this section, we will choose A to be the $n \times n$ identity matrix.

Remark 9.4.6 The above synthesis algorithm will certainly result in a space-invariant cloning template and a space-invariant bias term with any learning rate $\eta > 0$ in the Perceptron Training Algorithm. Considering the fact that all the desired patterns are bipolar vectors, the convergence of the training iteration can also be proved following similar steps as in Theorem 8.5.1. For the present design problem, a trivial solution, i.e., a template with only a center non-zero element, always exists. Our simulation results show that one can always obtain non-trivial solutions by choosing either zero initial weights or random initial weights in the perceptron training algorithm. ∎

Remark 9.4.7 Applying Theorems 9.3.1 and 9.3.2 to cellular neural network (9.4.1), we obtain for the present case the optimal constraints given by $T_{ii} = a_i = 1$ for $i = 1, \cdots, n$. It can easily be

9.4. CELLULAR NEURAL NETWORK SYNTHESIS

proved that a cloning template design with the diagonal elements of the connection matrix T satisfying $T_{ii} = 1$, for $i = 1, \cdots, n$, can be obtained from Synthesis Procedure 9.4.2 if and only if $w_c < 0$. If the algorithm terminates with $w_c \geq 0$, then one can repeat the perceptron training with an initial weight W chosen as

$$W = \left(w_1, \cdots, w_{c-1}, -\xi, w_{c+1}, \cdots, w_{(2r+1)^2+1}\right)$$

with $\xi > 0$. Experiments show that in this case we usually end up with $w_c < 0$ if such a solution exists. ∎

Synthesis Procedure 9.4.2 presented above will usually result in a non-symmetric coefficient matrix T since the resulting cloning template is normally not with the special structure required to render a symmetric T.

Next, we present a design algorithm of cellular neural networks with symmetric connections and with a space-invariant cloning template. In the sequel, the following notation will be used. For a matrix $H = [h_{ij}] \in \Re^{n \times n}$, denote

$$H^\sigma \triangleq \Sigma H \Sigma \qquad (9.4.15)$$

where $\Sigma = [\sigma_{ij}] \in \Re^{n \times n}$ with

$$\sigma_{ij} = \begin{cases} 1, & \text{if } i+j = n+1 \\ 0, & \text{otherwise.} \end{cases}$$

For example, if

$$H = \begin{bmatrix} h_{11} & h_{12} & h_{13} \\ h_{21} & h_{22} & h_{23} \\ h_{31} & h_{32} & h_{33} \end{bmatrix}$$

then

$$H^\sigma = \Sigma H \Sigma = \begin{bmatrix} h_{33} & h_{32} & h_{31} \\ h_{23} & h_{22} & h_{21} \\ h_{13} & h_{12} & h_{11} \end{bmatrix}.$$

The following result provides a simple criterion for symmetric cellular neural networks to have a space-invariant cloning template. Its proof is straightforward.

Theorem 9.4.1 Matrix T with space-invariant cloning template P_T is symmetric if $P_T^\sigma = P_T$. ∎

For the P_T determined from Synthesis Procedures 9.4.2 with $\mu > 1$, choose
$$\Delta P_T = \frac{P_T^\sigma - P_T}{2}.$$
Then,
$$\overline{P}_T \triangleq P_T + \Delta P_T = \frac{P_T + P_T^\sigma}{2}$$
satisfies $\overline{P}_T^\sigma = \overline{P}_T$ and the matrix T_s which is computed from $\overline{P}_T$ will be symmetric (according to Theorem 9.4.1). From Theorem 6.6.1, we know that if $\|\Delta T\|_\infty = \|T_s - T\|_\infty < \nu - 1$, where ν is obtained as
$$\nu = \min_{1 \leq k \leq m} \{\delta(\beta^k)\} > 1$$
with
$$\beta^k = T\alpha^k + I, \ k = 1, \cdots, m$$
then the neural network (9.4.1) with symmetric connection matrix T_s will also store all the desired patterns as memories. The notation $\delta(x) = \min_{1 \leq i \leq n} \{|x_i|\}$ for $x \in \Re^n$ was used in the preceding.

Based on the above observations, after obtaining the cloning template P_T and the bias vector I from Synthesis Procedure 9.4.2, we can proceed as follows to generate a symmetric design of cellular neural networks.

Synthesis Procedure 9.4.3

1) Use Synthesis Procedure 9.4.2 to obtain a space-invariant cloning template P_T.

2) Compute P_T^σ as in (9.4.15) from the cloning template P_T. If $P_T^\sigma = P_T$, stop.

3) Generate the connection matrix T using P_T. Generate T_1 using P_T^σ in the same manner.

9.4. CELLULAR NEURAL NETWORK SYNTHESIS

4) Compute $\beta^k = T\alpha^k + I$ for $k = 1, \cdots, m$ and let

$$\nu = \min_{1 \leq k \leq m} \{\delta(\beta^k)\}.$$

5) If $\nu \leq 1 + \eta$, stop. Here η is a small positive number (e.g., $\eta = 0.01$). Otherwise, go to step 6.
6) Compute $\Delta T = T_1 - T$. If $\|\Delta T\|_\infty < \nu - 1$, choose $\lambda = 1$. Otherwise, choose

$$\lambda = \frac{\nu - 1}{\|\Delta T\|_\infty} - \varepsilon$$

where ε is a small positive number (e.g., $\varepsilon = 0.001$).

7) Determine the cloning template $\overline{P}_T$ as

$$\overline{P}_T = P_T + \lambda \frac{P_T^\sigma - P_T}{2}.$$

8) Replace P_T by $\overline{P}_T$. Go to step 2.

If the algorithm terminates with $P_T^\sigma = P_T$, a solution has been determined for the symmetric design problem. If the algorithm terminates with $\nu \leq 1+\eta$ and $P_T^\sigma \neq P_T$, the symmetric design algorithm is not successful in solving a symmetric T for the given problem. ∎

We note that Synthesis Procedure 9.4.3 can also be applied after Synthesis Procedure 9.4.1 to obtain a symmetric cellular neural network design based on the Eigenstructure Method.

Remark 9.4.8 The robustness analysis result (Theorem 6.6.1) is applied repeatedly in Synthesis Procedure 9.4.3. The idea is to approach the cloning template which renders a symmetric connection matrix gradually (steps 6 and 7). Theorem 6.6.1 guarantees that after the parameter perturbation given by $\lambda(P_T^\sigma - P_T)/2$ in step 7, the desired patterns $\alpha^1, \cdots, \alpha^m$ will still be stable memory vectors of the neural network. ∎

9.5 Illustrative Examples

To demonstrate the applicability of the analysis results and synthesis procedures presented in the preceding sections, we consider several specific cases. The examples in this section concern neural networks described by (9.1.1) with constraints imposed on the interconnecting structure. One such set of constraints is in the form of sparsity requirements for the connection matrix T while another is in the form of specific values for the diagonal elements of matrix T. In particular, we consider several examples where the sparsity requirements for the connection matrix T lead to cellular neural networks described by (9.4.1).

Example 9.5.1 We use Synthesis Procedure 9.2.1 to synthesize a neural network (9.1.1) with $n = 12$ neurons. The network structure is depicted in Fig 9.5.1. We first note that the structure in Fig 9.5.1 renders neural network (9.1.1) a cellular neural network (9.4.1) with $M = 4$, $N = 3$, and $r = 1$ (neighborhood radius). Given are $m = 4$ vectors specified by

$$\alpha^1 = (1, -1, 1, 1, -1, 1, 1, 1, 1, -1, -1, 1)^T,$$
$$\alpha^2 = (1, 1, 1, 1, -1, -1, 1, -1, -1, 1, 1, 1)^T,$$
$$\alpha^3 = (1, -1, 1, 1, -1, 1, 1, -1, 1, 1, 1, 1)^T,$$

and

$$\alpha^4 = (1, -1, -1, 1, -1, -1, 1, -1, -1, 1, 1, 1)^T.$$

It is desired that these vectors be stored as memory vectors of system (9.1.1).

We determine the index matrix S according to the structure shown in Fig 9.5.1 as

9.5. ILLUSTRATIVE EXAMPLES

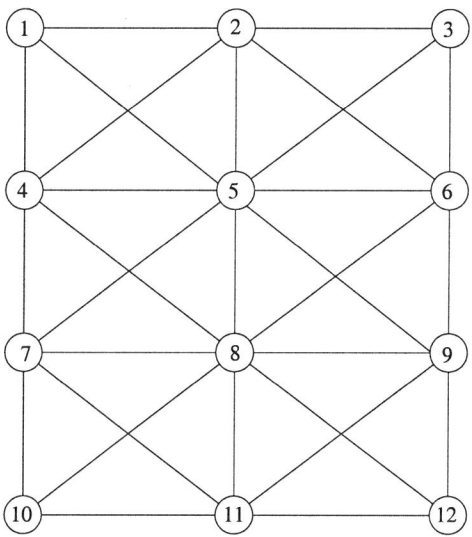

Figure 9.5.1: Interconnecting structure of a cellular neural network

$$S = S^T = \begin{bmatrix} 1 & 1 & 0 & 1 & 1 & 0 & 0 & 0 & 0 & 0 & 0 & 0 \\ 1 & 1 & 1 & 1 & 1 & 1 & 0 & 0 & 0 & 0 & 0 & 0 \\ 0 & 1 & 1 & 0 & 1 & 1 & 0 & 0 & 0 & 0 & 0 & 0 \\ 1 & 1 & 0 & 1 & 1 & 0 & 1 & 1 & 0 & 0 & 0 & 0 \\ 1 & 1 & 1 & 1 & 1 & 1 & 1 & 1 & 1 & 0 & 0 & 0 \\ 0 & 1 & 1 & 0 & 1 & 1 & 0 & 1 & 1 & 0 & 0 & 0 \\ 0 & 0 & 0 & 1 & 1 & 0 & 1 & 1 & 0 & 1 & 1 & 0 \\ 0 & 0 & 0 & 1 & 1 & 1 & 1 & 1 & 1 & 1 & 1 & 1 \\ 0 & 0 & 0 & 0 & 1 & 1 & 0 & 1 & 1 & 0 & 1 & 1 \\ 0 & 0 & 0 & 0 & 0 & 0 & 1 & 1 & 0 & 1 & 1 & 0 \\ 0 & 0 & 0 & 0 & 0 & 0 & 1 & 1 & 1 & 1 & 1 & 1 \\ 0 & 0 & 0 & 0 & 0 & 0 & 0 & 1 & 1 & 0 & 1 & 1 \end{bmatrix} \quad (9.5.1)$$

where "1" at location (i, j) in the matrix represents a connection from the jth neuron to the ith neuron and "0" represents no such connection.

Using Synthesis Procedure 9.2.1, we determine A as the 12×12 identity matrix,

$$T = \begin{bmatrix} -1.0000e+01 & 0.0000e+00 & 0 & -1.0000e+01 \\ -1.0000e+01 & -2.0000e+00 & 4.0000e+00 & -1.0000e+01 \\ 0 & -2.6667e+00 & 4.6667e+00 & 0 \\ -1.0000e+01 & 0.0000e+00 & 0 & -1.0000e+01 \\ -1.0000e+01 & -4.0000e+00 & 4.0000e+00 & -1.0000e+01 \\ 0 & -4.4000e+00 & 4.4000e+00 & 0 \\ 0 & 0 & 0 & -1.0000e+01 \\ 0 & 0 & 0 & -1.0000e+01 \\ 0 & 0 & 0 & 0 \\ 0 & 0 & 0 & 0 \\ 0 & 0 & 0 & 0 \\ 0 & 0 & 0 & 0 \end{bmatrix}$$

9.5. ILLUSTRATIVE EXAMPLES

$$
\begin{aligned}
&\begin{array}{cccc}
-1.0000e+01 & 0 & 0 & 0 \\
-1.0000e+01 & -4.0000e+00 & 0 & 0 \\
-1.0000e+01 & -2.6667e+00 & 0 & 0 \\
-1.0000e+01 & 0 & -1.0000e+01 & 0.0000e+00 \\
-1.0000e+01 & -2.0000e+00 & -1.0000e+01 & -1.0888e-14 \\
-1.0000e+01 & -1.2000e+00 & 0 & -2.1826e-15 \\
-1.0000e+01 & 0 & -1.0000e+01 & -1.3333e+01 \\
-1.0000e+01 & -4.4409e-16 & -1.0000e+01 & -1.2667e+01 \\
-1.0000e+01 & 1.0000e+00 & 0 & -1.0000e+01 \\
0 & 0 & -1.0000e+01 & -1.4000e+01 \\
0 & 0 & -1.0000e+01 & -1.4000e+01 \\
0 & 0 & 0 & -1.0000e+01 \\
\end{array}\\[6pt]
&\begin{array}{cccc}
0 & 0 & 0 & 0 \\
0 & 0 & 0 & 0 \\
0 & 0 & 0 & 0 \\
0 & 0 & 0 & 0 \\
-2.0000e+00 & 0 & 0 & 0 \\
-1.2000e+00 & 0 & 0 & 0 \\
0 & -6.6667e+00 & -6.6667e+00 & 0 \\
-1.3323e-15 & -7.3333e+00 & -7.3333e+00 & -1.0000e+01 \\
1.0000e+00 & 0 & -1.0000e+01 & -1.0000e+01 \\
0 & -6.0000e+00 & -6.0000e+00 & 0 \\
-2.2538e-15 & -6.0000e+00 & -6.0000e+00 & -1.0000e+01 \\
-7.8505e-16 & 0 & -1.0000e+01 & -1.0000e+01 \\
\end{array},
\end{aligned}
$$

and

$$
\begin{aligned}
I = (\ &1.2000e+01,\ 6.0000e+00,\ -1.2667e+01,\ 2.2000e+01,\\
&1.4000e+01,\ -1.4444e+01,\ 1.2000e+01,\ 2.0000e+01,\\
&-8.8818e-15,\ 1.0000e+01,\ 2.0000e+01,\ 1.2000e+01)^T.
\end{aligned}
$$

In the above computations, we choose $\mu = 2$ in step 2 and $W_i = -10 \times O_{m_i} \times U_{i2}$ in step 8 of Synthesis Procedure 9.2.1, where $O_{m_i} = (1, \cdots, 1) \in \Re^{1 \times m_i}$ and $m_i = \sum\limits_{j=1}^{n} S_{ij}$.

Using Lemma 6.6.1, we verify that $\alpha^1, \cdots, \alpha^4$ are memory vectors of the synthesized system (9.1.1) with $\{A, T, I\}$ given above. This was also confirmed by simulation runs of the synthesized neural network.

By Lemma 6.6.1, we determine that system (9.1.1) has 2 additional memory vectors in B^n given by

$$\alpha^5 = (1,\ -1,\ -1,\ 1,\ -1,\ -1,\ 1,\ 1,\ -1,\ -1,\ -1\,,1)^T,$$

and
$$\alpha^6 = (1,\ 1,\ 1,\ 1,\ -1,\ -1,\ 1,\ 1,\ -1,\ -1,\ -1,\ 1)^T.$$

Their corresponding asymptotically stable states are given by $\beta^5 = 2\alpha^5$ and $\beta^6 = 2\alpha^6$, respectively. Using a procedure similar to that of Theorem 4.4.1, we determine that system (9.1.1) designed above has 1 additional memory vector in $D^n - B^n$, given by

$$\alpha^7 = (-0.7273,\ -1,\ -1,\ 1,\ 1,\ -1,\ -0.7273,\ -1,\ -1,\ 1,\ 1,\ 1)^T.$$

Its corresponding asymptotically stable state is given by

$$\beta^7 = (\ -0.7273,\ -4.7273,\ -22,\ 16.5455,\ 12.5455,\ -22,$$
$$-0.7273,\ -4.7273,\ -22,\ 19.2727,\ 19.2727,\ 2\ )^T.$$

Similarly, we also determine that system (9.1.1) has 5 unstable equilibrium points. ∎

Example 9.5.2 In order to ascertain how typical the results of Example 9.5.1 are, we repeated the above example twenty times, using different sets of desired vectors to be stored as memory vectors. Each set contains $m = 4$ vectors in B^n which are generated randomly. For each given set of vectors, we synthesize system (9.4.1) using Synthesis Procedure 9.2.1. Table 9.5.1 summarizes our findings. Also shown in Table 9.5.1 are the results for system (9.1.1) synthesized by the Eigenstructure Method developed in Section 8.3 (cf. Synthesis Procedure 8.4.1) *for the same sets of desired vectors* to be stored as memories.

9.5. ILLUSTRATIVE EXAMPLES

Table 9.5.1: Results of Example 9.5.2.

	Cellular neural networks with $r=1$ using Synthesis Procedure 9.2.1	Fully connected neural networks using Synthesis Procedure 8.4.1
average of total number of memory vectors in B^n	12.2	4.5
average of total number of undesired memory vectors in B^n	8.2	0.5
average of total number of memory vectors in $D^n - B^n$	3.1	0.4
average of total number of unstable equilibrium points in $\Re^n$	64.65	14.25
total number of desired patterns which are not stored as memory vectors	0	0

From Table 9.5.1 we see that in the present example, implementations of associative memories using neural networks with sparse interconnecting structure (i.e., cellular neural networks) have more spurious states than using the fully connected networks. Also, there are more unstable equilibrium points in the synthesized cellular neural networks than in the fully connected networks. ∎

Example 9.5.3 We now present several problems which to the best of our knowledge cannot be addressed by other existing synthesis

456   CHAPTER 9. INTERCONNECTION CONSTRAINTS

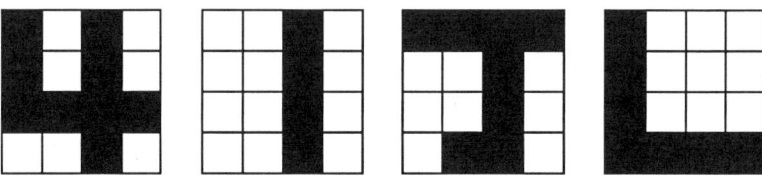

Figure 9.5.2: The four desired patterns used in Example 9.5.3.

procedures for associative memories. In all cases, we consider a neural network with 16 neurons ($n = 16$) and in all cases our objective is to store the four patterns shown in Fig. 9.5.2 as memories. As indicated, sixteen boxes are used to represent each pattern (in $\Re^{16}$), with each box corresponding to a vector component which is allowed to assume values between -1 and 1. For purposes of visualization, -1 will represent white, 1 will represent black, and the intermediate values will correspond to appropriate grey levels shown in Fig. 9.5.3.

The four cases which we consider below, are synthesized by Synthesis Procedure 9.2.1. These cases involve different prespecified constraints on the interconnecting structure of each network.

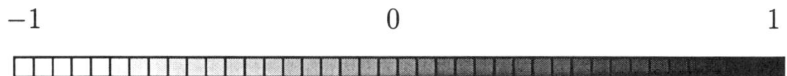

Figure 9.5.3: Grey levels.

Case I: Cellular neural network. We design a cellular neural network with $r = 1$, $M = 4$, and $N = 4$. (Due to space limitations, we will not display the interconnecting matrix T for the present case, as well as for the three subsequent cases.) The performance of this

9.5. ILLUSTRATIVE EXAMPLES

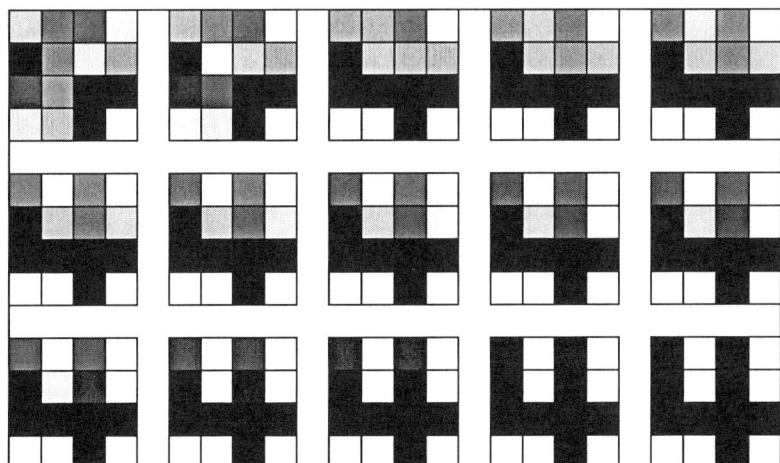

Figure 9.5.4: A typical evolution of pattern number 1 of Fig. 9.5.2.

network is illustrated by means of a typical simulation run of equation (9.1.1) [or equation (9.4.1)], shown in Fig. 9.5.4. In this figure, the desired memory pattern is depicted in the lower right corner. The initial state, shown in the upper left corner, is generated by adding to the desired pattern zero-mean Gaussian noise with a standard deviation SD=1. The iteration of the simulation evolves from left to right in each row and from the top row to the bottom row. The desired pattern is recovered in 14 steps in the simulation of equation (9.1.1). All our simulations are performed on a Sun SPARC Station using MATLAB.

Case II: Reduction of line-crossings. We arrange the 16 neurons in a 4×4 array and we consider only horizontal and vertical interconnections. For this case, the index matrix $S = Q = [S_{ij}] \in \Re^{16 \times 16}$, and $Q = [Q_{ij,kl}] \in \Re^{(4 \times 4) \times (4 \times 4)}$ assumes the form

$$Q_{ij,kl} = \begin{cases} 1, & \text{if } i = k \text{ or } j = l \\ 0, & \text{otherwise.} \end{cases} \quad (9.5.2)$$

A typical simulation run for the present case is depicted in Fig. 9.5.5. In this figure, the noisy pattern is generated by adding to the desired

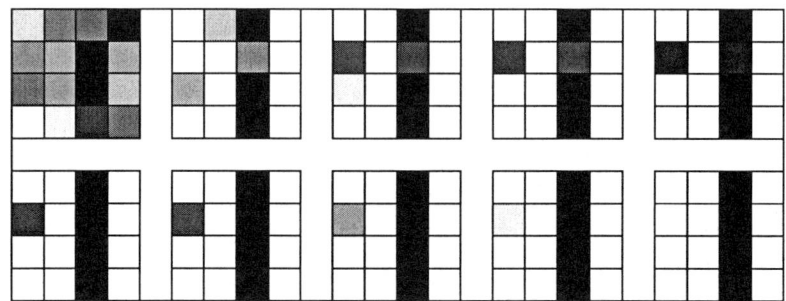

Figure 9.5.5: A typical evolution of pattern number 2 of Fig. 9.5.2.

pattern uniformly distributed noise defined on $[-0.7, 0.7]$. Convergence occurred in 9 steps.

We emphasize that by choosing the index matrix as in (9.5.2), we are able to reduce significantly the number of line-crossings, which is of great concern in VLSI implementations of artificial neural networks.

Case III: Two rows of S identical (see Remark 9.2.3). In this case, we choose an index matrix $S = [S_{ij}] \in \Re^{16 \times 16}$ of the form

$$S_{ij} = \begin{cases} 1, & \text{if } i = 1 \text{ or } i = 16 \text{ or } j = 1 \text{ or} \\ & \quad j = 16 \text{ or } |i - j| \leq 1 \\ 0, & \text{otherwise.} \end{cases}$$

This requires that the T matrix has zero elements everywhere except in its first and last rows, its first and last columns, and in its tridiagonal elements.

Rows 2 to 15 are designed by using Synthesis Procedure 9.2.1, step by step. Since the first row S_1 and the last row S_{16} of S are identical, we can design the rows T_1 and T_{16} of T simultaneously. To see this, we take in step 5 of the design procedure $y_{I1}^l = \left(y_{\sigma(1)}^l, \cdots, y_{\sigma(m_1)}^l \right)^T$ and $y_{I16}^l = \left(y_{\sigma(1)}^l, \cdots, y_{\sigma(m_{16})}^l \right)^T$ for $l = 1, \cdots, m - 1$. Clearly, $m_1 = m_{16} = n = 16$ and $y_{I1}^l = y_{I16}^l$ for $l = 1, \cdots, m - 1$, since $S_1 = S_{16} = (1, \cdots, 1) \in \Re^{1 \times 16}$. In step 6, we

9.5. ILLUSTRATIVE EXAMPLES

take $Y_1 = \left(y_{I1}^1, \cdots, y_{I1}^{m-1}\right)$ and the $2 \times (m-1)$ vector

$$Z_1 = \begin{bmatrix} z_1^1 & \cdots & z_1^{m-1} \\ z_{16}^1 & \cdots & z_{16}^{m-1} \end{bmatrix}.$$

In step 7, we perform a singular value decomposition of Y_1 and obtain U_{11}, U_{12}, D_1, and V_{11}. In step 8, we compute $G_1 = Z_1 V_{11} D_1^{-1} U_{11}^T + W_1 U_{12}^T$, where W_1 is an arbitrary $2 \times (m_1 - p_1)$ real matrix and $p_1 = \text{rank}(Y_1)$. In step 9, we determine T_1 from the first row of G_1 and T_{16} from the second row of G_1, using (9.2.3).

A typical simulation run for this network is shown in Fig. 9.5.6. In this case, the noisy pattern is generated by adding Gaussian noise $N(0, 0.5)$ to the desired pattern. Convergence occurred in 24 steps.

We can generalize the above case to design problems for which the index matrix S has several identical rows. In particular, if in $S = [S_{ij}]$, $S_{ij} = 1$ for all i and j, Synthesis Procedure 9.2.1 reduces to a procedure for a *fully connected* neural network (9.1.1). In the reduced synthesis procedure all rows of T are determined simultaneously and this reduced synthesis procedure will be more general than Synthesis Procedure 8.4.1 developed in Section 8.4. To see this, note that the reduced design procedure will generally result in a nonsymmetric T and by special choice of matrix W in step 8, the reduced design procedure will become Synthesis Procedure 8.4.1.

Case IV: Quinquediagonal matrix S resulting in an interconnecting structure without line-crossings. We choose $S = [S_{ij}] \in \Re^{16 \times 16}$ as

$$S_{ij} = \begin{cases} 1, & \text{if } |i-j| \leq 2 \\ 0, & \text{otherwise.} \end{cases} \quad (9.5.3)$$

This will result in a quinquediagonal matrix S, enabling us to arrange the $n = 16$ neurons in the configuration shown in Fig. 9.5.7. Note that in this figure there are no line-crossings. Furthermore, note that this configuration can be generalized to arbitrary n.

A typical simulation run for this case is depicted in Fig. 9.5.8. In this figure, the noisy pattern is generated by adding Gaussian noise $N(0.1, 0.7)$ to the desired pattern. We can see that convergence occurred in 13 steps. ∎

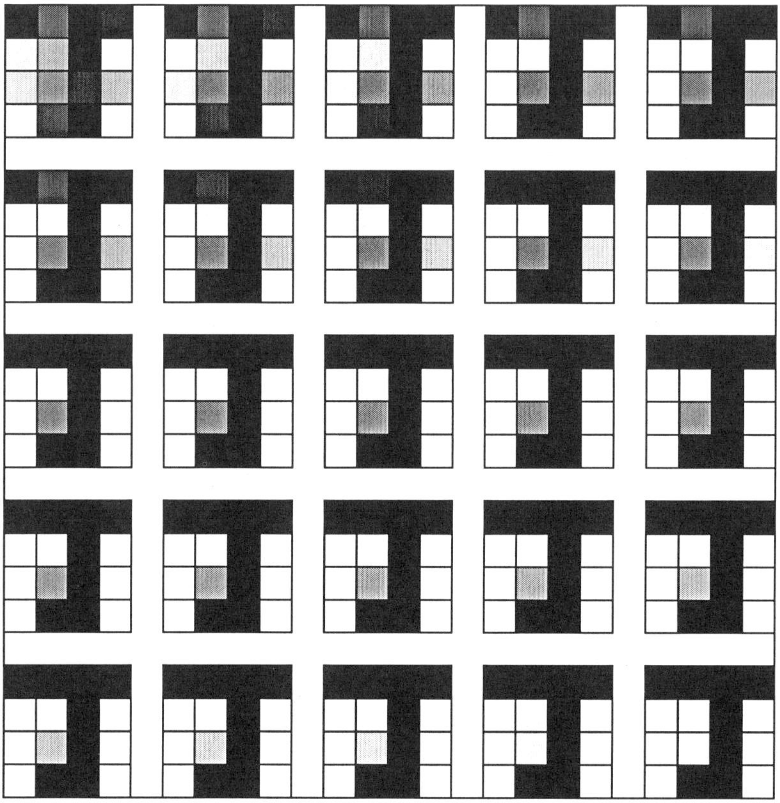

Figure 9.5.6: A typical evolution of pattern number 3 of Fig. 9.5.2.

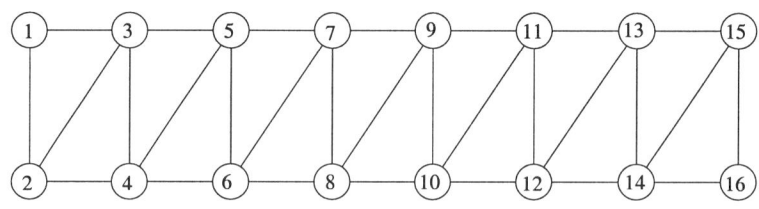

Figure 9.5.7: A possible structure for a neural network without line-crossings in the interconnecting structure.

9.5. ILLUSTRATIVE EXAMPLES

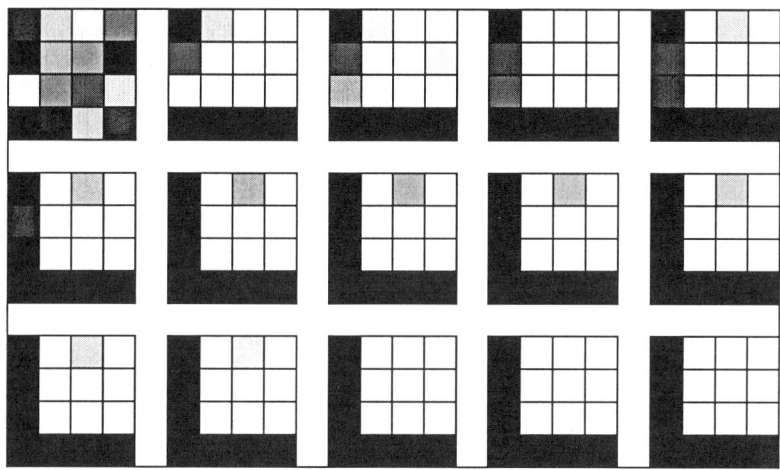

Figure 9.5.8: A typical evolution of pattern number 4 of Fig. 9.5.2.

We note that for the above example, many other interesting design cases can be addressed in a *systematic* manner, including a neural network (9.1.1) with lower or upper triangular matrix T, combinations of Cases I, II, III, and IV given above, and so forth.

Example 9.5.4 In this example, Synthesis Procedure 9.3.1 is used in the design of a neural network with configuration given in Fig. 9.5.1 and with the objective of storing the first four patterns $(\alpha^1, \alpha^2, \alpha^3, \alpha^4)$ in Fig. 8.7.6 as memories (see Section 8.7). In both cases, a neural network design for (9.1.1) with A equal to the identity matrix and with the network satisfying the optimal constraints [i.e., with every diagonal element of T equal to 1 $(T_{ii} = a_i = 1)$], will be part of the design objectives.

Case I: Sparse Design. The index matrix for this interconnecting structure is given in (9.5.1). Synthesis Procedure 9.3.1 is utilized with Remark 8.5.12. After each perceptron training, choose $T_{ii} = 1$ and $\mu_i = 1 - w_i^i$ whenever $w_i^i < 0$. Matrix T is obtained as

$$T = \begin{bmatrix} 1 & -2.2 & 0 & 8.6 & -3.2 & 0 & 0 & 0 & 0 & 0 & 0 & 0 \\ -0.6 & 1 & -0.6 & -0.6 & -6.2 & -4.4 & 0 & 0 & 0 & 0 & 0 & 0 \\ 0 & -1.1 & 1 & 0 & -6.1 & 4.9 & 0 & 0 & 0 & 0 & 0 & 0 \\ 5.7 & -0.3 & 0 & 1 & -2.7 & 0 & 5.7 & -2.5 & 0 & 0 & 0 & 0 \\ -2.1 & -4.7 & -2.1 & -2.1 & 1 & 0.9 & -2.1 & -1.7 & 0.9 & 0 & 0 & 0 \\ 0 & -3.2 & 3.2 & 0 & 0 & 1 & 0 & 2.2 & 8.6 & 0 & 0 & 0 \\ 0 & 0 & 0 & 4.8 & -2.4 & 0 & 1 & -2.4 & 0 & 4.8 & -2.4 & 0 \\ 0 & 0 & 0 & -1.7 & -2.1 & 1.1 & -1.7 & 1 & 1.1 & -1.7 & -1.1 & -8.7 \\ 0 & 0 & 0 & 0 & 0.1 & 6.5 & 0 & 0.1 & 1 & 0 & -6.5 & -0.1 \\ 0 & 0 & 0 & 0 & 0 & 0 & 7.9 & -3.7 & 0 & 1 & -3.5 & 0 \\ 0 & 0 & 0 & 0 & 0 & 0 & -1.9 & -1.3 & -9.7 & -1.9 & 1 & 1.3 \\ 0 & 0 & 0 & 0 & 0 & 0 & 0 & -9.8 & 0 & 0 & 0 & 1 \end{bmatrix}$$

and bias vector I is obtained as

$$I = (3.2,\ 6.4,\ 6.1,\ 2.7,\ 6.5,\ 0,\ 2.4,\ 2.1,\ -0.1,\ 3.5,\ 1.3,\ 0)^T.$$

In the above, $\eta = 0.1$ is used as the learning rate in the perceptron training. Even though the rank condition in Theorem 8.5.4 is not satisfied for $i = 2, 3, 5$, it is still possible to obtain a neural network design with every diagonal element of T equal to 1 using Synthesis Procedure 9.3.1 with Remark 8.5.12. Using Lemma 6.6.1, one can determine that system (9.1.1) has in this case a total of 8 spurious

9.5. ILLUSTRATIVE EXAMPLES

memories in B^n. From Corollary 5.7.1 we see that these 8 vectors are the only spurious memory vectors in D^n in this case since $T_{ii} \geq a_i$ for $i = 1, \cdots, n$ are satisfied. From Theorem 6.6.1, one can determine that $\nu = 7$.

Case II: Sparse and Symmetric Design. Starting with T and I obtained in Case I, one can obtain a neural network with symmetric interconnection matrix T for the same network structure using Synthesis Procedure 9.3.2. Matrix T is obtained as

$$T = \begin{bmatrix} 1 & -1.40 & 0 & 7.15 & -2.65 & 0 & 0 & 0 & 0 & 0 & 0 & 0 \\ -1.40 & 1 & -0.85 & -0.45 & -5.45 & -3.80 & 0 & 0 & 0 & 0 & 0 & 0 \\ 0 & -0.85 & 1 & 0 & -4.10 & 4.05 & 0 & 0 & 0 & 0 & 0 & 0 \\ 7.15 & -0.45 & 0 & 1 & -2.40 & 0 & 5.25 & -2.10 & 0 & 0 & 0 & 0 \\ -2.65 & -5.45 & -4.10 & -2.40 & 1 & 0.45 & -2.25 & -1.90 & 0.50 & 0 & 0 & 0 \\ 0 & -3.80 & 4.05 & 0 & 0.45 & 1 & 0 & 1.65 & 7.55 & 0 & 0 & 0 \\ 0 & 0 & 0 & 5.25 & -2.25 & 0 & 1 & -2.05 & 0 & 6.35 & -2.15 & 0 \\ 0 & 0 & 0 & -2.10 & -1.90 & 1.65 & -2.05 & 1 & 0.60 & -2.70 & -1.20 & -9.25 \\ 0 & 0 & 0 & 0 & 0.50 & 7.55 & 0 & 0.60 & 1 & 0 & -8.10 & -0.05 \\ 0 & 0 & 0 & 0 & 0 & 0 & 6.35 & -2.70 & 0 & 1 & -2.70 & 0 \\ 0 & 0 & 0 & 0 & 0 & 0 & -2.15 & -1.20 & -8.10 & -2.70 & 1 & 0.65 \\ 0 & 0 & 0 & 0 & 0 & 0 & 0 & -9.25 & -0.05 & 0 & 0.65 & 1 \end{bmatrix}$$

and I is the same as in the previous case. The network in this case has 8 spurious memories and one can determine that $\nu = 3.9$ from Theorem 6.6.1.

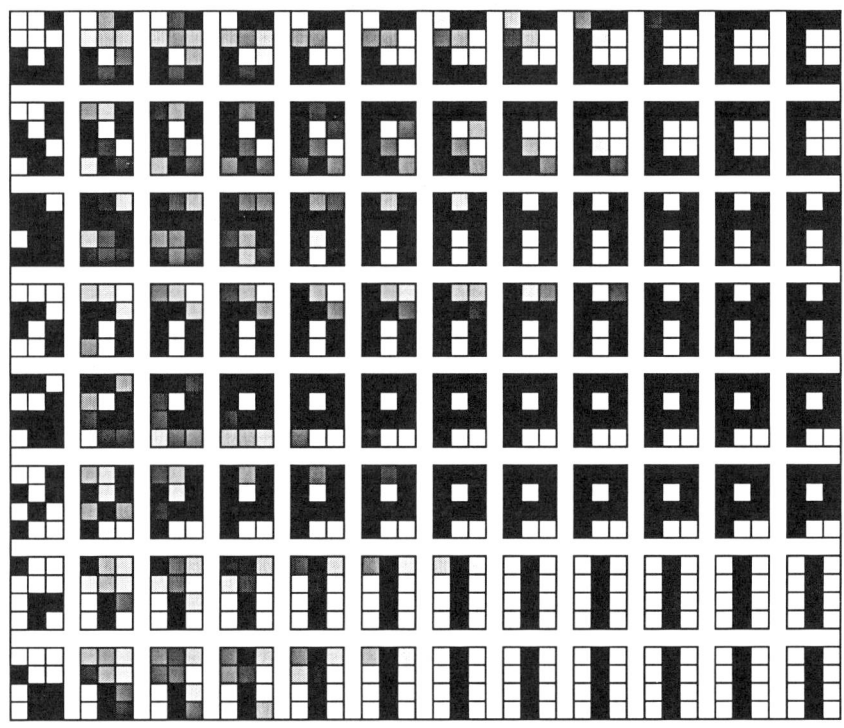

Figure 9.5.9: Typical evolutions of the four patterns in Example 9.5.4.

9.5. ILLUSTRATIVE EXAMPLES

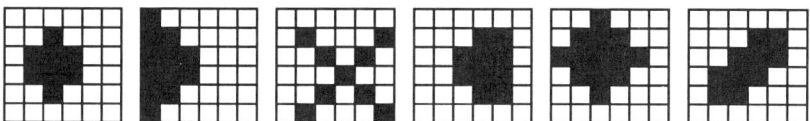

Figure 9.5.10: The six desired memory patterns

The performance of this network is illustrated by means of typical simulation runs of equation (9.1.1), shown in Fig. 9.5.9. In this figure, the desired memory pattern is depicted in the last column. The initial states, shown in the first column, are generated by randomly reversing 4 to 5 bits of each desired pattern. The iteration of the simulation evolves from left to right. The desired pattern is recovered in less than 11 steps in all cases in simulations of (9.1.1). ∎

Example 9.5.5 The present example demonstrates the applicability of Synthesis Procedure 9.4.1. To this end, the example in [12] is used. Consider a design of a cellular neural network (9.4.1) [or (9.1.1)] with 36 neurons ($n = 36$) with $M = 6$, $N = 6$, and $r = 1$. The objective is to store the six patterns shown in Fig. 9.5.10 as stable memories (black $= 1$ and white $= -1$).

Case I: Nonsymmetric Design. In this case, we utilize Synthesis Procedure 9.4.1 to design a cellular neural network (with $I = 0$). The matrix T obtained has a cloning template

$$P_T = \begin{bmatrix} 0.6582 & 0.9458 & 0.5621 \\ 0.3777 & 4.9381 & 0.4499 \\ 0.5230 & 0.9710 & 0.6495 \end{bmatrix}.$$

A comparison study between the present space-invariant cloning template design and the space-varying designs (cf. Section 9.4B and [12]) indicates that the cellular neural network with space-invariant cloning template has smaller basins of attraction for each desired pattern than those designed with space-varying cloning template.

Case II: Symmetric Design. Using Synthesis Procedure 9.2.2, we first determine a symmetric matrix T_1 for the present design. Starting with this symmetric T_1, we obtain a matrix T which is also

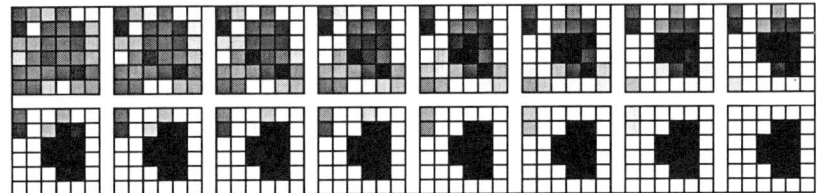

Figure 9.5.11: A typical evolution of pattern No. 4

symmetric using the Synthesis Procedure 9.4.1 (cf. Remark 9.4.4). Matrix T has in this case a cloning template given by

$$P_T = \begin{bmatrix} 0.7139 & 1.0520 & 0.5912 \\ 0.4517 & 5.2901 & 0.4517 \\ 0.5912 & 1.0520 & 0.7139 \end{bmatrix}. \tag{9.5.4}$$

It can be verified by Lemma 6.6.1 that the four desired patterns are also stable memory vectors for system (9.1.1) with the symmetric connection matrix determined above. Notice that the structure of the cloning template in (9.5.4) is a typical one for $r = 1$, i.e., $P_T^\sigma = P_T$ according to Theorem 9.4.1, which yields a *symmetric interconnection matrix*. We can see that this cloning template requires symmetric connections in vertical, horizontal, as well as diagonal directions from any cell unit.

The performance of this network is illustrated by means of a typical simulation run of equation (9.1.1), shown in Fig. 9.5.11. ∎

Example 9.5.6 The objective of this example is to demonstrate the capability of Synthesis Procedure 9.4.2 to satisfy the constraints on the diagonal elements if such a solution exists. It also illustrates the effect of diagonal elements on the number of spurious memories. Results are compared to fully connected neural networks designed using Synthesis Procedure 8.5.1.

In this example, a cellular neural network (9.1.1) with 12 neurons ($n = 12$) is required for the realization of an associative memory. The cellular neural network is arranged in a 4×3 array as in Fig. 9.5.1. Four desired patterns (Fig. 9.5.12) are to be stored in the

9.5. ILLUSTRATIVE EXAMPLES

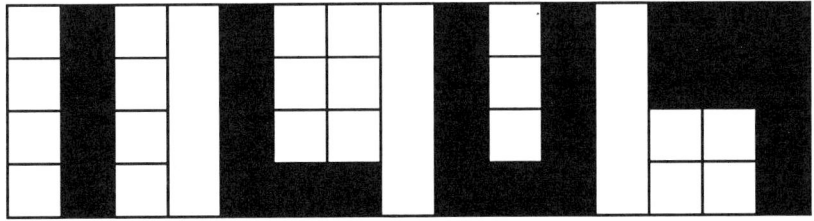

Figure 9.5.12: The four desired memory patterns for Example 9.5.6.

network designed by using Synthesis Procedure 9.4.2 combined with Remark 9.4.7. A cloning template whose center element is 1 can be determined as

$$P_T = \begin{bmatrix} -2.205 & 5.980 & -2.550 \\ 5.255 & 1 & 4.755 \\ -5.345 & 7.120 & -3.990 \end{bmatrix}$$

and $I_i = 1.825$ for $i = 1, \cdots, n$. The above cloning template guarantees that $T_{ii} = 1$ for $i = 1, \cdots, n$.

The performance of this network is illustrated by means of a typical simulation run of equation (9.1.1), shown in Fig. 9.5.13. In this case, the (noisy) initial pattern is generated by reversing five bits in the desired pattern. Convergence occurs in 14 steps.

Choosing the diagonal component T_{ii} to be $0, 1, 2, 3$ and 4, respectively, the number of spurious memory vectors for each case can be computed using the results developed in Chapter 4. One can see that the number of spurious memory vectors decreases as $T_{ii} \geq 1$ decreases. Table 9.5.2 summarizes the experimental results. It is noted that in Table 9.5.2, the number of spurious memories is for the entire 12-dimensional space (4 × 3 array). The comparison with fully connected neural networks designed using Synthesis Procedure 8.5.1 is also shown in the table. One can see that the number of spurious memories in a fully connected neural network is significantly smaller than that in a cellular neural network.

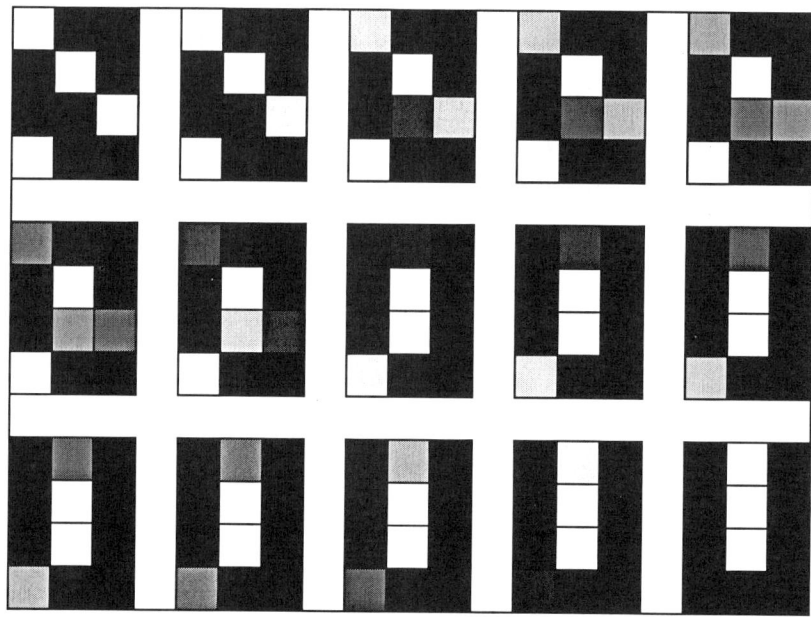

Figure 9.5.13: A typical evolution of pattern No. 3 of Fig. 9.5.12.

Table 9.5.2: Results of Example 9.5.6.

T_{ii}	0	1	2	3	4
Total number of spurious memories (Synthesis Procedure 9.4.2)	22	22	50	81	111
Total number of spurious memories (Synthesis Procedure 8.5.1)	4	4	4	5	6

We note in Table 9.5.2 that in order for the comparison to be meaningful, we must choose to design neural networks using the two algorithms with the same $\mu = \mu_i$, which is a parameter that controls the robustness of the neural network design (see Theorem 6.6.1). We also note that when $T_{ii} < 1$ in Table 9.5.2, non-bipolar spurious memories exist in the designed cellular neural networks. Although the performance of the cellular neural network (9.1.1) is excellent when the diagonal elements of T are all equal to 1, this design is not always attainable. ∎

9.6 Summary

In the present chapter, we addressed the synthesis problem of associative memories realized by neural networks that are subjected to constraints on the interconnecting structure. These constraints are expressed as sparsity conditions, and sometimes as symmetry constraints on the interconnection coefficient matrix T.

We first introduced the index matrix $S \in \Re^{n \times n}$, defined by $S = [S_{ij}]$ where $S_{ij} = 1$ or 0. This matrix specifies a specific interconnecting structure, letting $S_{ij} = 1$ indicate a connection from the jth neuron to the ith neuron and letting $S_{ij} = 0$ indicate no such a connection. Next, we defined the restriction of a matrix $W \in \Re^{n \times n}$ to an index matrix S as $W|S = [h_{ij}] \in \Re^{n \times n}$, where

$$h_{ij} = \begin{cases} W_{ij}, & \text{if } S_{ij} = 1 \\ 0, & \text{otherwise.} \end{cases}$$

With these conventions, the sparse design of neural networks requires that matrix T must satisfy the condition

$$T = T|S$$

for a given index matrix S.

Throughout the chapter, we considered neural networks described by equations of the form

$$\begin{cases} \dot{x} = -Ax + Ty + I, & T = T|S \\ y = \text{sat}(x). \end{cases} \quad (9.6.1)$$

We first modified the Eigenstructure Method (developed in Chapter 8) to solve the present sparse design problem. We showed that solutions to this problem always exist as long as $S_{ii} = 1$, $i = 1, \cdots, n$. That is to say, if we allow each neuron to have self feedback, a solution for the sparse design problem, using the Eigenstructure Method, for any sparsity constraints and for any number of desired bipolar patterns in the prototype set will always exist.

To design a neural network (9.6.1) with symmetric and sparse interconnection matrix, we employed the robustness analysis results of Section 6.6 to develop a synthesis procedure which will lead to a sparse and symmetric design, provided that such a solution exists.

To solve the design problem described above, we also modified the synthesis approach based on the perceptron training algorithm (developed in Section 8.5). The results of the present chapter indicate that both the Eigenstructure Method and the approach based on the perceptron training algorithm can easily be modified to design neural networks with sparsity and/or symmetry constraints in the interconnecting structure.

One of the reasons for studying neural networks described by (9.6.1) is that for such networks, a special choice of the index matrix S, describes a class of cellular neural networks. Cellular neural networks are characterized by local connections constrained to a neighborhood, called a cell. When the connection weights maintain the same values from cell to cell, a cellular neural network is said to have a space-invariant cloning template. Otherwise, the cellular neural network has space-varying cloning templates. Now since (9.6.1) becomes equivalent to cellular neural networks by a special choice of the index matrix S, the sparse design procedure presented herein can directly be applied in the design of cellular neural networks with space-varying cloning template. We developed two different approaches for the design of cellular neural networks with space-invariant cloning template. The first approach is an application of the robustness analysis results of Section 6.6, utilizing an iterative algorithm to gradually approach a potential target of space-invariant cloning template. The second approach is an application of the synthesis approach based on the perceptron training algorithm. By reformulating the linear inequalities used in the design problem on hand, we were able to devise a cellular neural network design with space-invariant cloning template by simply training one perceptron. We also devised a synthesis procedure for cellular neural networks with space-invariant cloning template and with symmetric interconnection matrix T (requiring that $S = S^T$). We noted that a space-invariant cloning template yields a symmetric connection matrix when the template is symmetric in horizontal, vertical, and both diagonal directions.

Finally, we used several examples to demonstrate the applicability of the synthesis procedures developed in the present chapter.

9.7 Notes and References

The material presented in Section 9.2 is based on [9], [10], and [17] while Section 9.3 relies on the material presented in [8]. Section 9.4 is based on [7] and [11]. Cellular neural networks which were originally introduced by Chua and Yang in [4], have found several applications. Our application domain for cellular neural networks concerns associative memory. For other applications of cellular neural networks, refer to [1]. The examples in Section 9.5 are taken from [7], [8], [10], and [11].

Bibliography

[1] LO Chua. CNN: A Paradigm for Complexity. Singapore: World Scientific, 1998.

[2] LO Chua, T Roska. Stability of a class of nonreciprocal cellular neural networks. IEEE Transactions on Circuits and Systems 37:1520–1527, 1990.

[3] LO Chua, T Roska. The CNN paradigm. IEEE Transactions on Circuits and Systems-I: Fundamental Theory and Applications 40:147–156, 1993

[4] LO Chua, L Yang. Cellular neural networks: Theory. IEEE Transactions on Circuits and Systems 35:1257–1272, 1988.

[5] LO Chua, L Yang. Cellular neural networks: Applications. IEEE Transactions on Circuits and Systems 35:1273–1290, 1988

[6] J Levendovszky. A possible transformation of fully connected neural nets into partially connected networks. Proceedings 1990 IEEE International Workshop on Cellular Neural Networks and Their Applications, Budapest, Hungary, 1990, pp 55–64.

[7] D Liu. Cloning template design of cellular neural networks for associative memories. IEEE Transactions on Circuits and Systems-I: Fundamental Theory and Applications 44:646–650, 1997.

[8] D Liu, Z Lu. A new synthesis approach for feedback neural networks based on the perceptron training algorithm. IEEE Transactions on Neural Networks 8:1468–1482, 1997.

[9] D Liu, AN Michel. Dynamical Systems with Saturation Nonlinearities: Analysis and Design. Lecture Notes in Control and Information Sciences, vol 195. Berlin, Germany: Springer-Verlag, 1994.

[10] D Liu, AN Michel. Sparsely interconnected neural networks for associative memories with applications to cellular neural networks. IEEE Transactions on Circuits and Systems-II: Analog and Digital Signal Processing 41:295–307, 1994.

[11] Z Lu, D Liu. A new synthesis procedure for a class of cellular neural networks with space-invariant cloning template. IEEE Transactions on Circuits and Systems-II: Analog and Digital Signal Processing 45:1601–1605, 1998.

[12] G Martinelli, R Perfetti. Associative memory design using space-varying cellular neural networks. Proceedings of the 2nd International Workshop on Cellular Neural Networks and Their Applications, Munich, Germany, 1992, pp 117–122.

[13] T Matsumoto, LO Chua, R Furukawa. CNN Cloning template: Hole-filler. IEEE Transactions on Circuits and Systems 37:635–638, 1990.

[14] T Matsumoto, LO Chua, H Suzuki. CNN Cloning template: Connected component detector. IEEE Transactions on Circuits and Systems 37:633–635, 1990.

[15] T Matsumoto, LO Chua, H Suzuki. CNN cloning template: Shadow detector. IEEE Transactions on Circuits and Systems 37:1070–1073, 1990.

[16] T Matsumoto, LO Chua, T Yokohama. Image thinning with a cellular neural network. IEEE Transactions on Circuits and Systems 37:638–640, 1990.

[17] AN Michel, D Liu. Theory and applications of sparsely interconnected neural networks. Neural, Parallel and Scientific Computations 4:305–324, 1996.

[18] Proceedings of the 1990 IEEE International Workshop on Cellular Neural Networks and Their Applications, Budapest, Hungary, 1990.

Index

Activation function, 1, 3, 17, 18, 216, 217, 228, 229, 250, 259, 266
   multi-threshold, 229
Address addressable memory, 35
   AAM, 35
Amplification function, 48, 49, 272
Analog Hopfield neural network, 3, 6, 7, 18, 23, 40–44, 50, 59, 170, 171, 180, 216, 224, 399
   circuit implementation, 41, 42
   symbolic representation, 42
Analog Hopfield neural network with infinite gain amplifiers, 3, 50–51, 85
Artificial neural network, 1, 4, 19, 34, 250, 292, 347
   sparsely interconnected, 427
Associative memory, 4, 5, 12, 26, 34–37, 347, 438
   storage capacity, 378
Asymptotically stable equilibrium, 3, 11, 21, 37, 73, 98, 122, 124–130, 133, 135–143, 145, 153, 169, 177, 178, 211, 220, 221, 226, 261, 262, 266, 323
Asynchronous mode, 6, 8, 23, 38, 45, 51, 59, 61, 107
Asynchronous solution, 11, 86, 106, 107

Back Propagation Algorithm, 1
Basin of attraction, 37, 196
Bias term, 1, 216, 271, 375, 430, 439, 444, 446
Bipolar vector, 19, 27, 361, 370
Brain-state-in-a-box (BSB) model, 58
Brouwer's Fixed-Point Theorem, 18, 243, 266, 269

Cellular neural network, 5, 27, 34, 37, 60, 427, 438–451, 455, 456, 466, 467, 469–471
   nonsymmetric, 439
   two-dimensional, 438
Class $\mathcal{K}$, 74, 146, 153, 169
Class $\mathcal{KR}$, 153
Cloning template, 440, 467

476 INDEX

space-invariant, 440, 444–449, 465, 466, 470, 471
space-varying, 465, 470, 471
Closed hypercube, 52
Cohen-Grossberg neural network, 7, 21, 49, 60, 111
  global stability, 294
  local stability, 302
  with multiple delays, 20, 22, 273, 291, 293, 294, 302, 335
Column dominance condition, 186
Comparison Principle, 190, 226
Comparison system, 190
Complete instability, 227
Completely continuous, 277
Completely unstable equilibrium, 16, 168, 179, 199, 227
Composite system, 174, 224, 225
Correlation memory, 348

Decomposition, 14, 174, 225
Delay equation, 272
Descendant, 108
Differential-difference equation, 277, 278
Directed acyclic graph, 108
Directed graph, 108, 109
Discrete-time Hopfield neural network, 7, 17, 44–47, 60, 206, 207, 228
Domain of attraction, 4, 10, 16, 22, 37, 109, 196, 275, 328, 402, 403, 411, 419

Eigenstructure Method, 24–26, 360–373, 411, 417, 418, 420, 433, 434, 449, 454, 469, 470
Energy function, 10–12, 21, 36, 43, 55, 70, 76, 80–84, 86, 100–107, 111, 117, 128–130, 139–142, 159, 160, 180, 201, 222, 349, 350, 365
Energy functional, 274, 280, 286, 295, 301, 304, 336, 338
Equilibrium, 73, 77, 97, 122, 133
  asymptotic stability, 14, 15, 73, 74, 98, 122, 124–130, 133, 135–143, 169, 178
  exponential stability, 14, 15, 167, 168, 178
  in the usual sense, 97
  instability, 14, 16, 74, 98, 122, 124, 126, 133, 135, 136, 138, 168, 169, 179, 197, 199, 227
  isolated, 73, 167, 190
  stability, 14, 73, 98, 122, 133, 169
  uniform asymptotic stability, 277
  uniform stability, 277
Error estimate, 257
Euclidean norm, 87, 277
Euler's method, 47
Existence Theorem, 91, 93, 95, 121
Exponentially stable equilibrium,

INDEX

167, 168, 178, 182, 187, 191, 238, 240, 245, 253, 256
Extraneous pattern, 37

Feedback neural network, 1, 37, 292
   fully interconnected, 37
Feedforward neural network, 1, 37
Filippov, 96
Free subsystem, 13, 14, 174, 209, 224
Functional differential equation, 276, 277
   autonomous, 277

Gain, 8, 23, 40, 51, 52, 59, 60, 322, 350
Gastinel-Kahan Theorem, 243, 269
Generalized Hopfield neural network, 7, 48–49, 60, 70, 75, 109
Globally asymptotically stable equilibrium, 13, 109, 145, 153, 154
Globally stable neural network, 4, 10, 20, 109, 273, 279, 294, 295, 336, 444
Grey levels, 405, 456

Hahn-Banach Theorem, 95
Hamming distance, 188, 212, 380, 382, 390, 391
Hard limiter activation function, 18, 19, 234, 259, 267

Hebb's hypothesis, 348
Hessian matrix, 288, 305
High gain limit, 201, 350
Ho-Kashyap recording, 414
Hopfield neural network, 1, 13, 20, 21, 36, 165, 348
   analog model, 40–44, 50, 59, 170
   continuous-time, 39
   discrete model, 44–47, 60
   equivalent linear representation, 219
   generalized model, 48–49, 60, 70, 75, 109
   global stability, 273
   implementation, 41, 42
   with delays, 20, 278, 285, 335
   with infinite gain amplifiers, 50–51, 85
   with multiple delays, 272
Hurwitz stable, 145, 240, 244, 253–255, 257, 266, 267, 322, 327, 329, 332, 340, 342

Implementation process, 4, 19
Index matrix, 26, 427, 470
   indexed design problem, 428
Instability, 197, 227
Interconnected system, 13–15, 174, 224
Interconnecting structure, 14, 22, 174, 209, 224, 225
Interconnection constraints, 1, 5, 14, 26, 378, 380, 382,

386, 395, 425, 435, 436, 450, 456, 466, 469
Invariance Theory, 277, 301, 336
Inverse Function Theorem, 78, 279
Isolated equilibrium, 73, 167, 190
Isolated subsystem, 174, 209

Jacobian matrix, 10, 72, 77, 110, 206, 237, 244

Kirchhoff's current law, 41

Leaf, 108
Linear separability, 374
Linear system operating on a closed hypercube, 3, 12, 24
   continuous-time, 52–57, 61, 116, 144, 159
   discrete-time, 57–58, 61, 131, 152, 160
   implementation, 53
   reduced linear system, 120, 132
Local minimum, 11, 21, 37, 101, 102, 111, 128–130, 139–142, 286, 304
Local solution, 95, 96, 120, 121, 129, 132, 140
Locally stable neural network, 20, 21, 302, 337
Lyapunov, 84
   first method, 206
   function, 14, 145, 147, 148, 154, 156, 160, 179, 184, 188, 192, 195, 196, 198, 210, 211, 213, 225, 226, 315
   functional, 310
   principal stability results, 168
   second method, 238
   stability theory, 84, 172
   vector Lyapunov function, 190, 192, 226

M-matrix, 15, 185, 211, 226
   properties, 185, 186
Matrix measure, 151
Matrix norm, 72, 118, 155, 167, 236, 251, 276
McCulloch and Pitts, 37, 38
McCulloch-Pitts model, 37, 51, 59
   asynchronous mode, 38, 59
   synchronous mode, 39
   threshold logic unit, 37
Memory vector, 221, 260, 375
Moore-Penrose pseudo-inverse, 24, 353, 368, 416
Multi-layer perceptron, 1

Neural cell, 40, 54
Neuron, 1, 6, 34, 35, 40
Nonlinear amplifier, 40, 51, 59

Operational amplifier, 52, 54
Optimal constraints, 382, 389–395, 419, 461
Ordinary difference equation, 168
   autonomous, 167, 168

INDEX 479

Ordinary differential equation, 72, 167
   autonomous, 72
   Existence Theorem, 91, 93, 95, 121
Orthonormal basis, 367
Outer Product Method, 1, 22, 23, 347–352, 368, 414–416, 419
Output sequence, 11, 104, 106
Output vector, 11, 86, 97, 99, 100, 111, 260
   stable, 11, 86, 99, 100, 105, 106
   unstable, 99

P-matrix, 151
Parameter perturbation, 17, 19, 249, 250, 265, 266, 269, 270, 392, 411, 419, 449
Perceptron, 25, 34, 373, 376, 420
   Convergence Theorem, 374, 420
   multi-layer, 1
   training algorithm, 347, 374, 417, 420, 445
Perceptron based training algorithm, 25, 27, 373–395, 417, 445–449, 470, 471
Permutation, 104, 120, 217
Perturbation model, 234, 260
Perturbed equilibrium, 241, 268
Perturbed system, 4, 260, 268
Projection Learning Rule, 23, 347, 352–360, 367, 368, 416, 417, 419
   extensions, 355–360
   iterative algorithm, 357–360, 417
Pseudo-inverse, 353, 357, 368, 416

Quasimonotonically increasing, 190
Quinquediagonal matrix, 459

Recurrent neural network, 1, 2, 4, 19, 34, 37, 271, 347
   fully interconnected, 34, 37
   partially interconnected, 34
   with multiple delays, 272
Reduced linear system, 120, 132, 223
Restriction to a matrix, 427, 469
Robust stability, 22, 236, 241, 275, 331
Robustness, 18, 250
   analysis, 27, 259–265, 389–395
Row dominance condition, 186

Sard's Theorem, 79, 279, 294
Saturated mode, 12, 116, 117, 120
Saturation function, 7, 19, 39, 44, 57, 60, 61, 131, 152, 216, 228, 234, 259, 267, 426

Sector condition, 22, 275, 322, 339
Sgn function, 6, 37–39, 45, 50, 59, 85, 201, 348
Sigmoidal function, 3, 6, 18, 39, 40, 170, 202, 233, 234, 250, 266, 271, 278, 389, 390
Singular value decomposition, 24, 366, 368, 396
Sliding mode, 10, 11, 85, 96, 97, 103, 111, 112
Small gain condition, 22, 322, 325
Sparse design problem, 27, 427–438
Sparsity constraints, 5, 450, 469, 470
Spurious state, 4, 24, 37, 44, 365, 412, 413, 417
Stable equilibrium, 21, 73, 98, 122, 133, 145, 153, 169
Stable memory, 19
Storage capacity, 4, 5, 378, 413–415
Structural perturbation, 17, 200
Symmetric design, 387, 388, 418, 448, 463, 465
Symmetric group, 118
Synchronous mode, 7, 17, 23, 39, 46, 47, 59, 206, 207, 228
Synthesis problem, 361, 427
Synthesis procedure, 26, 366, 370, 376, 387, 391, 428, 434, 435, 437, 443, 446, 448
Synthesis strategy, 362
System $(\mathcal{S})$, 174
System $(\mathcal{S}_i)$, 174
System (Ω_i), 209
System (Σ_i), 173
System $(\tilde{S})$, 234
System (A), 190
System (C), 193
System (D), 168
System (E), 72, 167
System (F), 276
System (FA), 277
System (H_i), 170
System (H'_i), 170
System (L), 70, 75, 109
System (M_{d_ξ}), 131
System (M_{d_i}), 131
System (M_d), 131, 160
System (M_ξ), 120
System (M), 116, 159
System (N_ξ), 88
System (N_d), 107
System $(N_{\xi i})$, 88
System (N), 85, 110
System (S), 233
System (VC), 190
System (W_i), 209
System (W), 208

Test matrix, 14, 15, 185, 225
Threshold logic unit, 37
Time delay, 4, 271–342
Time sequence, 104
Trajectory, 16, 75
 bounds, 16, 193, 213

Transmission delay, 19
Transportation delay, 272

Uniformly asymptotically stable equilibrium, 277
Uniformly stable equilibrium, 277
Unsaturated mode, 147
Unsaturated region, 390
Unstable equilibrium, 74, 98, 122, 124, 126, 133, 135, 136, 138, 168, 169, 176, 179, 199, 227
    completely unstable, 168, 179, 199, 227

Variable structure system, 3, 8, 10, 60, 110, 112
Vector Lyapunov function, 190, 192, 226

Weak-coupling conditions, 185